Godfrey Hounsfield: Intuitive Genius of CT

Written by Stephen Bates, Liz Beckmann, Adrian Thomas, and Richard Waltham

and including many recollections from his family, friends, and colleagues

BIR
The British Institute of Radiology

First published 2012

British Library Cataloguing in Publication Data

A catalogue record for this book is available from the British Library

ISBN-13 978-0-905749-75-4

ISBN-10 0-905749-75-8

Published by The British Institute of Radiology, 36 Portland Place, London W1B 1AT, UK (www.bir.org.uk)

Typeset by The British Institute of Radiology

Printed on acid-free paper by Henry Ling Ltd, Dorchester

BIR

The British Institute of Radiology

The authors were friends of Godfrey. Stephen, Liz and Richard worked with Godfrey at EMI during his CT work. Adrian, Liz and Godfrey were active together at the British Institute of Radiology, where Adrian is Honorary Archivist and Liz is a past president. Adrian is a consultant radiologist and Clinical Director of Diagnostic Radiology for South London Healthcare NHS Trust, and has written and broadcast extensively on the history of radiology. The proceeds of this book go to charities associated with Godfrey, and the authors and contributors will collect no fees or royalties. Richard did most of the writing and the others corrected the text and provided support, advice, knowledge and the vision of what book Godfrey deserved.

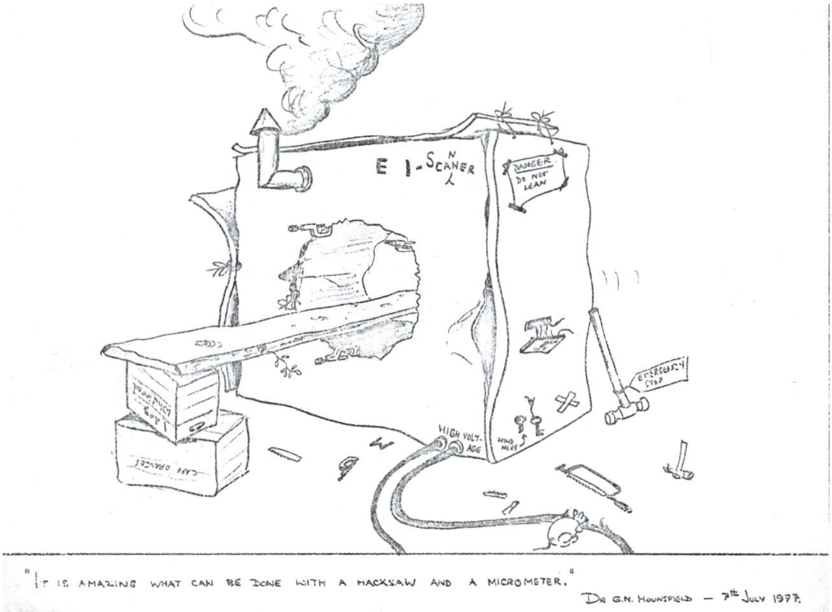

"It is amazing what can be done with a hacksaw and a micrometer." Cartoon by Tony Williams based on a casual remark by Godfrey

Dedications

Stephen Bates

This book is dedicated to all those people who worked with Godfrey during the formative years of CT, many of whom (but not all by any means) are mentioned in the book. But primarily this book is dedicated to Richard Waltham who did most of the work in writing it. Without his energy and perseverance the story of Godfrey would not have been properly told.

Liz Beckmann

In memory of Neil and my father who inspired me to have an enquiring mind. And for Godfrey, without whom my life, like so many other peoples', would have been very different.

Adrian Thomas

For my son Gareth. He has taught me more than he will ever know.

Richard Waltham

For my wife Jean, who undertook much of the research. For my father who, among many other things, showed me that a boy from a farm could write a book, and that it is better to write it with friends, as he did with Frank Raymond. And for Godfrey, who showed me that a boy from a farm can do **anything**.

Contents

Acknowledgements

We thank the BIR for support and encouragement in preparing and publishing this book.

We thank the following organisations for permission to study and use material from their archives: EMI Music (formerly EMI), the Department of Health (formerly the DHSS), the Royal Society, and the Institute of Engineering and Technology. Special thanks go to Anthony Strong and the late Colin Woodley who kept their own copies of many EMI-owned items that might otherwise not have survived. We also thank the RAF, Magnus school, City & Guilds, the National Museum of Computing, the Computer Conservation Society, Sutton on Trent Local History Society, and the Faraday House Old Students Association for their help.

The Nobel Foundation kindly allowed us to quote from Godfrey's autobiography, and William Ellis Ingham (known as "Bill" hereafter) allowed us to quote extensively from his excellent unpublished history of the early research on CT scanning at EMI.

Professor John Hendry kindly lent us a copy of his book about the early history of computers, in which field Godfrey was active between 1956 and 1967.

Godfrey liked walking, skiing and travelling and he joined clubs where he met friends with similar interests. Roger Voles and Maggie Knox-Scott kindly helped to put us in contact with many of those friends.

Many of Godfrey's friends, family and former colleagues have contributed invaluable memories, photographs and documents. These contributors are mentioned by name at appropriate points in the book. With their help, we hope that the book describes what made Godfrey unique as a person and is not simply a description of his technical work. Further contributions for a possible second edition are welcome via the BIR. We are also grateful to Godfrey for all that he meant to us, and for the times that we shared.

While we are very grateful to all of the above, they do not bear responsibility for any errors or omissions.

Stephen Bates	Punched tape photo in Chapter 6
David Bosomworth	Photo of IVC ramble in Chapter 5 and on the front cover
BIR	Extract from article by Gordon Higson in Chapter 6, awards photo in Appendix 3
Pat Cassidy	Photo in chapter 3
City & Guilds	Photo of the Prince Philip Medal in Chapter 7, exam details in Appendix 5
Kitty Cook	Ramblers photo in Chapter 4
Computer Conservation Society	Quote from Ron Clayden in Chapter 4
Kathleen Dix	Loire valley photos in Chapter 11
EMI Music	Photos and images in Chapters 4–12, Appendix 8, and on the front cover
Susan Edwards	Quotes from Paul Hounsfield's wartime diaries in Chapter 2
Pat and Gordon Ellis	Photo of the Lyric Cinema in Chapter 2
Elsevier Ltd	Extracts and photos in Chapter 6 reprinted from Bull J. History of computed tomography. In *Radiology of the skull and brain: Technical aspects of computed tomography.* Newton TH, Potts DG, editors. St Louis, MI: C.V. Mosby Co; 1981. pp. 3835–49.
Ian Fairbairn	Photo of Godfrey at his bench in the laboratory in Chapter 7
Pauline Figgins	Loire valley picnic photo in Chapter 11
Eric Foxley	Frightful tangles photo in Chapter 4
Mac Gollifer	Photos of RSNA 1972 in Chapter 8

Ian M. Green	Photo of the student notes of Douglas Foster in Appendix 5
Ruth Harston	Photos in Chapters 2 and 3
Hackenthorpe Hall Nursery	Hackenthorpe Hall photo in Chapter 2
Andrew Hounsfield	Photos and images in Chapters 2, 3, 10–12
Lynda Hounsfield	Photos and images in Chapter 3. Paintings in Chapter 11
Imperial Tobacco	Photo by Desmond O'Neill Features in Chapter 10 from the 1977 Genius Exhibition sponsored by the John Player Foundation
Joanna Irvin	Skiing photo in Chapter 4
Matt King	Photo in Chapter 10, e-mails in Chapter 11
Lasker Foundation	Photo and citations in Chapter 8
Mike Leith	EMIDEC back-plane photo in Chapter 4
Geoff Lewis	Photos from Italy in Chapter 4
Keena Millar	Opening Sir Godfrey's path in Chapter 11
François Mémeteau	Photos of EMIDEC 1100 in Chapter 4
Newark Advertiser	Ninety-ninth birthday photo of Blanche Hounsfield and family in Chapter 11
Nobel Foundation	All quotes from Godfrey's autobiography and photos of his medal. ® © The Nobel Foundation; 1979
Royal Society	Bill Ingham has assigned copyright in his document to the Royal Society. Chapters 5–10 and Appendix 4
Raymond Schulz	Photo from 1995 Röntgen Centenary in Chapter 11

Geoff Spurr	Diagrams and extract from a letter in Chapter 2
Studio D Photography	Knighthood photo in Chapter 10
Don Tyzack	Diagram of reading a book in Chapter 5
Peter Walters	Photos of lathe bed and caged Godfrey, Chapters 6 and 11
Jean Waltham	Photos of Palmer House and Magnus school in Chapter 2
Richard Waltham	Photos of core store and Terry Froggatt's punched tape in Chapter 4
Reverend A. M. Williams	Cartoons in front pages and in Chapter 10
Wimbledon Guardian	Photo of Atkinson Morley Hospital in Chapter 6
Andrew Wylie	Photos of an EMIDEC 1100 logic card in Chapter 4

We have made best efforts to obtain permission to use all copyright items. In some cases, it is difficult to identify the correct copyright owner with certainty, and we apologise to both parties if our identification is incorrect. In other cases, we have not been able to contact the copyright owner, and we offer our apologies, including to those listed below. We invite those affected to contact us via the publisher and we will rectify matters as soon as is reasonably possible.

David Clarke	The letter in Chapter 6
Jeanne Hancock	Extract from a letter quoted in Chapter 8
Leslie H. Hounsfield	The family history in Chapter 2
Albert Hutchinson	The letter in Chapter 9
A&A Kamerabild Ronny Karlsson	Our best efforts have been unable to contact the owner of a photo in Chapter 9
Dr David G. Kilpatrick	Possible owner of the photo of Harold N. Potts Award in Chapter 8
Judith Rook	The letter in Chapter 9
Unknown	Best efforts did not identify the owner

Foreword by Professor Ian Isherwood, CBE

Banquo asked of the witches in "Macbeth":

If you can look into the seeds of time
And say which grain will grow and which will not
Speak then to me.

If that request had been made by Banquo at the British Institute of Radiology's meeting in 1972, then the response would have been unequivocal. There was no doubt that computed tomography (CT) – scanning of the brain – was destined to be a fundamental advance of the greatest importance in diagnostic medicine. I was fortunate to have been an enthusiastic witness even earlier in 1971. Some would say, in retrospect, that CT had as great an impact on medicine and surgery as Röntgen's earlier discovery of X-rays in 1895. With its first step, it liberated the brain of both patient and doctor from the constraints of traditional imagery. Medicine is a continuous search for the resolution of uncertainty, and CT provided the stimulus and scientific environment for other major developments to follow. Painful and disturbing experiences for the hapless patient became, thankfully, things of the past. The marriage of science and medicine was, on this occasion, a total success, and Godfrey Hounsfield was the perfect broker.

Godfrey Hounsfield had already made notable advances in computer design, increasing the speed of the machine from the, then very slow, transistor to compete with the valve, when his thoughts were drawn to the idea that images of the living brain might be achievable using X-rays, computer technology and the notion of the skull as a closed box.

As Poincaré, the French mathematician, said:

Thought is only a flash between two long nights
But that flash is everything.

With inspired support from Gordon Higson and others at the Department of Health, and the scientific expertise of EMI, Hounsfield's EMI-scanner was enabled to become a reality. Neither EMI nor the medical community had any experience in this new technological field, and the learning curve for both was steep.

One of the first patients we scanned in Manchester in 1973 was a lady who had suffered a severe head injury falling down her cellar steps. She was admitted deeply unconscious and would, under normal circumstances, have been subjected to multiple surgical and painful procedures to reveal the symmetrical blood clots in her brain. Instead she was scanned immediately on admission and taken straight to theatre for definitive surgery. It gave us all the greatest pleasure and encouragement to see her make a total recovery and return to her previous occupation as a correspondent on a national newspaper. By any standards of journalism such an outcome must surely be regarded a success. Certainly, it changed forever the clinical management of head injuries. The skull was no longer a barrier to the radiological investigation of brain disorders including head injuries, tumours and strokes. This novel diagnostic method enabled significant advances to be made in improving the quality of life and treatment of these brain-damaged patients. The public's imagination was captured and the patient's response was one of enthusiastic gratitude.

In 1975, at an international conference that I attended, Godfrey announced his latest development of a general purpose body scanner that could provide access to parts of the rest of the body that other techniques could not reach. The announcement was greeted with a standing ovation – and a queue of Americans wielding cheque books. It was clear that the enhanced diagnostic possibilities of this general purpose scanner could provide crucial visual and quantitative information about body organs and diseases that had previously remained hidden during life. Whereupon, of course, it then became possible to plan and apply more effective treatment programmes for a wider variety of patients.

I had many opportunities to travel around the world with Godfrey and to witness his total lack of interest in power, position or possessions. His unusual habit of retaining Greenwich Mean Time wherever we went in the world could be disconcerting for the uninitiated but meant, on occasion, that he could work in the dead of night and be unavailable for prying reporters, and even sometimes for lectures he disliked giving, in the day time. Awards, a Nobel Prize and a Knighthood, followed, yet Godfrey remained as always the retiring bachelor.

There can be few individuals of whom it can be claimed that, by their thoughts and their actions, they influenced medical progress and permanently improved the clinical care of patients.

Voltaire said:

> *Men who are engaged in the restoration of health to other men by the joint exertions of skill and humanity are above all the great of the world.*

Of such greatness was Godfrey Hounsfield.

Chapter 1 Introduction

From Newark to the Nobel Prize

On 10 December 1979, an unassuming British engineer – Godfrey Hounsfield – received the Nobel Prize in Stockholm. The award was for the "Development of computer assisted tomography". He had pioneered an entirely new machine which became a household name, the CT scanner. It was a remarkable event. Godfrey had no previous experience of working in the medical field but was an engineer who had spent his working life, prior to X-ray scanners, developing computers and radar.

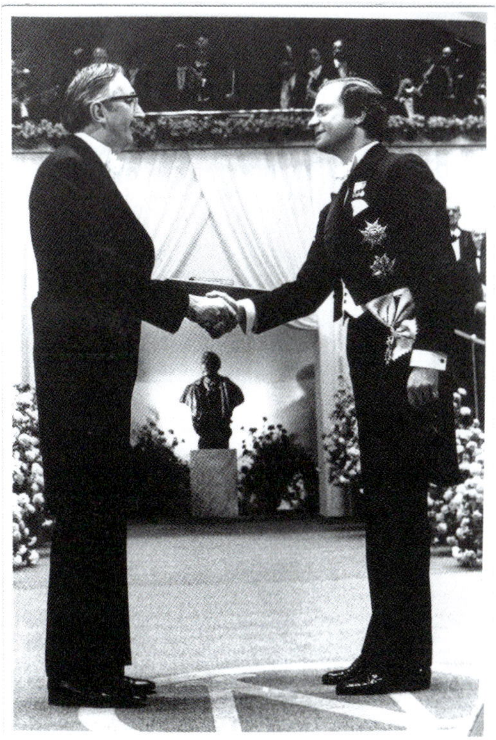

Carl XVI Gustaf, King of Sweden, presents the Nobel Prize
(Photo ownership unknown)

Godfrey grew up on a small farm near Newark and left school with no academic qualifications. So his early years did little to suggest that he would pioneer such a great medical breakthrough or be awarded the highest honour in science.

Godfrey ushered in a whole new era of medical imaging when he published the first clinical CT scan pictures in April 1972. Many previous medical tests were made obsolete by his innovation, including painful and risky tests in which patients felt as if they had been kicked in the head by a horse. His method was fast, pain-free, and made the most efficient use of the allowable X-ray dose. Forty years on from his great breakthrough, CT scanners are still in use all around the world, and millions of people have benefited from better diagnosis. Modern scanners have few features that were not first envisaged by Godfrey in 1968.

CT stands for computed tomography, in which a computer works out the 3D structure inside the patient from X-ray beams that pass through the patient from many different angles.

How did this happen? Many accounts have been written about the development of CT scanning which went on to have such a profound impact on medical diagnostic techniques. None of them has told the real story of the way that Godfrey worked and developed his ideas. We describe his life both before and after the CT scanner development. The dozens of contributors to this book knew Godfrey well, and help to give an insight into how his unique way of seeing the world led to one of the greatest medical advances. We attempt to answer questions such as:

- What was his background?
- How were the attributes that led to his discovery formed?
- How did he work and what was he like to work with?
- What was the driving force that led to his many inventions?
- What were the obstacles that he had to overcome?
- What led to the countless awards and recognition given to him?
- What was he like as a person: what would it be like to meet him?

Above all, this book will attempt to provide an insight into the way in which inventions grow from initial conception and become reality through the sheer perseverance and determination of one remarkable individual.

Sir Godfrey Hounsfield rarely used his title, so we called him Godfrey, as we do in this book. He was gentle, generous, modest and unambitious, but doggedly persistent in his work. He liked working in small teams, but he was always slightly outside the formal structure – a man who set his own rules. Although some people of his seniority rarely talked to those beneath them, he would talk to anybody who was interested in his work, whether it was the cleaner, the panel-beater or the managing director.

But most of all, he thought in an unusual way that he described as *you've just got to use the absolute minimum of maths but have a tremendous lot of intuition.* This is easy to say, but very hard to get right. He used a lot of pictures and mental models, a lot of analogies, and he had a lot of curiosity about how everything in the world worked. This was uncomfortable for academics. How could this highly mathematical field be opened up by someone who was not an academic, not a mathematician, but a man who used the subversive art of intuition? Describing how he thought is a big challenge, partly because he found it hard to describe himself.

Part of his story is already in the historical record, but many interesting aspects have been omitted or have not previously been drawn together. The reasons for this were that Godfrey was modest and did not want to draw extra attention to himself, that technical areas were kept under wraps to avoid helping competitors, and that commercial aspects were not published unless they aligned with the public relations plan. Another factor is that from April 1972, events unfolded at a tremendous pace – writing the history could always be left until tomorrow.

From his teenage years he was interested in how things worked, and in how science and engineering could help to improve the world. He wanted to pass this enthusiasm on to the next generation. Although he dreaded public speaking, he agreed to speak to pupils at his former school. He wanted to tell them that *each new discovery brings with it the seeds of other, future, inventions. There are many discoveries, probably just around the corner, waiting for someone to bring them to life. Could this possibly be you?* What an inspirational message!

It was a pleasure to know him. We hope that this book will give readers a picture of the whole person, and perhaps encourage them to look around the corner and seek new discoveries.

Chapter 2
Early years in Nottinghamshire

Life at school and on the farm

Godfrey was born in Sutton on Trent near Newark on 28 August 1919. He grew up on a farm and, although he was unsuccessful at school, he taught himself to test scientific ideas in a very practical way. Godfrey's father Thomas was born near Sheffield in 1877. He was a farmer in Sutton on Trent from 1919 to 1939. His mother was born Sophia Blanche Dilcock in Sheffield, in 1885.

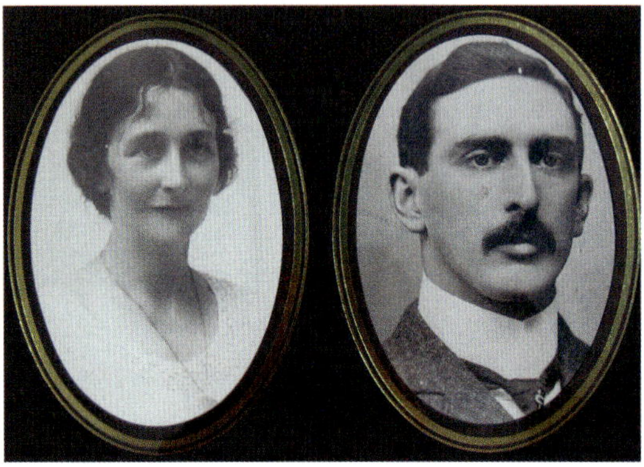

Thomas and Blanche Hounsfield
(Courtesy of Andrew Hounsfield)

Thomas's grandfather James Hounsfield lived in Hackenthorpe Hall, which is now a children's nursery. It is a substantial building. Several members of the Hounsfield family lived in the Hackenthorpe and Beighton region, about six miles from Sheffield, near the border between Derbyshire and Yorkshire.

Hackenthorpe Hall
(Courtesy of Hackenthorpe Hall Nursery)

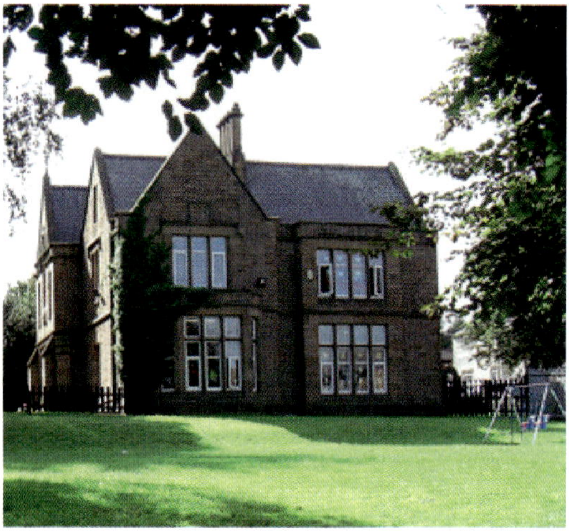

Godfrey's nephew Andrew Hounsfield says, *Grandfather (Thomas) had a birth certificate saying he was a 'gentleman'. He came from a wealthy family in Sheffield, and had a trust fund invested in heavy industry, but it all went wrong. He ended up with a 50 acre farm in Sutton on Trent, which he found very difficult to make a living out of, with five children to support. My father was in constant trouble with grandfather, for getting in the way or breaking tools. He used to have to 'single' sugar beet seedlings, which he hated. He was paid by the row. They had a few cattle and chickens, almost subsistence farming. Grandfather employed one man but it was a real struggle to pay his wages.*

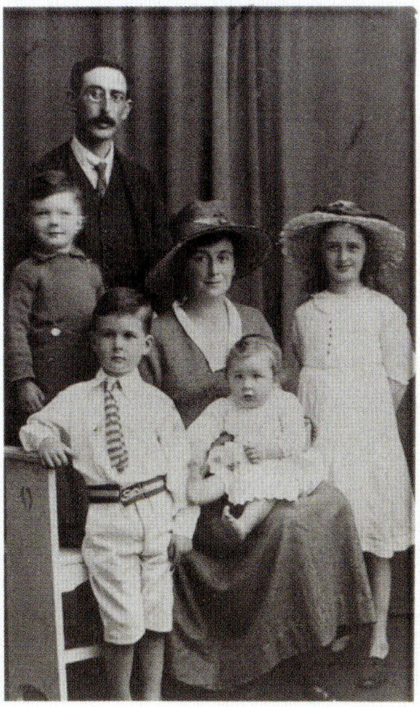

Family group, about 1920
(Courtesy of Ruth Harston)
The children are, from left to right, Michael, Paul, Godfrey, and Joan. Godfrey's eldest sister, Molly, is not in the photo. Godfrey became the most like his father in looks. Thomas was firmly in charge: Blanche had a wonderful contralto voice, but he would not let her sing except in church. Blanche had strong views on what was best for the children, and how they should behave.

Godfrey's sister Molly wanted to marry a man from South Africa but their mother said that he wasn't good enough for her. Molly stayed single and ended up spending a lot of her life looking after her mother, who lived to age 100.

In his excellent short autobiography on the Nobel Foundation's website (www.nobelprize.org), Godfrey allocates a lot of space to his rural childhood: *I was born and brought up near a village in Nottinghamshire and in my childhood enjoyed the freedom of the rather isolated country life. After the first world war, my father had bought a small farm, which became a marvellous playground for his five children. My two brothers and two sisters were all older than I and, as they naturally pursued their own more adult interests, this gave me the advantage of not being expected to join in, so I could go off and follow my own inclinations.*

The farm offered an infinite variety of ways to do this. At a very early age I became intrigued by all the mechanical and electrical gadgets which even then could be found on a farm; the threshing machines, the binders, the generators. But the period between my eleventh and eighteenth years remains the most vivid in my memory because this was the time of my first attempts at experimentation, which might never have been made had I lived in a city. In a village there are few distractions and no pressures to join in at a ball game or go to the cinema, and I was free to follow the trail of any interesting idea that came my way. I constructed electrical recording machines; I made hazardous investigations of the principles of flight, launching myself from the tops of haystacks with a home-made glider; I almost blew myself up during exciting experiments using water-filled tar barrels and acetylene to see how high they could be waterjet propelled. It may now be a trick of the memory but I am sure that on one occasion I managed to get one to an altitude of 1000 feet!

Acetylene lamps were in use in the 1930s. Acetylene gas was made by dripping water onto calcium carbide. It burns brightly and it can, as Godfrey describes, make an explosive mixture with air.

Godfrey put a tar barrel upside down in a trough that held drinking water for the farm animals. The trough contained about the same amount of water as you might use when having a bath, but it had rectangular metal sides. Godfrey rigged everything up, lit the fuse and withdrew to what he hoped was a safe distance. One of his experiments caused a big explosion that broke the drinking trough, and his father was not very pleased that it had been flattened out into a useless sheet of metal!

For Godfrey, these experiments were a very vivid way of testing whether he understood how things worked. As he says himself: *During this time I was learning the hard way many fundamentals in reasoning. This was all at the expense of my schooling at Magnus Grammar School in Newark, where they tried hard to educate me but where I responded only to physics and mathematics with any ease and moderate enthusiasm.*

Some of his persistence and determination may have come from thinking like a self-employed person – the man working alone on his farm who needs to find all of his own answers. The farm kindled his interest in understanding how things worked. He enjoyed testing his understanding and putting it to practical use. He says that the farm gave him opportunities to experiment, but there was something special in Godfrey – few farmers' sons conduct such spectacular and dangerous experiments. Not many are allowed to take such liberties with expensive new machinery as were described by his nephew Andrew at Godfrey's funeral: *My first recollection of Goffa was of this mysterious scientist uncle who lived far away in London and drove a great big Jag: now how cool is that to a lad of age seven. The thing I found very appealing was that he wasn't politically correct, well according to my parents anyway.* (He was called Goffa at home from the 1930s.)

He took me down the A1 at 100 mph in that Jag. When I was being badgered into mowing the lawn, he agreed with me that mowing the lawn was boring. He told me not to worry about exams, as passing exams wasn't important, and that getting up before 9 am was not to be recommended, and as you can imagine all of this horrified my parents.

Later on when I was working on the farm with my father, his visits were tinged with a little apprehension. Goffa would come to the farm, see a new machine and immediately want to know how it worked and what it did. If I could not tell him all the answers, which was invariably the case, bits would start to be removed from the said machine, with me nervously looking over his shoulder waiting for my father to come around the corner.

We used to be livestock farmers and it normally fell to me to feed them on Christmas Day. One year I managed to spill about four tons of corn on the floor and was busy shovelling it up when Goffa came through the door: without a second thought he got another shovel and started to help me. I can safely say I am the only person in this world to have shovelled corn on Christmas day with the help of a Nobel Prize winner!

When the great diagnostic benefits of the CT scanner became evident, I know that Goffa was very moved, and got great pleasure from the thousands of letters he was sent from people whose lives had been transformed because of his invention. It is not just his family or the village he grew up in or even the country he lived in but the whole of mankind that has gained and benefited from Uncle Goffa's life.

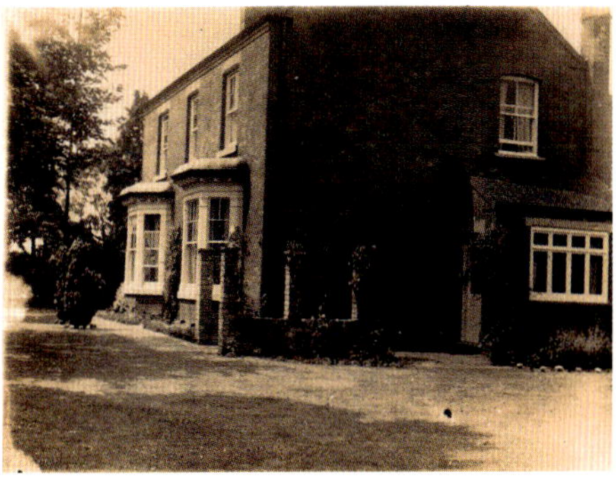

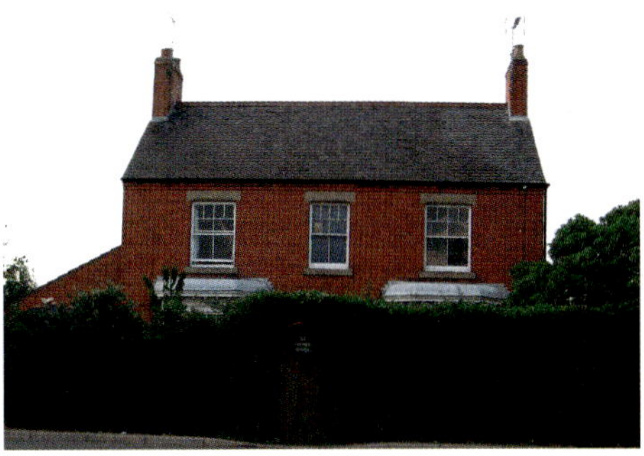

Boyhood home
(Courtesy of Andrew Hounsfield and Jean Waltham)
The upper photo shows the house in Godfrey's time and the lower photo shows it in 2011.

Godfrey's family lived and farmed on the south side of the village of Sutton on Trent. The nearest large town was Newark, and Godfrey went to school there at the Lilley and Stone preparatory school, and from age nine onwards attended Magnus school, which in those days was a grammar school. Magnus is about nine miles away from Godfrey's house, and London is a further 120 miles beyond Newark.

Godfrey's niece Lynda Hounsfield says, *When Godfrey was very small Grandma saw something in him, by the way he put his building bricks together, just little things. Her grandfather clock hadn't worked for ages, and when he was five he took it to pieces and put it back together and it worked! I heard this first-hand from Grandma. He was not good at school: his concentration was poor and he was very dyslexic, but they didn't call it that then, they just called you thick.*

Whether or not dyslexia is the correct diagnosis, there is no doubt that Godfrey thought in a different way to most people, and that he learnt best by being self-taught rather than in a classroom.

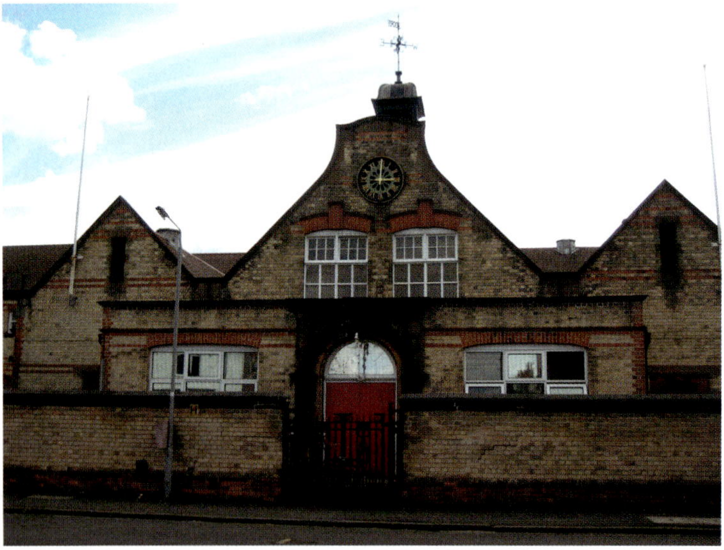

Magnus school
(Courtesy of Jean Waltham)

Godfrey's school report card shows that he started at Magnus in September 1928 at age nine and left in April 1936 at age sixteen and a half with no qualifications. This was due, in Godfrey's own words, to a lack of ease with subjects apart from physics and maths. Those subjects included Latin, which was compulsory at Magnus until it was dropped for pupils below age sixteen in 1939.

His report card shows average form positions for his first four years of eleventh, third, sixth, and twenty-sixth. After being demoted to the B stream in February 1932, his form positions were tenth, twentieth, and twelfth. He was not doing well at school, but demoting him did not produce much change.

Two notes on the report card may have been written by Godfrey's house master, and both record visits by his father. On 13 February 1932:

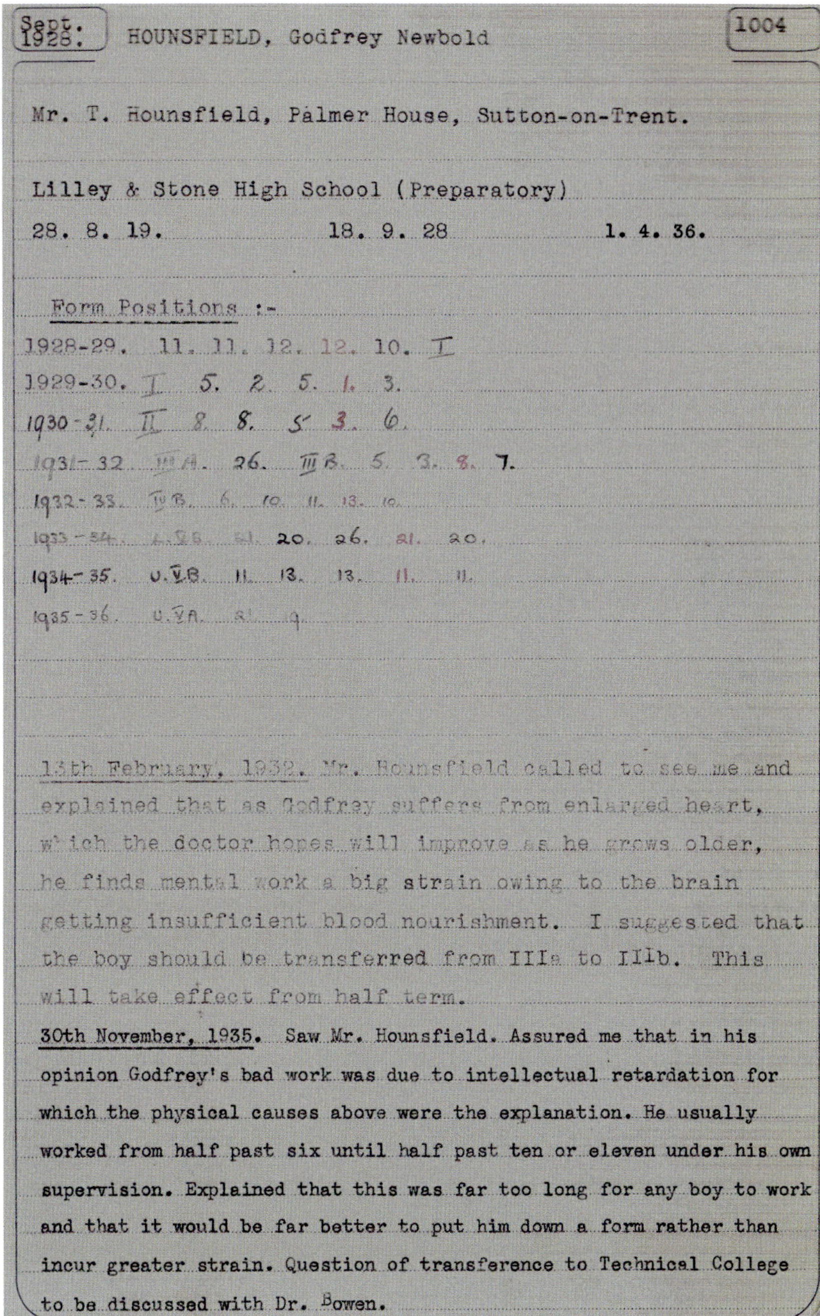

Sept. 1928. HOUNSFIELD, Godfrey Newbold 1004

Mr. T. Hounsfield, Palmer House, Sutton-on-Trent.

Lilley & Stone High School (Preparatory)

28. 8. 19. 18. 9. 28 1. 4. 36.

Form Positions :-

1928-29. 11. 11. 12. 12. 10. I

1929-30. I 5. 2. 5. 1. 3.

1930-31. II 8. 8. 5 3. 6.

1931-32 III A. 26. III B. 5. 3. 8. 7.

1932-33. IV B. 6. 10. 11. 13. 10.

1933-34. L.V B. 21. 20. 26. 21. 20.

1934-35. U.V B. 11. 13. 13. 11. 11.

1935-36. U.V A. 21. 9.

13th February, 1932. Mr. Hounsfield called to see me and explained that as Godfrey suffers from enlarged heart, which the doctor hopes will improve as he grows older, he finds mental work a big strain owing to the brain getting insufficient blood nourishment. I suggested that the boy should be transferred from IIIa to IIIb. This will take effect from half term.

30th November, 1935. Saw Mr. Hounsfield. Assured me that in his opinion Godfrey's bad work was due to intellectual retardation for which the physical causes above were the explanation. He usually worked from half past six until half past ten or eleven under his own supervision. Explained that this was far too long for any boy to work and that it would be far better to put him down a form rather than incur greater strain. Question of transference to Technical College to be discussed with Dr. Bowen.

School report

(Kindly provided by Jane Johnson of Magnus library, by permission of Andrew Hounsfield)

Mr Hounsfield called to see me and explained that as Godfrey suffers from enlarged heart, which the doctor hopes will improve as he grows older, he finds mental work a big strain owing to the brain getting insufficient blood nourishment. I suggested that the boy should be transferred from IIIa to IIIb. This will take effect from half term.

On 30 November 1935, when Godfrey was age 16, his report card says, *Saw Mr Hounsfield. Assured me that in his opinion Godfrey's bad work was due to intellectual retardation for which the physical causes above were the explanation. He usually worked from 6:30pm to 10:30 or 11pm under his own supervision. Explained that this was far too long for any boy to work and that it would be far better to put him down a form rather than incur greater strain. Question of transference to Technical College to be discussed with Dr Bowen.* Dr Bowen was head of Newark Technical College. Godfrey left school the following April.

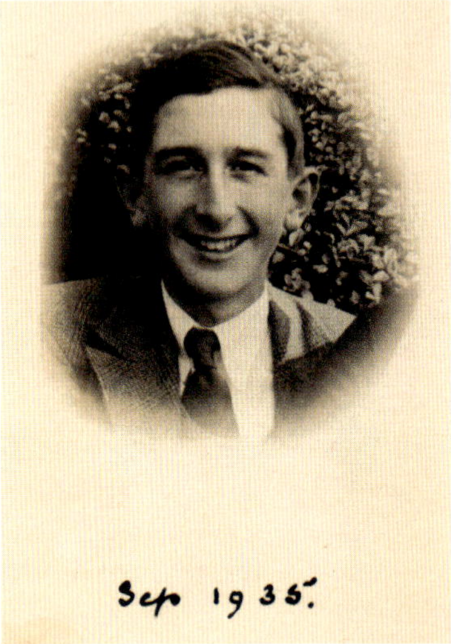

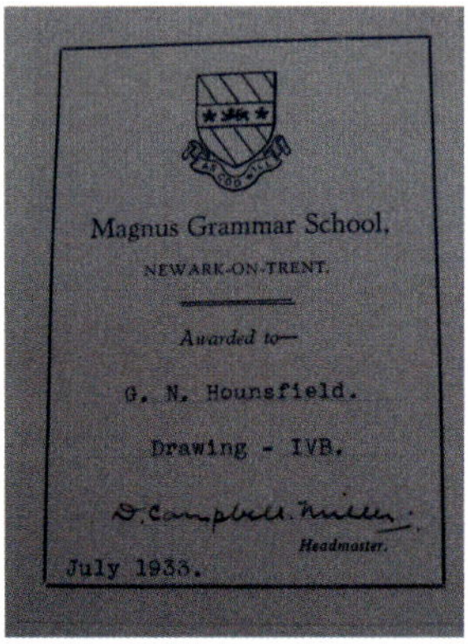

Magnus Grammar School,
NEWARK-ON-TRENT.
Awarded to—
G. N. Hounsfield.
Drawing - IVB.
D. Campbell Miller.
Headmaster.
July 1933.

Above: Award for drawing
Left: Photo shortly after his sixteenth birthday
(Courtesy of Andrew Hounsfield)

The records do not show whether or not Godfrey passed an exam to enter the school. In the 1930s, the funding of grammar schools was changing: some pupils still paid fees, while a new group of scholarship pupils had their education funded by the government.

Godfrey won three awards from Magnus for drawing. His nephew Andrew recalls, *He used to hate school and think it was a total waste of time. He didn't get his matriculation, like O-levels or GCSE now, which included Latin. He left school soon after that. He used to hate sport: he thought it a great waste of time.*

The December 1930 photo shows Godfrey at age eleven. His brother John Michael (known as Michael) was two years older. He wanted to become a farmer, but the farm was not able to support him in addition to his father. So initially he worked in a bank, and then volunteered for the Army during the war. After the war he rented some ex-RAF land, and became a farmer. His brother Thomas Paul (known as Paul) was four

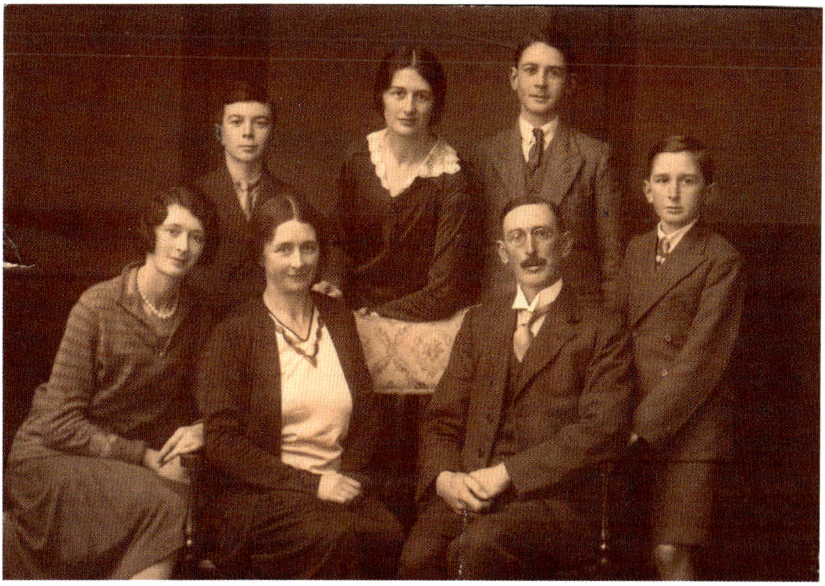

December 1930. Back: Michael, Joan, and Paul
Front: Molly, Mother, Father, and Godfrey
(Courtesy of Ruth Harston)

years older than Godfrey. Paul was very good at sports, and was Victor Ludorum – the best at sports and games – at Durham University. He was ordained in 1947 and served in the parish of Treeton from 1950, and then in Donington in Shropshire from 1961 to 1980. Godfrey's sister Joan was eight years his senior, and she won a scholarship to Oxford to read English, and spent much of her working life in the USA at the John Tracy Clinic for deaf children, which was set up by the film actor Spencer Tracy and his wife Louise, and is named after their deaf son. His other sister Blanche (known as Molly) was eleven years older than Godfrey, and she was a teacher.

A distant relative called Leslie Haywood Hounsfield made contact with Godfrey's father Thomas. Leslie was updating the family tree, and he has many interesting similarities to Godfrey. Leslie produced a seventy-eight-page bound book "The Hounsfield Family", containing charts showing each part of the family tree in detail, and text to record whatever is known about previous generations.

Leslie's book is a **very** thorough study, whereas the family tree on the following page shows only the link between Godfrey and Leslie. The entry for Godfrey's father Thomas says, *Thomas Hounsfield was born 26-3-1877 at Cotleigh House and was educated at Sheffield Royal Grammar School and Repton. From 1984 to 1907 he was on the staff of a steel manufacturer but had to retire owing to failing eyesight. Since 1919 he has been farming in Sutton on Trent near Newark. His interests are cricket, football, shooting and tennis; he has always taken an active part in the work of the Church having, in the past, held office*

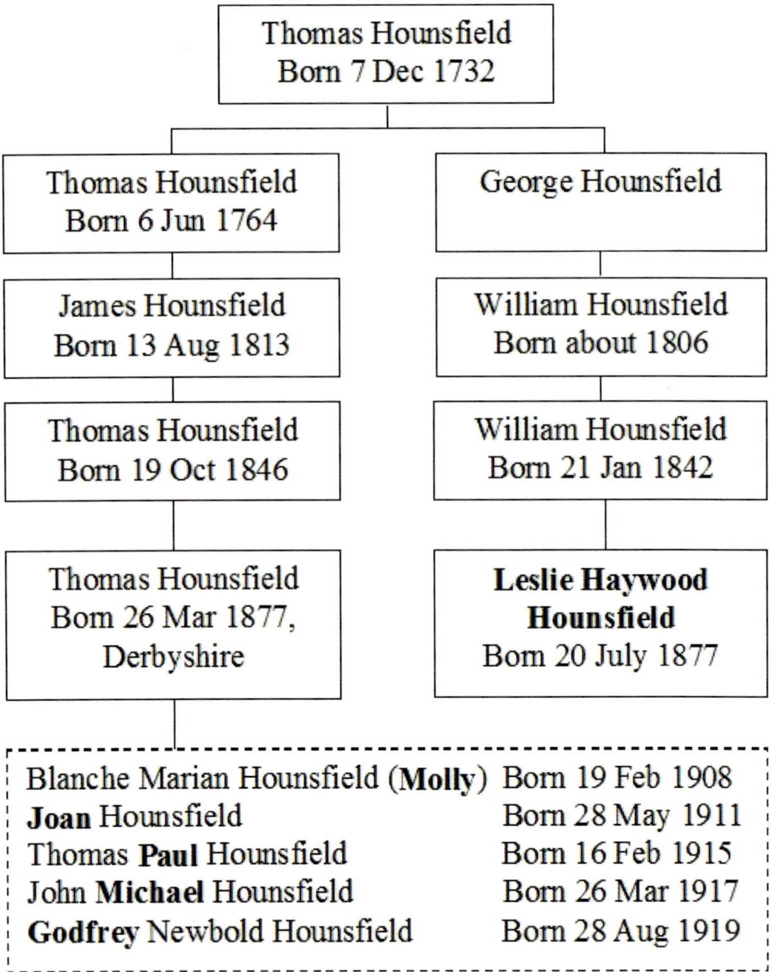

Family tree, showing the relationship to Leslie Haywood Hounsfield

as Churchwarden for eleven years, as Diocesan Conference member for eight years and as Ruri-Decanal Conference member for eleven years. On 4-5-1907 [...] he married Sophia Blanche, second daughter of the late Thomas Dilcock, of Broomhill Sheffield. (Cotleigh House was near Hackenthorpe in Derbyshire.)

The entry for Leslie Haywood Hounsfield includes the following: *He went to Brighton Grammar School. He was put to engineering 'because he could never pass an examination' so he attended engineering day-school at the Battersea Polytechnic. Here he passed the first of a long series of examinations, coming out top of the school the first year. He got a job at James Simpson & Company, the Worthington Pump Manufacturers of Pimlico. After three years' evening study he won a Whitworth Exhibition and came second on the list of Royal Exhibitioners which enabled him to take the three years course at the Royal College of Science and obtain his ARCS.*

Being in the Electrical Engineers Volunteers, he volunteered for the South African War in 1899, in the middle of the College course. This diversion upset his studies and he had to abandon his ambition to get the DSc.

In 1904 he started in business in Clapham, where he developed his designs for a poor man's car; this eventually became known as the 'Trojan'. [...] After the war Leyland Motors Limited manufactured the Trojan car at their Ham Works, near Kingston where he acted as chief engineer on the Trojan section. All went well until the demand for heavy vehicles caused Leyland Motors to pass the Trojan back to Trojan Ltd with all production equipment under very favourable conditions.

The business policy of the other directors of Trojan Ltd deteriorated so he resigned in 1930 [...] to manufacture his Tensometer testing machine and other apparatus for testing materials. At the same time he cancelled the license with Trojan Ltd to manufacture his patent camp-bed which in their hands had been a financial failure.

Both the testing machine business and the camp-bed factory prospered so greatly that in 1939 a large proportion of the work had to be done by subcontractors to meet the demand.

(Both quotations copyright the estate of Leslie Haywood Hounsfield.)

After retirement, Leslie continued to develop his scientific and engineering ideas in a workshop he built in his garden.

Nothing about Leslie's Trojan car was conventional. The engine had only seven moving parts, and the advertising was based on the fact that it was cheaper to travel by Trojan car than the cost in shoes and socks to walk the same distance.

There are several parallels between Godfrey and Leslie Haywood Hounsfield, from not getting on very well at grammar school to continuing work into their retirement. They were both engineers with an interest in pioneering new markets and a talent for unconventional and economical design. In later life Godfrey owned two of Leslie's camp beds, one of which was in Godfrey's lab and the other was in a holiday home belonging to the IVC.

At about age fifteen, Godfrey and his brothers and other local lads held motorbike races on the farm fields. There was some home advantage because the Hounsfield boys knew which corners had been watered and where the track was especially slippery! Whenever a motorbike broke it was handed to Godfrey to repair. He certainly was not always on his own on the farm, but he could quietly immerse himself in experiments there when he wanted to.

Years later Godfrey talked about his childhood to Richard Waltham: *on the long flight to Chicago he mentioned that as a youngster on the farm he climbed unsupported ladders. I had no idea what he meant, so he explained that the aim was to climb up a ladder, keeping it balanced while climbing over the top and down the other side. Sadly I didn't ask him what was the tallest ladder which he climbed in this way. We shared an interest in farming: when he interviewed me to join his team we somehow spent most of the time discussing pig farming, which his brother and my father were then involved with. Maybe I got the job on the basis of our shared experience of growing up on a farm!*

Paul's eldest daughter, Ruth Harston, says, *My father used to take Godfrey to all sorts of places on the back of his motorbike. They went camping in the Lake District. They were very close when they were younger. Godfrey could tinker with the motorbikes and make them go faster. My father would buy a really old bike and Godfrey would get it going, and would fix tractors for my grandfather, and improve them. He was also keen on music and played a double bass in a jazz group when he lived at Sutton on Trent and he would 'honky-tonk' on my parents' grand piano when he came to visit.*

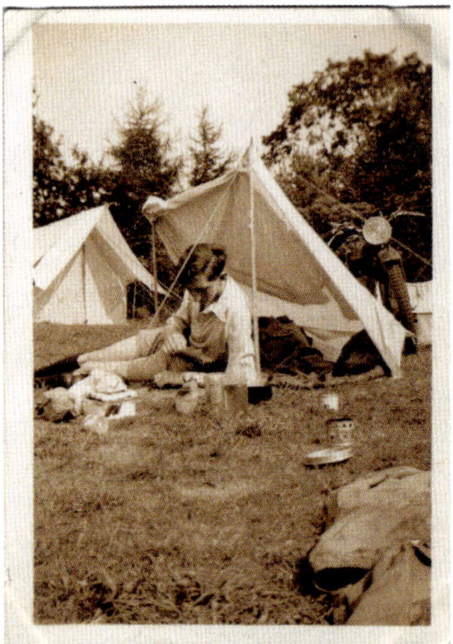

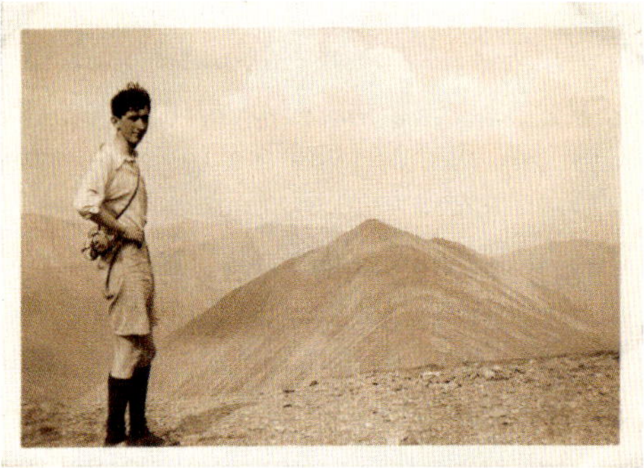

Above: Lake District – on top of Helvellyn
Left: making tea at Keswick
(Photos courtesy of Ruth Harston)

There was a room at Palmer House which was called the Nursery. Godfrey and the other children used it when they were young and we played in it, too. There were lots of electric wires in there and a microphone which Godfrey had made from a bicycle lamp!

After leaving school, Godfrey did various jobs such as running a cinema and drawing plans for a local builder. His brother Paul's second daughter, Susan Edwards, remembers, *My father told me when we were walking in Sutton on Trent when I was a child that this building, this village-hall, was where my uncle Godfrey showed films. All of the villagers used to come and watch them.*

He was running a little cinema at about age 18, being the projectionist and everything else, and showing the Keystone Cops and other films. He built his own radio and fixed an aerial wire onto a nearby telegraph pole by climbing up like a boy in the tropics climbing a palm tree.

Godfrey was enthusiastically involved with the cinema that was set up by Geoffrey Walton. They were good friends, and both lived in Sutton on Trent.

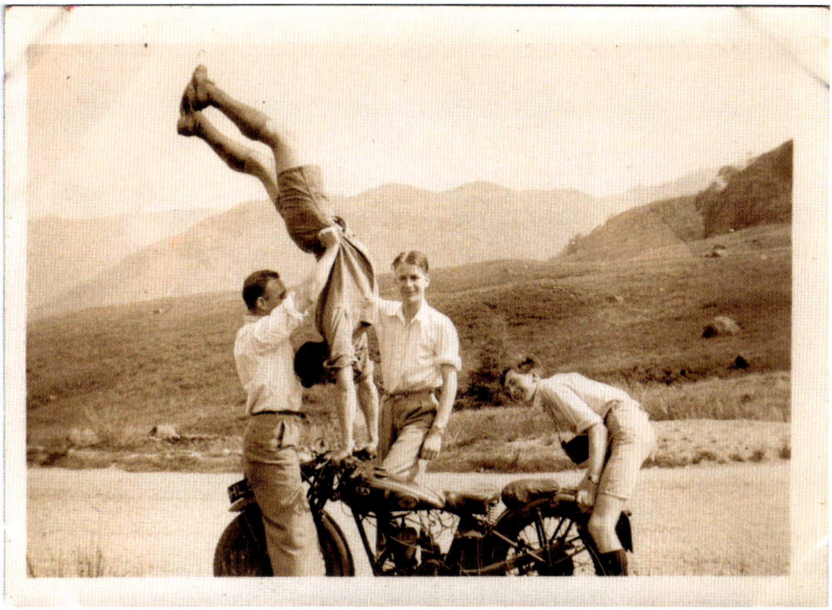

Above: Paul does a handstand while Godfrey steadies the back mudguard. Below: Helvellyn
(Photos courtesy of Ruth Harston)

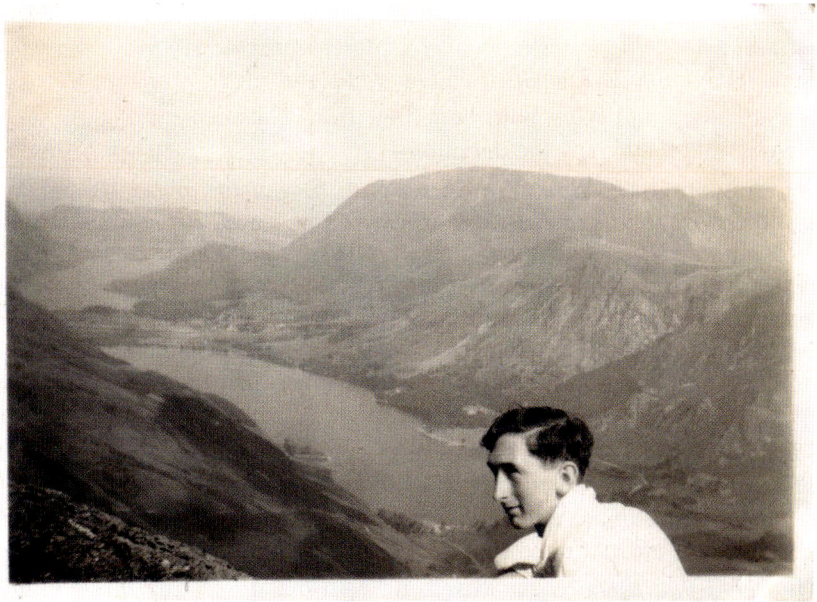

Members of the Sutton on Trent Local History Society say that the cinema was initially in the garage at the house where Geoffrey Walton and his parents lived, and then it moved to the building shown in the photograph, which was a birthday present to Geoffrey – his family made timber buildings. At one stage, Godfrey and Geoffrey ran the cinema at Sutton on Fridays and Saturdays and took the equipment to nearby villages on a trailer on other days. Local lads helped to set up the benches and earnt a penny or two for that.

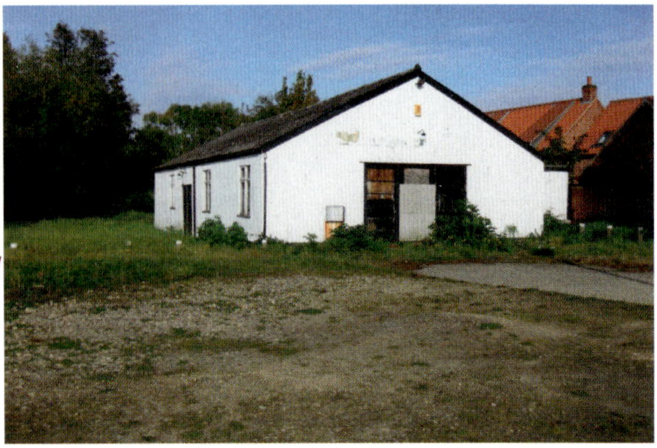

The Lyric Cinema, Sutton on Trent (Courtesy of Pat and Gordon Ellis, who took the photo shortly before the building was removed)

When Godfrey won the Nobel Prize, two of his school friends wrote to congratulate him and to reminisce about their youth. Geoff Spurr wrote, *You may have to cast your mind back about 45 years to remember the Spurr brothers, Alan and I, when we were at Magnus and used to come over to Sutton on Saturday nights for film shows in Geoffrey Walton's garage, and ride old jalopies between the poultry runs on the Walton chicken farm, and your old TDC and the twin cylinder JAP motor-bikes around your field, opposite your house. Perhaps you will also remember the notched film device which you made for our own Coronet projector.*

Geoff's wife and Alan both benefited from CT scans, and they were pleased that they knew the inventor.

Geoff Spurr says, *Alan, Goffa and I all owe a lot to Mr Ashton, an inspirational physics teacher at Magnus. There was nothing deficient in Godfrey's intellect. Like most boys of that age, including me, he had not yet woken up to the importance of hard work in furtherance of a future career, and aimed to get by doing as little as possible. 'How to escape prep by Professor G Hounsfield' was a quip in the school magazine, probably put in by some other boy. He worked at what interested him: physics and maths.*

The cinema started with 20 seats in the garage. When it moved into the bigger building there was a 16mm projector in a wooden projectionist's booth. We were in there once talking with Goffa and we forgot to change the reel until the audience called out!

He found that a cocoa tin was a tight fit into a Tate and Lyle golden syrup tin. With a hole punched into the side of the cocoa tin near the up-turned bottom, a little water and calcium carbide in the bottom of the syrup tin as in the sketch, waiting until some gas was generated and with a lighted taper applied at the hole. With a perfect mixture strength he calculated that the cocoa tin would be blown to a height of 80 feet. The height actually achieved was a matter of judgement and luck. Sometimes

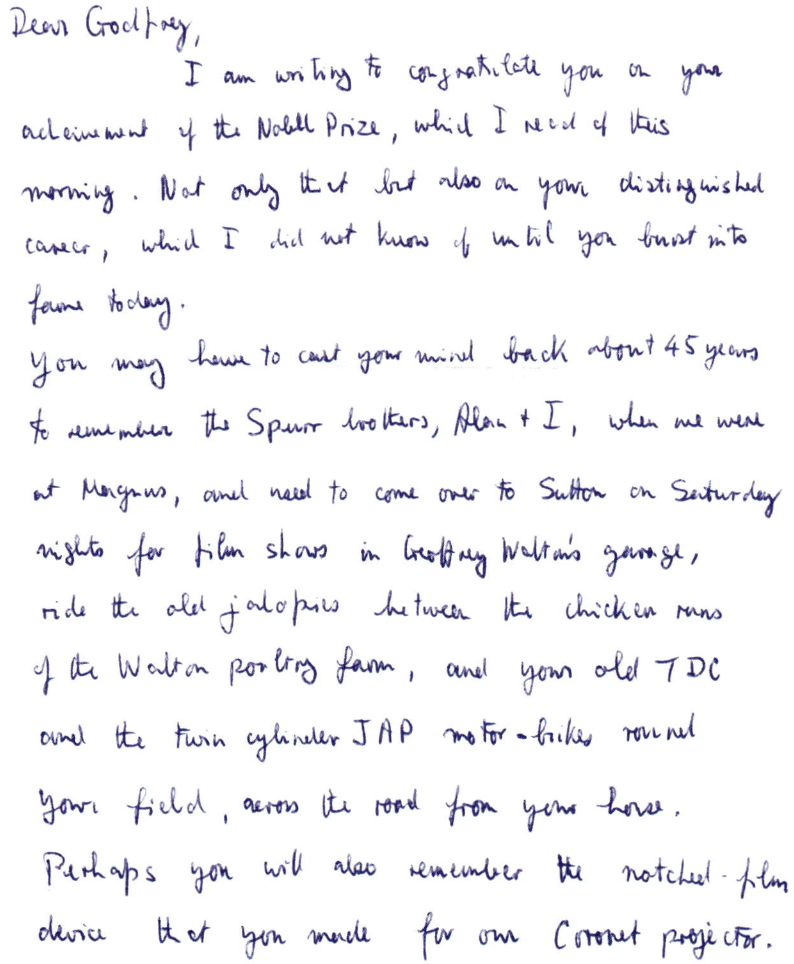

Dear Godfrey,

I am writing to congratulate you on your achievement of the Nobel Prize, which I read of this morning. Not only that but also on your distinguished career, which I did not know of until you burst into fame today.

You may have to cast your mind back about 45 years to remember the Spurr brothers, Alan + I, when we were at Magnus, and used to come over to Sutton on Saturday nights for film shows in Geoffrey Walton's garage, ride the old jalopies between the chicken runs of the Walton poultry farm, and your old TDC and the twin cylinder JAP motor-bike round your field, across the road from your house.

Perhaps you will also remember the notched-film device that you made for our Coronet projector.

October 1979 letter from Geoff Spurr
(Courtesy of Geoff Spurr)

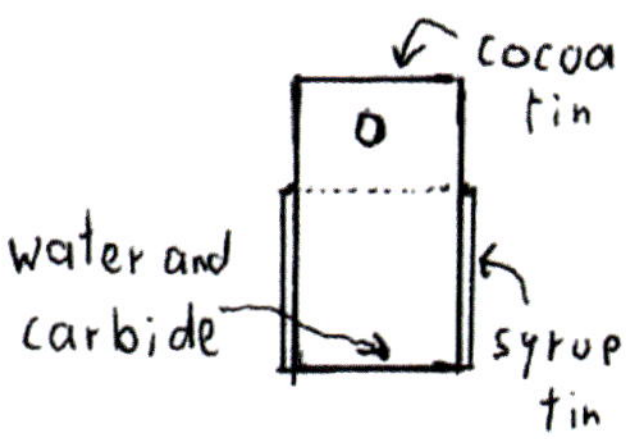

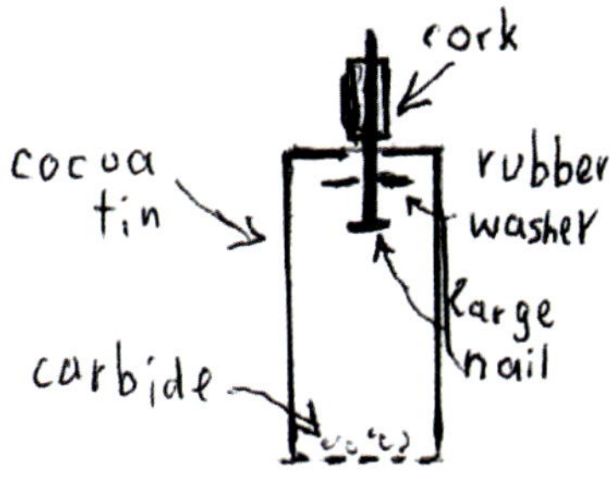

Risky cocoa and syrup tin rocket. Submarine
(Sketches courtesy of Geoff Spurr)

it would pop out only a few feet. The best result was when it shot high over our house and clattered onto what was then the main Newark to Mansfield road, just outside. There was not much traffic in those days.

Godfrey was adept in the use of acetylene gas. He devised a submarine that would submerge and resurface in succession and tested it in our water tub at Averham. The sketch shows what it consisted of. When put in the tub the contraption would sink, the cork would pull up the nail, the hole would be sealed by the washer, made from bicycle inner tube. Gas would be generated, and the assembly rise to the surface, the nail would drop, releasing the gas, and it would sink again.

Two of the many other letters congratulating Godfrey on his Nobel Prize came from people who knew him at RAF Cranwell during the war: Frank Durden and John Whinneral and his wife Mary (née Oxley).

Chapter 3
Royal Air Force and college
A significant turning point

Godfrey left the farm in 1939. The Second World War had started, and he volunteered for the Royal Air Force (RAF). The RAF, like the farm, gave Godfrey many opportunities, but again he took those opportunities in his own special way. The time in the RAF broadened his skills, made him an expert in radar and increased his confidence. His Nobel autobiography says, *Aeroplanes interested me and at the outbreak of the second world war I joined the RAF as a volunteer reservist. I took the opportunity of studying the books which the RAF made available for Radio Mechanics and looked forward to an interesting course in Radio. After sitting a trade test I was immediately taken on as a Radar Mechanic Instructor and moved to the then RAF-occupied Royal College of Science in South Kensington and later to Cranwell Radar School. At Cranwell, in my spare time, I sat and passed the City and Guilds examination in Radio Communications. While there I also occupied myself in building a large-screen oscilloscope and demonstration equipment as aids to instruction, for which I was awarded the Certificate of Merit.*

It was very fortunate for me that, during this time, my work was appreciated by Air Vice-Marshal Cassidy. He was responsible for my obtaining a grant after the war [to go to college].

City & Guilds is an organisation with a focus on vocational qualification and it has helped many people to overcome initial setbacks in education. They are rightly proud to have helped Godfrey to get his first qualification. Godfrey studied their Telecommunications syllabus, passing the Grade II exam in Radio Communications in 1944. More detail on this can be found in Appendix 5.

A certificate from July 1944 (on page 21) mentions devotion to duty, which was a quality that Godfrey showed in later years as well as in the RAF. Perhaps this is the certificate that Godfrey mentions in his autobiography, and calling it a Certificate of Merit (rather than Appreciation) was a lapse in memory. The certificate is dated a week after a letter from Air Vice-Marshal Cassidy.

Godfrey's RAF service records show that he spent the first half of his war years in places that he does not mention in his autobiography. This included a year in Taunton, close to the Quantock Hills, which he visited many times in later years with his friends. He was salvaging parts from crashed aircraft before he became a radar instructor. Presumably, he regarded the years during which he was a radar instructor (in Air Vice-Marshal Cassidy's 27 Group at South Kensington and at Cranwell) as the most important part of his time in the RAF.

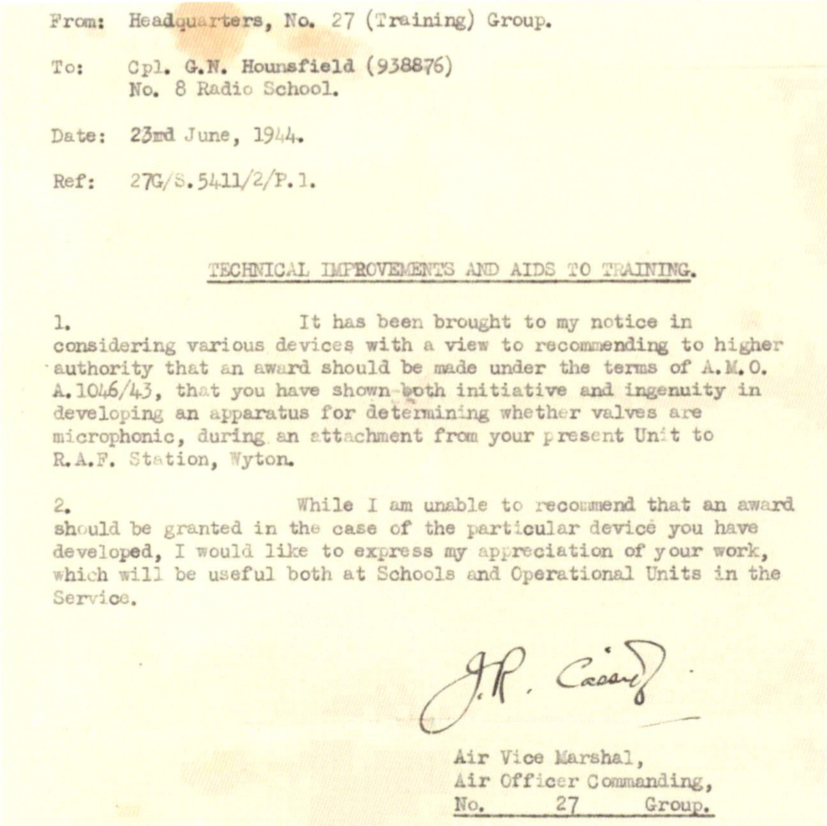

From: Headquarters, No. 27 (Training) Group.

To: Cpl. G.N. Hounsfield (938876)
No. 8 Radio School.

Date: 23rd June, 1944.

Ref: 27G/S.5411/2/P.1.

TECHNICAL IMPROVEMENTS AND AIDS TO TRAINING.

1. It has been brought to my notice in considering various devices with a view to recommending to higher authority that an award should be made under the terms of A.M.O. A.1046/43, that you have shown both initiative and ingenuity in developing an apparatus for determining whether valves are microphonic, during an attachment from your present Unit to R.A.F. Station, Wyton.

2. While I am unable to recommend that an award should be granted in the case of the particular device you have developed, I would like to express my appreciation of your work, which will be useful both at Schools and Operational Units in the Service.

J.R. Cassidy

Air Vice Marshal,
Air Officer Commanding,
No. 27 Group.

Letter to Godfrey from Air Vice-Marshal J. R. Cassidy
(Courtesy of Andrew Hounsfield)

TECHNICAL IMPROVEMENTS AND AIDS TO TRAINING

1. It has been brought to my notice in considering various devices with a view to recommending to higher authority that an award should be made under the terms of A.M.C. A.1046/43, that you have shown both initiative and ingenuity in developing an apparatus for determining whether valves are microphonic, during an attachment from your present Unit to RAF Station, Wyton.

2. While I am unable to recommend that an award should be granted […] I would like to express my appreciation of your work which will be useful both at Schools and Operational Units in the Service.

An Air Vice-Marshal is a senior rank, only three grades below the top, so this letter shows that Godfrey's work was appreciated at a high level.

Godfrey's RAF records show that he spent the first half of the war in Maintenance Units, and the second half working with radar mostly at Cranwell, or on attachment from Cranwell to stations including RAF Wyton. The dividing line between the two halves is 27 May 1942.

Godfrey joined the RAF on 20 October 1939. The recording of the dates is patchy in the middle years of his movement records. For example, the only indication of his time at Prestwick is that it comes between lines dated May and October 1942.

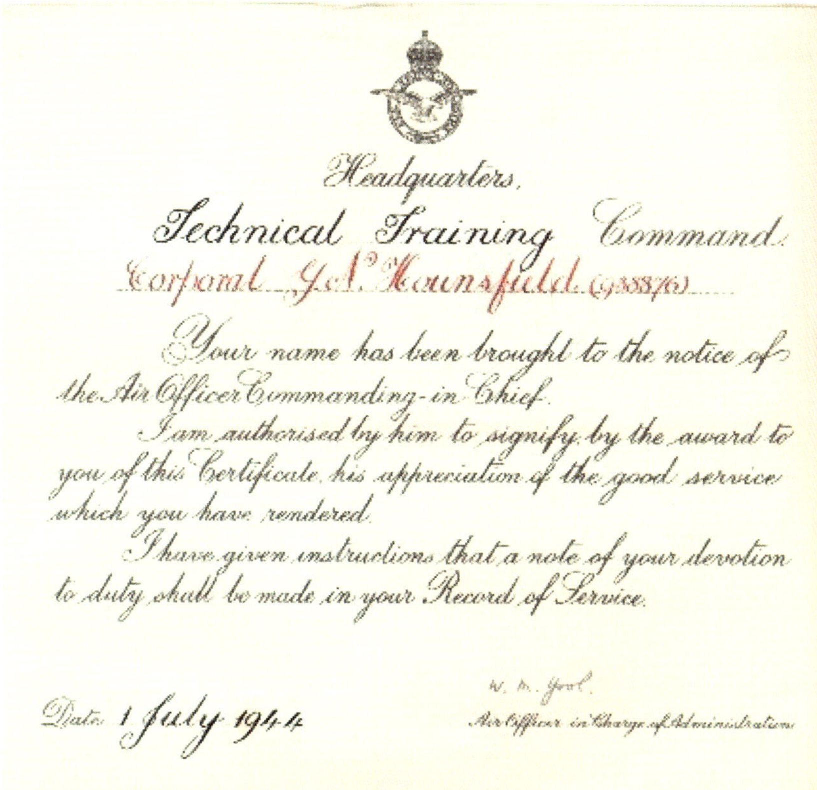

Headquarters,
Technical Training Command.
Corporal G. N. Hounsfield (938876)

Your name has been brought to the notice of the Air Officer Commanding-in-Chief.

I am authorised by him to signify by the award to you of this Certificate his appreciation of the good service which you have rendered.

I have given instructions that a note of your devotion to duty shall be made in your Record of Service.

Date 1 July 1944

W. M. Yool.
Air Officer in Charge of Administration

Certificate of Appreciation
(Courtesy of Andrew Hounsfield)

Godfrey's brother Paul kept a wartime diary from which his daughter Susan Edwards provided extracts that show an undated address for Godfrey at Number 7, Cell of Signals, Albert Court, South Kensington, London. "Cell of Signals" should be "School of Signals" and Godfrey was there from 1 October 1942. The diary includes the following notes about Godfrey: *Feb 10th 1941 – TPH home on leave and went to Eric Taylor's and then skating with Godfrey, who has now been promoted LAC.*

TPH is Godfrey's brother Paul – Thomas Paul Hounsfield. LAC is Leading Aircraftman. Godfrey joined the RAF as an Aircraftman 2. He was promoted to Aircraftman 1 in July 1940, to Leading Aircraftman in January 1941, and to Corporal in May 1943.

Apr 27th 1941 – Wrote letter to Godfrey to arrange combined leave for the 18th to take Mum and Dad to Lake District.

May 27th 1941 – TPH and Godfrey went to visit Godfrey's old landlady and then went for tea with Godfrey, Marion and Richard Forshaw at Clarks.

It seems likely that Godfrey stayed with a landlady while he was based at the RAF's number 58 Maintenance Unit in Newark from July 1940 to March 1941. Many RAF staff at the unit were billeted with local landladies. The

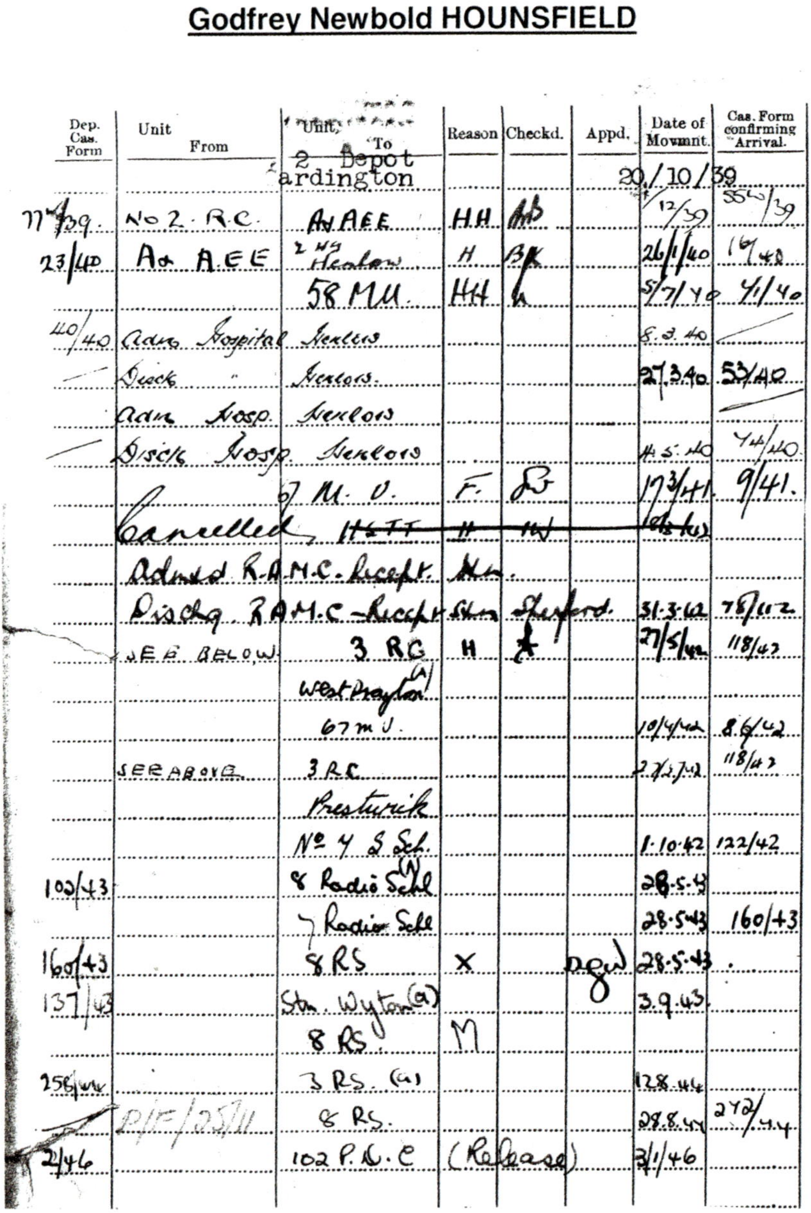

Godfrey Newbold HOUNSFIELD

Dep. Cas. Form	Unit From	Unit To	Reason	Checkd.	Appd.	Date of Movmnt.	Cas. Form confirming Arrival.
		2 Depot Cardington				20/10/39	
77/39	No 2. R.C.	At A.E.E.	HH	[illegible]		12/39	554/39
23/40	At A.E.E	2 MG Heaton	H	BK		26/1/40	16/40
		58 MU	HH	[illegible]		5/7/40	41/40
40/40	Adm Hospital	Henlow				8.3.40	
	Disch "	Henlow				27.3.40	53/40
	Adm Hosp.	Henlow					
	Disch Hosp	Henlow				4.5.40	74/40
		67 M.U.	F.	[illegible]		17/3/41	9/41.
	Cancelled	HSTT	H	[illegible]		[illegible]	
	Admd R.A.M.C. Recept.		[illegible]				
	Disch R.A.M.C. Recept		[illegible]	Shefford		31.3.42	78/42
	SEE BELOW	3 RC	H	[illegible]		27/5/42	118/42
		West Drayton (A)					
		67 MU				10/4/42	8.6/42
	SEE ABOVE	3 R.C.				27/2/42	118/42
		Prestwick					
		No 4 S Sch.				1.10.42	122/42
100/43		8 Radio Sch (W)				28.5.43	
		7 Radio Sch				28.5.43	160/43
160/43		8 RS	X		DGW	28.5.43	
137/43		Stn. Wyton (a)				3.9.43	
		8 RS	M				
256/44		3 RS. (a)				12.8.44	
	P/F/2511	8 RS.				28.8.44	272/44
2/46		102 P.D.C.	(Release)			3/1/46	

Godfrey's movement records, 1939–46

main role of this Maintenance Unit was to recover and dismantle aircraft that had crashed, and to salvage those parts that could be reused.

May 29th 1941 – The Keal family came to tea and everyone danced to Godfrey's piano playing. Godfrey's last day on leave.

July 19th 1941 – Received news that Godfrey has been passed unfit for duties abroad.

Aug 8th 1941 – Letter from Mum saying Godfrey is ill with a cough and is spending his leave in York with Geoffrey. This was Geoffrey Walton, Godfrey's friend from Sutton on Trent.

Sept 30th 1941 – Letter from Mum saying that Godfrey is home on leave and has gone to the Nottingham Empire.

April 13th 1942 – Letter from Mum saying Godfrey is in hospital.

Godfrey's movement records show that he was discharged from the Royal Army Medical Corps hospital at Sherford near Taunton on 31 March 1942, so the news took two weeks to reach Paul.

July 17th 1942 – Letter from Mum saying that Godfrey has finished second on a course and has a job as an instructor in Kilmarnock. (Dankeith House, Symington, Kilmarnock, Ayrshire.) Symington is two miles from Prestwick, and this lines up with Godfrey's movement records showing him at Prestwick in 1942. Prestwick was the base of No. 3 Radio School, which became No. 3 Radio Direction Finding School in August 1942.

Feb 14th 1943 – Saw Godfrey off. His absentmindedness made him pick up a woman's parcel by mistake at the station. He needs a firm guide.

Feb 25th 1943 – reference to TPH and Godfrey walking at Lodore Falls in the Lakes 7 years earlier. (Lodore Falls is near Keswick.)

Sept 27th 1943 – Letter from Dad saying Godfrey is flying at 30,000ft testing apparatus.

Godfrey was flying from RAF Wyton. His movement records show that he arrived at Wyton on 3 September 1943.

Feb 13th 1944 – TPH and Godfrey walked around Ossington – 'he is still very shy with girls and seems to live in another world with his job'. (Ossington is two and a half miles west of Sutton on Trent.)

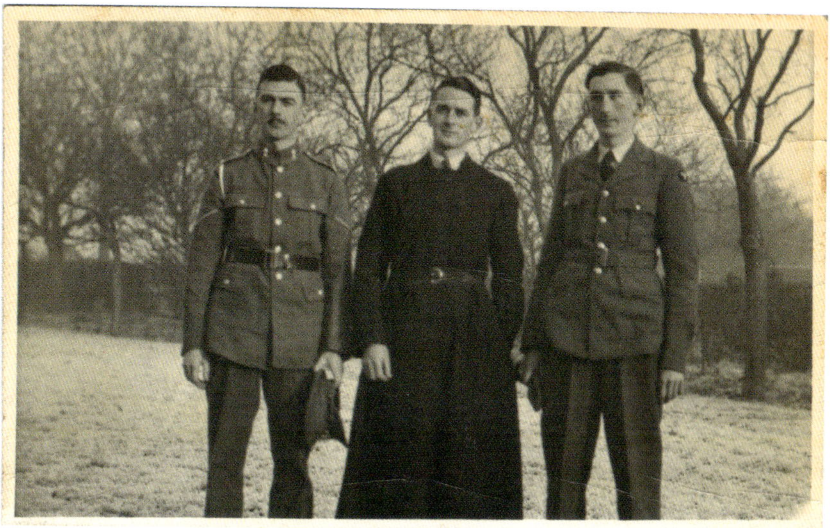

Michael, Paul, and Godfrey, 1939
(Courtesy of Ruth Harston)

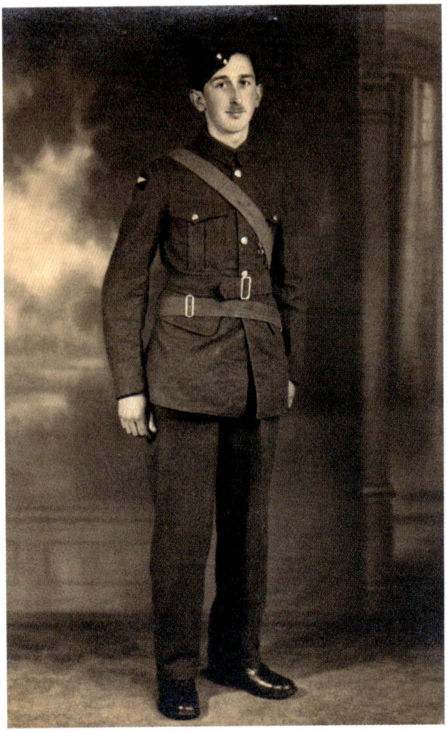

Godfrey as a "rookie" in the RAF in October 1939
(Courtesy of Andrew Hounsfield)

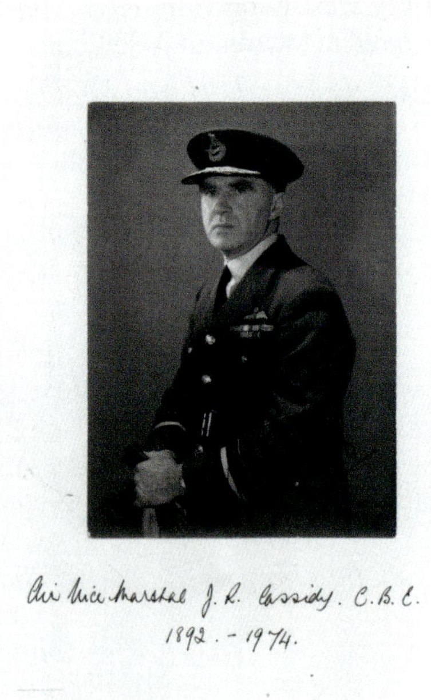

Air Vice-Marshal John Reginald Cassidy (1892–1974)
(Courtesy of Pat and Sheila Cassidy. The owner of this photo is either RAF, in which case it is UK Crown Copyright, or the Cassidy family. Both have kindly given consent for it to be used here)

In 1943, Godfrey was posted to RAF Cranwell as a radar instructor in a group commanded by Air Vice-Marshal Cassidy.

John Cassidy was born in Australia and won a Rhodes Scholarship to study at Oxford University. During the 1914–18 war, he served as a volunteer in the British Army before transferring to the RAF in April 1918 and taking an early interest in radio. He commanded the No 27 (Signals Training) Group from 1941 until his retirement in May 1946. Andrew Hounsfield says that Godfrey was full of praise for Air Vice-Marshal Cassidy.

Cranwell is twenty-two miles from Sutton on Trent, so Godfrey could visit his parents reasonably easily, and he could travel by bicycle if no petrol was available owing to wartime rationing.

Ian Dadley knew Godfrey through the MGR (Merry Go Round) social club, and had also served in the RAF, so they chatted about it. *During the war, he was a radar instructor at Cranwell, where he was lecturing to officers. Wing Commanders and Group Captains were being taught by Godfrey, although they would have lunch in the officer's mess and Godfrey would eat with the other sergeants.* (Many of his students were "other ranks" rather than officers, but he was at ease with everyone, and interested in people with ideas rather than in their status.)

He was made 'orderly sergeant' for the usual 24 hour period, and for some reason he was needed but couldn't be found. Eventually he was found asleep in his bed in the barracks, and he was given a rocket, a real telling off! Afterwards his commanding officer told him 'in the circumstances, Hounsfield, I don't think we will make you orderly sergeant again'.

One night Godfrey was called out to a nearby airfield where there was a problem with the newly arrived radar kit in the nose cone of the aircraft. Up they went for some flight tests in the Lancaster bomber. Much to the consternation of the two crewmen watching him, Godfrey started to dismantle this equipment, with sparks flying everywhere, although fortunately it was relatively safe because they were in the front of the aircraft. By the time they landed he had fixed the fault and the technical people on board with him were able to copy his modification into the radars in other Lancaster bombers.

The story about the Lancaster bomber links with stories from two of Godfrey's colleagues in the 1970s. John Ryan says: ... *around the time of the Nobel Prize, Godfrey was invited to Philips, Hamburg, where they made X-ray tubes. It was a courtesy visit because everybody wanted to meet him. Bob Froggatt asked me and Steve to accompany Godfrey and told us that we were not expected to do any work. He jokingly added that we were 'minders' and I think Godfrey may have known this. Near the centre of Hamburg there are two lakes (Aussenalster and Binnenalster) which I believe were formed in medieval times by damming a stream. Godfrey told me and Steve that it had been his job in the war to put a cross on the map of Hamburg to indicate to the bomb aimer when he should press the button to release the bombs. The cross was at the juncture of the two lakes so that the bombs landed on the ammunition dump beyond the second lake. We told Godfrey that if he did not behave himself we would tell our hosts what he did in the war. It was a beautiful evening and our hosts took us on a boat trip on the Elbe around the Freeport with a running commentary. Some of war damage to the quays was pointed out. When no-one was listening we asked Godfrey whether he was responsible.*

Anthony Strong, who was a colleague of Godfrey's from 1972, talks of a visit to Philips, probably in 1981: *When I was working at Philips Godfrey was to make a visit. He rang me up to enquire if people at the company would remember. I assured him that no one would know the past and I would not tell them. In his Air Force days he had been involved in planning a raid on one of the Philips factories. A group of Mosquitoes went in at treetop height to destroy the place where the Germans were developing radar.*

The letter from Air Vice-Marshal Cassidy in July 1944 and his service records show that Godfrey went on attachment to RAF Wyton. It was one of the airfields from which Pathfinder squadrons flew, and it was probably where he worked on bomb aiming. What may have been interesting work to a youngster in 1944 probably looked very different to him forty years later, when the full horror of the bombing by both sides was well known.

Cassidy's letter said that Godfrey had developed equipment to test whether or not valves were microphonic. An electronic valve is like a light bulb, in that it is a glass tube that contains a wire that gets hot when electricity is passed through it, and there is a vacuum inside.

In a valve, the hot wire is called the cathode, and its purpose is to emit electrons into the vacuum. The cathode and other metal electrodes inside the valve are "microphonic" if they are not rigidly mounted. If they move about as a result of noise from the aircraft engines then the output signal will include an unwanted contribution from the engine noise. This sometimes happens in guitar amplifiers as unwanted "feedback", particularly if the valve amplifier is inside the loudspeaker case. It can be caused by a manufacturing fault, or by wear and tear. Godfrey's test circuit would have put the valve into a known state and then checked that adding vibration did not alter the output, and it shows that he had taught himself a lot about electronics.

Andrew Hounsfield says, *Anything which interested him he just grabbed hold of, and would not let it go. When I was talking to him about the RAF I asked him how he had got into radar, and he said 'well, I just read a book about it, and then got a position in radar because of my knowledge'.*

Godfrey's answer is characteristically modest. Radar was a new and highly secret field. The available books were about radio, which would not make him a very strong candidate for radar work. His enthusiasm and persistence made him stand out. As Andrew says: if he was interested, he grabbed hold and would not let go.

There was a famous raid to try to capture some German radar equipment to dismantle the equipment and bring it back to be examined. Godfrey didn't know it at the time but he was being considered to go on the raid. He didn't do very well in the physical test at the obstacle course, so he wasn't taken on the trip. That was a great joke to my father. (Godfrey's brother Michael.) We have been unable to discover which raid this was. Operation Biting on 27 February 1942 was a raid on a radar installation in Bruneval on the northern coast of France. However, Godfrey's movement records suggest that he was not trained in radar until after that date.

Lynda Hounsfield, Andrew's sister, is sure that Godfrey would have got on well socially during these years: *The ladies loved him you know. They liked him because he wasn't bothered, he was just there, and he would take it or leave it. He was charming but he didn't know he was being charming, and they thought oh gosh, isn't he lovely. He hadn't realised what he had done... he hadn't realised that he had caused them to fancy him. It was sort of easy going charm and not really noticing he'd done it. That is how I saw him as a little girl: his smile was wonderful. He used to be sort of so smooth and relaxed. In would come this lanky man – everything just sort of rolled over him. That's my first impression of him at the beginning.*

Godfrey continued his interest in jazz while in the RAF. This photocopy shows him playing his home-made double bass.

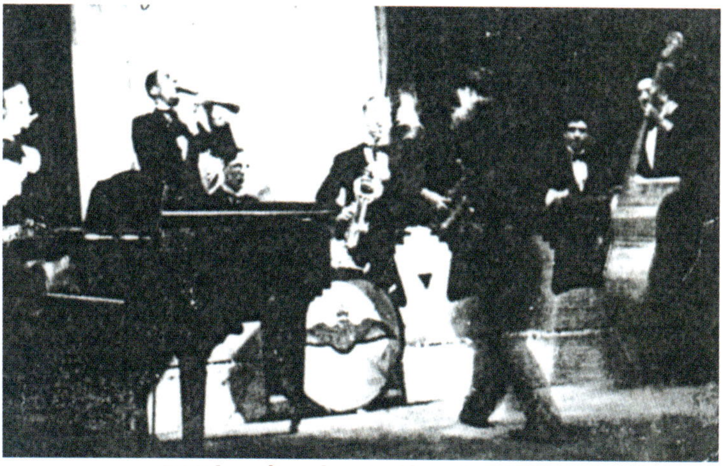

RAF jazz band – Godfrey far right
(Courtesy of Lynda Hounsfield)

He learnt music by ear in the NAAFI, which organises clubs, bars, restaurants, and shops for the UK armed services.

Godfrey's records show that he started with seven weeks at the Recruit Centre at Cardington, eight weeks at the Aeroplane and Armament Experimental Establishment at Boscombe Down and then five months at Henlow where his unit is not clearly written (if it is 2WG, this is Number 2 Training Wing, which trained aircraft riggers). Then he worked in

Newark and Taunton, salvaging parts from crashed aircraft, so he was probably trained for that work while at Henlow. He was at Newark for eight months in Maintenance Unit 58MU. Then he spent over a year in Taunton in 67MU, which was based in Marshalsea Garage in Wellington Road, and was operated by Morris Motors Ltd on behalf of the RAF. We have found no evidence of whether Godfrey had any specialised role at this stage. His pre-war record suggests that he would have happily repaired most mechanical items and radios.

He had a cancelled posting to No. 11 School of Technical Training on 18 March 1942. It is tempting to speculate whether the cancellation was related to his discharge from Sherford hospital two weeks later, or to being considered for a raid on a radar station overseas as mentioned by his nephew Andrew earlier in this chapter, but there is no definite evidence.

27 May 1942 marks the end of Godfrey's time in Maintenance Units, as he moved to Unit 3RC (possibly a transit point) and from there to Prestwick. Four months later, on 1 October 1942, he moved to No. 7 Signal School in South Kensington where he stayed for nine months. He transferred to No. 8 School of Signals in Cranwell in May 1943. He was sent on attachment from Cranwell to RAF Wyton in September 1943, and he may have remained there until shortly before the June 1944 letter from AVM Cassidy. He was attached to 3RS for part of August 1944, and was then back at Cranwell for his last 16 months in the RAF.

He spent nineteen days in hospital in May 1940. The records do not show the lengths of his other two stays in hospital.

Godfrey was demobilised from the RAF on 3 January 1946. He had learnt many new skills and obtained a grant for further education. Getting involved with radar in 1942 in the RAF was a real turning point in his life.

Godfrey's autobiography says that Air Vice-Marshal Cassidy *was responsible for my obtaining a grant after the war which enabled me to attend Faraday House Electrical Engineering College in London, where I received a diploma.*

Godfrey studied at Faraday House from 1946 to 1949. The course covered electrical and mechanical engineering. A course programme for 1947 and the lecture notes of a contemporary of Godfrey are stored in the archives of the IET and are summarised in Appendix 5. The four-year course consisted of three terms in college as "Juniors", then eight months in industry followed by five terms in college as "Seniors" and a further year of practical experience in industry.

Candidates for Faraday House either showed their school exam results, or they sat an entrance exam. It seems likely that Godfrey sat the exam, because he had no school qualifications.

The course programme shows a four-year course, but Godfrey spent about three years there. It looks as if his contemporary Douglas Foster obtained an exemption from the first year, which mostly repeated the

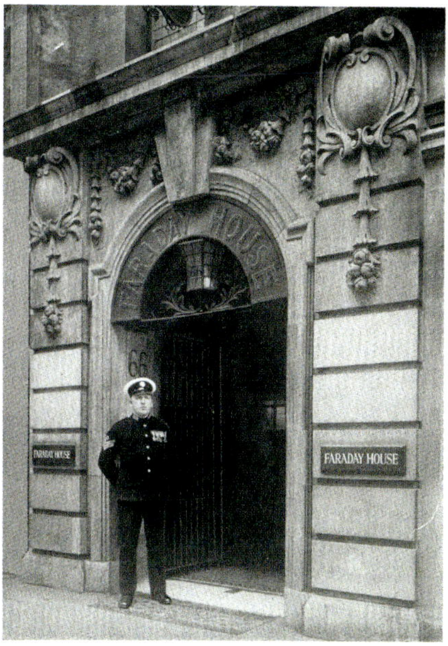

Faraday House College
(Copyright unknown, possibly expired)
The college was in Southampton Row in London. It closed in 1967, owing to difficulty in competing with universities, and the information that survives from the 1940s is sparse.

maths and science that was studied between the ages of sixteen and eighteen at school. Godfrey's RAF experience far exceeded an industrial placement, so he may have been exempted from those placements, or from the first year. He started at Faraday House no earlier than January 1946 when he left the RAF, and finished before joining EMI in October 1949. David Ollington of the Faraday House Old Students Association kindly confirmed that Godfrey was awarded the Faraday House Diploma in the Michaelmas term of 1949.

There is surprisingly little overlap between his studies at Faraday House and his subsequent work in designing electronic systems, although this is not a criticism of Godfrey or of Faraday House. They did not know how his career would develop, and colleges aim to teach students how to think, not merely how to use a set of techniques. The course covered how to generate electricity in power stations, how to transmit electric

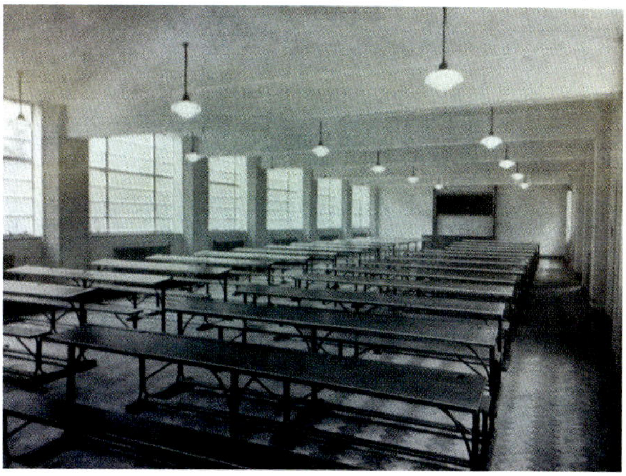

Inside Faraday House
The photograph comes from a 1939 brochure. The rooms look rather austere.

power, how to design electric motors and how magnetism works. It was a very thorough course if you wanted to know how to design electric motors, but it did not cover radio or television. So he was not taught how to design the electronic circuits that he subsequently used in his work on radar, computers and CT scanners. His knowledge of electronics relied on what he had learnt in the RAF and what he taught himself for his City & Guilds Radio Communications exam.

The mathematics was significantly below the level of a university engineering course. Godfrey did not subsequently show any liking for university-level mathematics.

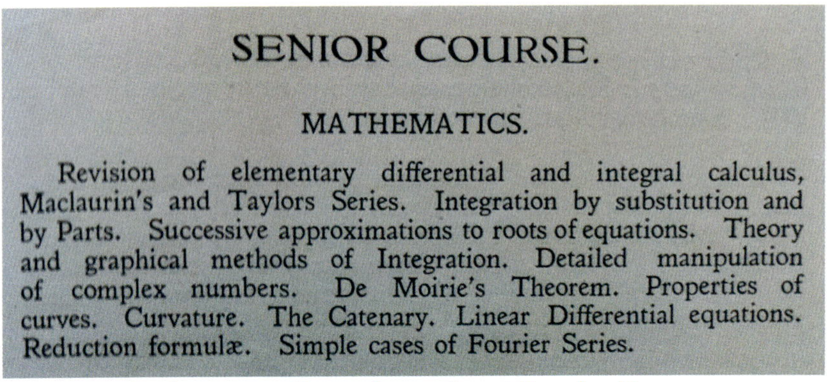
SENIOR COURSE.

MATHEMATICS.

Revision of elementary differential and integral calculus, Maclaurin's and Taylors Series. Integration by substitution and by Parts. Successive approximations to roots of equations. Theory and graphical methods of Integration. Detailed manipulation of complex numbers. De Moirie's Theorem. Properties of curves. Curvature. The Catenary. Linear Differential equations. Reduction formulæ. Simple cases of Fourier Series.

Senior course in mathematics at Faraday House

Godfrey may have chosen Faraday House as one of the few institutions that would accept him with his existing qualifications and because it would give him a Diploma of Faraday House (DFH), which made him eligible for Associate Membership of the Institute of Electrical Engineers (AMIEE, now known as the IET). At that stage he had a City & Guilds certificate but he did not have the exam results that universities required. Perhaps he chose Faraday House as a route to qualification by the age of thirty, rather than because he wished to spend his life designing electric motors.

Andrew Hounsfield says, *Godfrey didn't think much of Faraday House. He didn't like anything institutionalised or disciplined, and he found it rather restricting, like a straightjacket. But he needed a qualification and he was very grateful to Air Vice-Marshal Cassidy for his help in getting the grant to go there*.

Having left school without any qualifications the RAF had been a highly significant turning point for Godfrey. He now understood radar and electronics and had a City & Guilds qualification. The RAF had helped him to go to college. Now he could add the letters DFH and AMIEE after his name, which was useful when applying to work at EMI.

Chapter 4
Radar and computers at EMI
The years 1949–67

Godfrey would have worked on EMI's radar equipment during the war, and perhaps that was why he joined EMI after getting his Diploma from Faraday House. The company was called Electric and Musical Industries Ltd from 1931, but it was often shortened to EMI and that became the official name in 1971. Godfrey's autobiography covers his work on radar and computers as follows: *I joined the staff of EMI in Middlesex in 1951, where I worked for a while on radar and guided weapons and later ran a small design laboratory. During this time I became particularly interested in computers, which were then in their infancy. It was interesting, pioneering work at that time: drums and tape decks had to be designed from scratch. The core store was a relatively new idea which was the subject of considerable experiment. The stores had to be designed and then plain-threaded by hand (causing a few frightful tangles on occasions). Starting in about 1958 I led a design team building the first all-transistor computer to be constructed in Britain, the EMIDEC 1100. In those days the transistor, the OC72, was a relatively slow device, much slower than valves which were then used in most computers. However, I was able to overcome this problem by driving the transistor with a magnetic core. This increased the speed of the machine so that it compared with that of valve computers and brought about the use of transistors in computing earlier than had been anticipated. Twenty-four large installations were sold before increases in the speed of transistors rendered this method obsolete.*

Godfrey wrote this about twenty years after the events, and he remembered details only if they really mattered to him. The date when he joined EMI was actually 10 October 1949, not 1951. The 1949 date comes from EMI Pensions, and is correct. The 1951 date may come from an off-the-cuff remark by Godfrey in 1972 that was propagated everywhere, but is definitely wrong. The 1949 date matches receiving his Diploma from Faraday House in 1949 and his twenty-five-year long-service award from EMI in autumn 1974.

The following photo shows the complex wiring in a store inside Godfrey's computer. It is part of a buffer that stored data on the way to the printers and tape decks. Each ferrite core is about two millimetres in diameter, and has many wires threaded through it. The "frightful tangles" mentioned in his autobiography seem very likely to happen.

Godfrey worked on defence projects for his first five years at EMI, and he started to file patents at a remarkably early stage. His first patent for EMI (patent GB707450) describes an improved amplifier circuit, with an

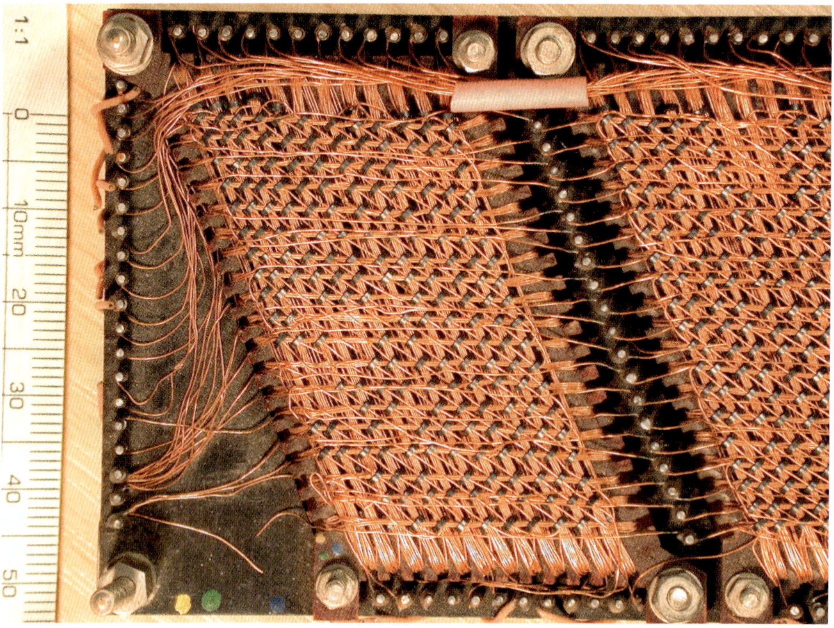

"Frightful tangles"
(Courtesy of Eric Foxley)

application date of 27 September 1950. The patent mentions computing, but in 1950 the word "computing" covered any method of calculating. Thus, a person using a mechanical calculator was called a computer. At that time EMI was using what are now called "analogue computers" in a number of defence programmes, but in those days they would simply have been called "computers". Godfrey's invention would have been used in such an analogue system.

Patents are a useful part of the historical record, but a patent does not guarantee that the invention was put to any significant use, and patents are written in legalistic language, which can be difficult to understand. In this book we mention patents when they contribute to the story. Relevant patents are listed in Appendix 6, and more detail is available from the European Patent Office website (http://ep.espacenet.com/numberSearch).

Godfrey had been living in London for four years, but his family were still mostly near Newark. At Christmas 1950 he was at his brother Michael's farm, as Richard Hounsfield recalls, *I first remember Godfrey one Christmas when I would be 4 years old, I had received a clockwork train set and I seem to remember that he spent more time playing with it, making bridges and tunnels, than I did. Anything mechanical or electronic was his world.*

I remember Christmas at home with father, Godfrey and the two sisters, Joan and Molly, where lively discussions took place on a multitude of subjects, usually with very little agreement.

One of Godfrey's colleagues on radar work was Don Tyzack, who says, *I started my engineering career as an electronic engineering trainee working for EMI Electronics. At that time there was an engineer also working there called Godfrey Hounsfield. He was a typically long haired, moustached and rather eccentric genius. Like many clever people he was anxious about his work, suffered from stomach trouble and took indigestion pills.*

I had an assignment as his assistant in those early days when he was designing the display system of a military radar called Red Indian. He would sketch out a circuit for his latest bit of invention and it was my job to solder the resistors, capacitors and inductors together with, in those days, some valves or vacuum tubes and then to try to adjust the values to make it all work.

Typical of the way Godfrey worked was the environment we worked in. In those days parts of the bare circuit were up at plus 300 volts while others were down at minus 300 volts. All this was often on a little circuit board of a few inches square.

So as you adjusted the values (of course while it was all switched on) your fingers were often low down in the bare terminals and many a time got their richly deserved shock and sometimes much remembered holes in the skin.

The valves described by Don Tyzack were the workhorse of the electronics industry for over fifty years. The work that used to be performed by valves is now carried out by 'semiconductors', such as transistors and collections of millions of transistors in silicon chips. The Red Indian radar project was designed for the Bofors gun, but it did not enter production.

Another colleague of Godfrey's was T. J. "Dick" Richards who says, *On a personal note, when I joined EMI as a student apprentice in September 1955 I had the good fortune to work in the radar and guided weapons development laboratories under the tutelage of the then Mr Hounsfield and found him to be a very kind and helpful person as well as a great engineer. An abiding memory will always be seeing Mr Hounsfield (no first names then for your elders and betters!) driving into the car park at Hayes in his scruffy dark green, mud spattered, swept back bodied Standard Vanguard. It never seemed to get cleaned! Sir Godfrey Hounsfield was a great man and engineer, who has left a lasting legacy for which millions must be thankful.*

Mac Gollifer first met Godfrey in the 1950s, and worked with him on CT scanners from 1972 onwards. Mac's wife June met Godfrey via the Ramblers Association before she met Mac, and the photo below shows them on a ramble in 1955. Mac says, *I joined the Ramblers in August 1956 and the first time I saw Godfrey on a ramble someone told me that he was a brilliant scientist who worked at EMI. Well I knew him as I worked in the next lab. I started at EMI in August 1954 working on a radar project in the Dawley 2 building.* [EMI had two buildings on Dawley Road, referred to as Dawley 1 and Dawley 2.] *Godfrey was in charge of the next lab working on a large screen radar display. He had just got it working so we went to have a look as you do. It was an orange circle with a wobble on it and my boss said 'that's the sort of thing that puts the customer off'.* Doubtless Godfrey fixed the wobble soon afterwards. The orange screen of the Red Indian radar was memorable because most screens used green phosphors in those days. Mac continues, *I remember that Godfrey wasn't with our Ramblers group very long after I joined as he joined the IVC for more stimulating conversation!* The IVC (Inter-Varsity Club) is a social and activities club started in 1947 by some undergraduates at Cambridge University who wanted to continue their social activities during vacations and after leaving university. Godfrey liked walking and lively conversation so the IVC was a good club to belong to. His friend Roger Voles introduced Godfrey to the IVC, having first met him a few years earlier: *It could have been in September 1948 when I had just joined EMI as a trainee and was working in the Marine Radar Laboratory or it may have been in the nearby Centimetrics Laboratory where I had my eighth placement in January 1951. Since then, Godfrey and I remained good friends although we never worked together on the same project and, before long, were always in different divisions within the Company and met only occasionally. From the late 1950s, we used to meet sometimes on the special Ramblers' Excursion trains that ran from London stations on Sundays.* (The 1948 date is possible if Godfrey went to EMI for a placement in industry as part of his Faraday House course.)

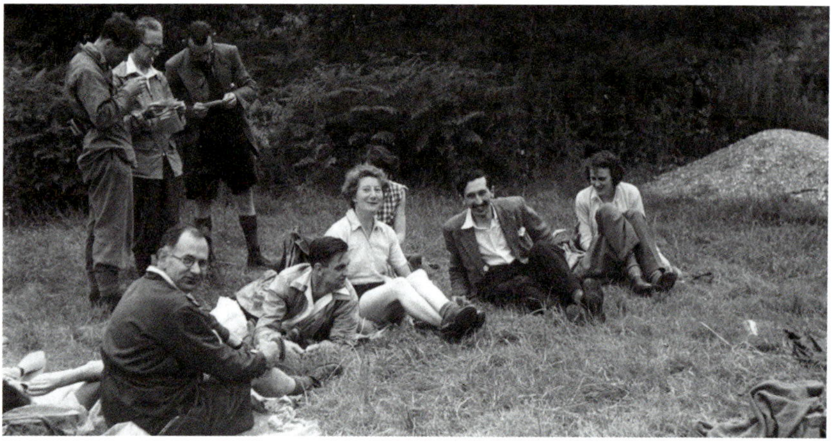

Littleworth Common, Godfrey and June are on the right
(1955 photo by Jack Cook, courtesy of Kitty Cook who is in the centre)

Mac's sister Rosemary Pegg says, *Godfrey was always a popular member of our IVC weekends exploring different parts of the country. I remember him as amiable, amusing, absent-minded and he often had problems with his car. The back seat was always strewn with papers, files and books which had to be swept into a heap if he gave anyone a lift.*

People who Godfrey met via the IVC remained an important part of his life for the next fifty years. Rosemary Pegg tells another story from the 1970s. *He was always reticent about his achievements and I remember on one occasion he turned up a day late on one of the weekends and it was only much later we discovered that he had in fact been in Spain receiving an award from the Spanish king. Godfrey didn't mention it.*

In his book "Thorn EMI: 50 Years of Radar", Derek Martin says that the Type 922 was the largest radar ever produced by EMI and that Godfrey designed the signal processing for it.

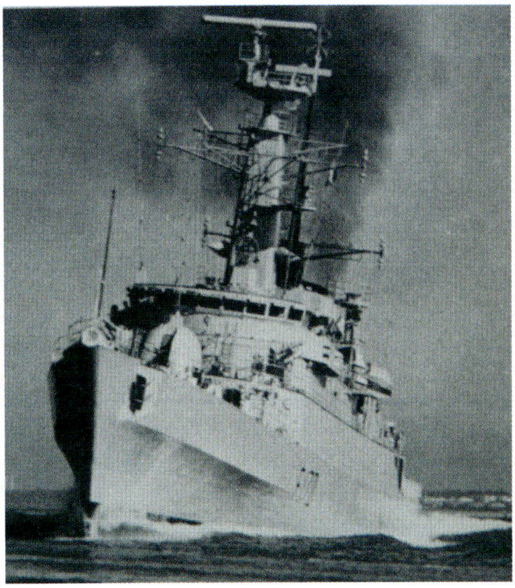

HMS Antelope with Type 992 radar mounted on the fore mast
(Copyright owner is unknown)
Godfrey designed part of the Type 992 radar that was fitted to several warships.

Godfrey worked on a mixture of radar and computer projects throughout the 1950s, and radar filled the majority of his time until 1956. After that, his main focus was on computers, but he still did some work on radar. On 24 October 1957 (in the middle of his computer work) he applied as joint inventor with Dr Eric White and Keith Huntley for a patent about improving "interscan" on radar displays. Eric White was a prolific inventor at EMI, so Godfrey had been noticed by a highly respected scientist in the company. Eric White was one of several people from the Cavendish Lab in Cambridge whom EMI recruited for the work leading up to the first 405-line television broadcasts in 1936.

Godfrey helped to design the first computer that EMI made, which was officially called the BMC Payroll Computer, or EMI Project 407, but was often called the "Austin" computer. This was a one-off design for the BMC, which made vehicles including Austin cars at its factory in Longbridge near Birmingham, UK. It was ordered in 1956 and delivered in 1957.

When Godfrey died, some photos of computers with a few words in his handwriting were found among his papers. It would be unlike Godfrey to write such notes for posterity, so perhaps he wrote them for EMI's press relations office in 1972 when he became world-famous for pioneering CT scanning. Godfrey wrote on this Austin drawing: *Despite the fact that I knew little about computers I was given half of the 'Austin' machine to design. I designed my half of the machine with transistors and magnetic cores (just emerging as new components). This persuaded management*

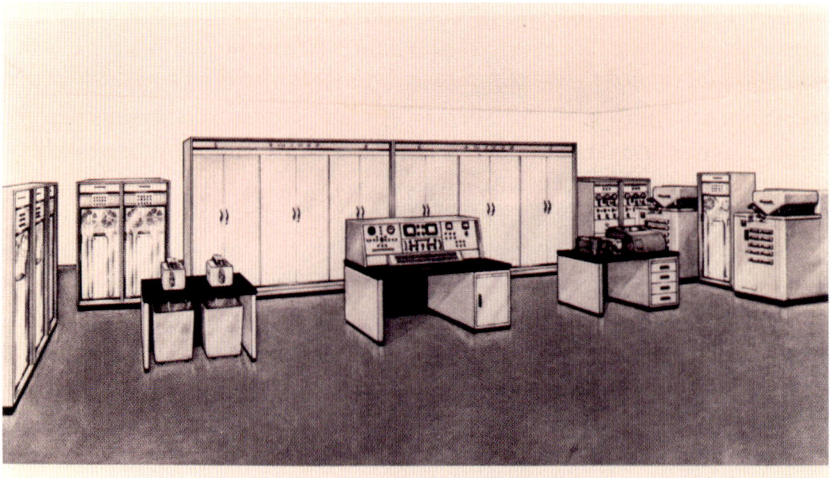

Artist's impression of the "Austin" computer
(Copyright EMI Music)

to give me a complete machine to design with the same cores and transistors, and this would be considerably faster.

The magnetic drum and the tape decks were developed by a team at EMI's site in Wells in Somerset. Godfrey's team designed the circuits to drive the punched card readers and the line printer. Ron Clayden's team designed the central processor, which carried out the arithmetic and logical calculations, and he ran the project.

The magnetic drum worked similarly to modern disks drives, but it played roles that today would be spread between the processor, the RAM and the disk. Every instruction involved reading from the drum and writing the result back to the drum.

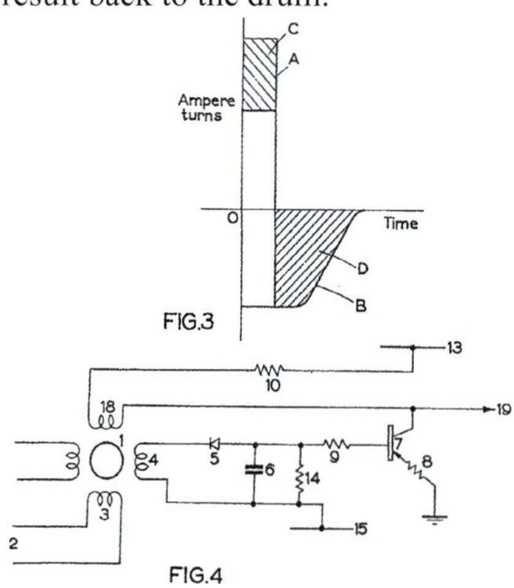

This diagram from Godfrey's patent GB893355 shows one of his ideas for using transistors and cores. The patent gives several other examples. It is not clear whether or not Godfrey used this exact circuit in the EMIDEC, but the patent gives an insight into his thinking in April 1957.

The Austin computer used both valves and transistors, which had been invented at Bell Labs in the USA a few years before. At that stage transistors were not as fast as valves. Godfrey invented a way of using magnetic "cores" to make the transistors faster. He first used this in the Austin computer, and subsequently in the central processor of the EMIDEC 1100.

Alan Thomson who worked on Ferranti computers during this period says, *the use of magnetic cores may have been partly motivated by the need to minimise the number of transistors which were used. This was due to a limited supply of transistors from the USA.*

One of the team who worked on the Austin computer with Godfrey was Robert "Bob" Froggatt, who played several important roles in Godfrey's working life over the next two decades.

Bob Froggatt in about 1976
(Copyright EMI Music)
Bob Froggatt wrote about the Austin computer in the "Journal of the Institute of Radio Engineers", as described in Appendix 9.

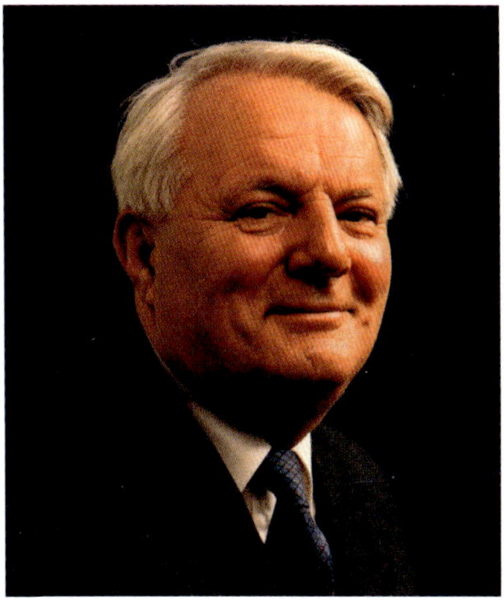

Each word of data in the Austin computer contained thirty-six binary bits, and by processing each bit in a serial manner the computer used far fewer valves than if it had tried to process all thirty-six bits at once.

The Austin computer was designed only for payroll calculations: it was not a general purpose computer. BMC and EMI worked in close partnership to define the detailed specification of the machine, and they decided that subsequent machines should be general purpose computers that could perform other tasks such as invoicing, production scheduling, and accounting, as well as payroll. Even before the BMC Payroll Computer had been delivered, BMC ordered an EMIDEC 1100.

On a photo of the EMIDEC 1100, Godfrey wrote that twenty-four machines were built. The total sales were about £6 million, which would be about the same as £100 million in 2012. The ICT company bought EMI's mainframe computer business in 1962. ICT continued to manufacture and sell this computer (as the ICT 1101) until 1966, rather than simply taking over the service and maintenance contracts from the machines that EMI had already sold. It was a substantial business over many years.

Professor Simon Lavington's book "Early British Computers" gives some sales figures that set the EMIDEC 1100 in context. In 1963, Ferranti had the joint highest sales figures in the installed base of UK-manufactured computing equipment. Ferranti's sales figures were as follows: the Pegasus 1 was launched in 1956 and sold twenty-six machines, Mercury launched in 1957 and sold nineteen machines and Pegasus 2 launched in 1959 and sold twelve machines. So selling twenty-four EMIDEC 1100s was more than respectable.

Godfrey's autobiography says that *Starting in about 1958 I led a design team building the first all-transistor computer to be constructed in Britain, the EMIDEC 1100.* Godfrey meant that the EMIDEC 1100 was the first to be commercially available: there had been earlier experimental machines. He was in charge of driving the design project, so it was his job to deliver the right result and to do so on time and on budget. Several other designers worked on this computer, and Godfrey led the design team.

After the prototype phase the manufacturing team was run by Norman Partridge. Godfrey's skills were in initial design, not in managing subsequent production. His instincts would have been to continue to improve the design, which runs counter to the need to have a stable design for easier production and maintenance.

The following photo shows a computer being assembled in EMI's factory. Godfrey has written, *EMIDEC – the largest installation at the time. There is an extra cabinet on the left containing 4 or 6 drums. It is probably the Boots machine installed 1959?* The sign above the computer says, "E.1 (Boots), Engineer in charge E.R. Randell".

A patent from February 1961 is an example of Godfrey's innovative approach. A general-purpose logic circuit would be sandwiched with capacitive coupling to a second circuit board, which defined whether it was (for example) a shift register or an adder. The second circuit board was just wiring, with no components, and so was highly unlikely to fail. This reduced the number of spare parts that were needed to only one or two boards. It is a similar idea to the configurable gate arrays that appeared about twenty years later. As far as we know, Godfrey's attempt was too early to be useful, but it is an example of his creativity and originality.

At weekends, Godfrey preferred outdoor activities. Vic Royce went on IVC outings with him and recalls his courteous and gentlemanly disposition, good humour, and self-effacement. *These qualities, combined with his physical appearance – the lean tallish figure, open and kindly facial expression and diminutive moustache – brought to mind the knightly figure one encounters on Medieval stone tombs, clad in armour, his sword by his side.*

During a walk we passed a late-eighteenth century watermill which had been restored and was open to the public. Godfrey immediately suggested we should look inside. While most of the rest of us stood staring incomprehensibly at a tangle of machinery, he made a brief

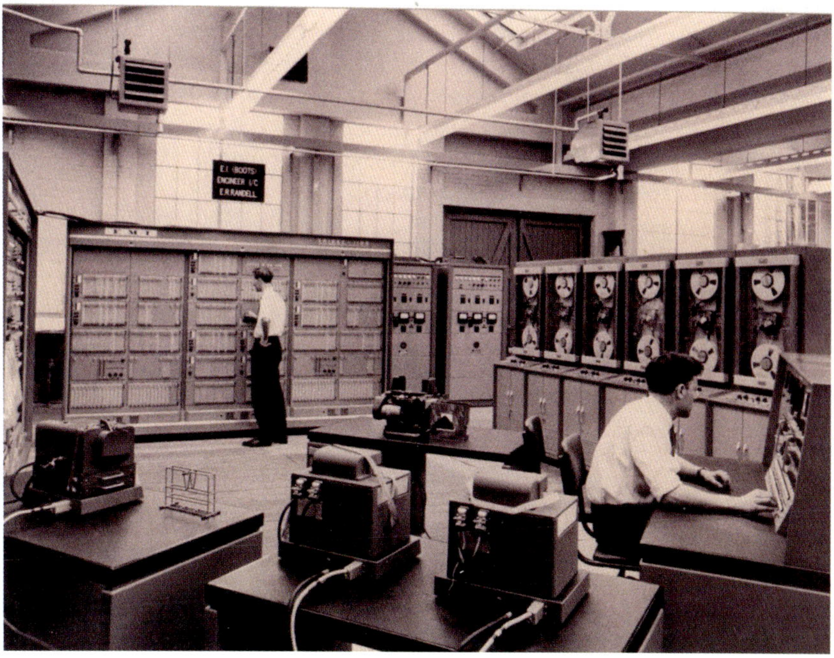

EMIDEC 1100 in the factory
(Copyright EMI Music)

but intense scrutiny of its intricacies, then, in his quiet way, explained in non-technical terms exactly how the system worked. Later, over tea back at the house, I happened to be sitting in a small group on the same table as Godfrey. In a matter-of-fact way, using a pencil and back of an envelope for illustration, he explained various gear ratios and leverages and thence what the efficiency of the mill had been in its working days. He then went on to calculate how, using the technology of its time, the design could have been changed to improve the efficiency substantially.

The transition from the BMC Payroll Computer to the EMIDEC 1100 is described by David Robinson, who worked as a logical designer on both machines: *Once the BMC machine was under construction I joined Bob Froggatt for a while, brainstorming a successor for the BMC machine. Bob was keen to use Hounsfield's core-transistor technique for as much as possible of the design, and for a while the new concept was christened 'Oxo', indicating the compactness and concentration that Bob felt should be achievable. The overall architecture of the new machine was Bob's and mine, a parallel machine with a 2-address instruction code and 1024-word memory, with magnetic drum as backing store. We felt that 1024 words of immediate access storage was ambitious enough for anyone! The basic computer would be as simple as possible with the more complicated operations, such as multiplication, being controlled by a hard-wired 'micro-program'. Bob succeeded in selling our ideas to senior management (Clifford Metcalfe) and 'Oxo' was born, later to be named EMIDEC 1100.*

At this point Godfrey was appointed as project engineer, with the job of making it all happen. There would of course have been numerous discussions before this between Bob and Godfrey on the detailed technology. When the project was under way I remember how hard Godfrey ('H' as we called him then) worked. He would always stay late in the lab working on the circuits himself.

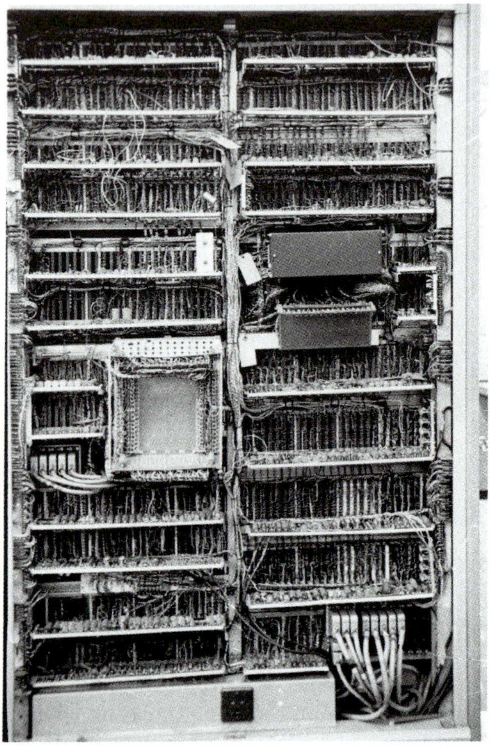

EMIDEC back-plane
(Courtesy of Mike Leith)
This shows the back of the computer. The flat rectangle on the left is the control matrix, also known as the microprogram store. Above to the right is the core store box.

The core of the control unit was a rectangular array of two-millimetre ferrite cores, mounted in a protective sandwich of Perspex. The microprogram for each function was set up by threading wires in and out of this array. The EMIDEC 1100 was faster than the Austin Computer. It operated in parallel and included magnetic core memory, which ran faster than the magnetic drum. Using transistors instead of valves made it much more reliable, as Ron Clayden explains, *If you assume a failure rate of 0.1% per 1,000 hours, a machine with 2,000 valves would on average break down every 500 hours. This was bad enough in itself, but while searching for the defective valve a second could fail, and even a third. That would lead to considerable downtime while the faults were found and rectified.* (From Computer Resurrection issue 16; 1996. p. 18; copyright Computer Conservation Society.)

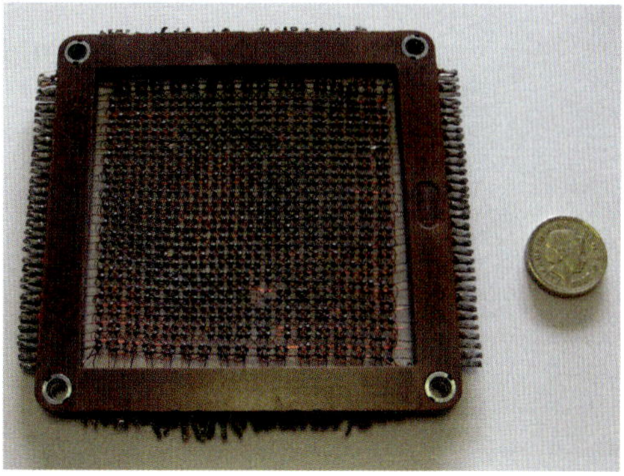

Core store
(Courtesy of Richard Waltham)
This shows 1024 bits of storage next to a £1 coin. Thirty-six of these stacked together made a store for 1024 words. Each word was thirty-six bits.

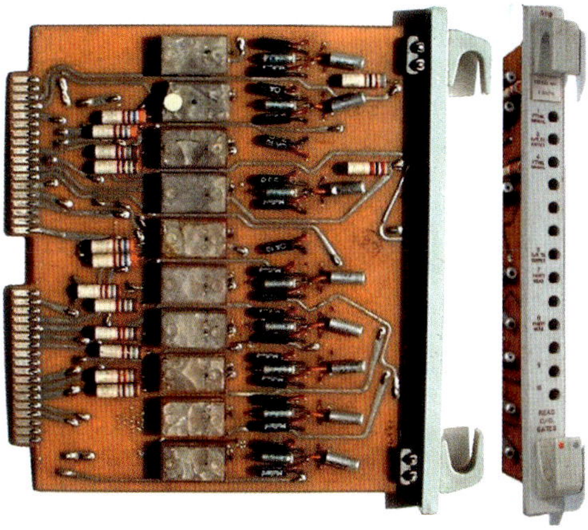

EMIDEC 1100 circuit card
(Courtesy of Andrew Wylie)

Each grey box on this circuit card is one logic gate. One gate might perform a logical AND function (in which the output is true if inputs 1 AND 2 are both true). The transistors are the grey metallic cylinders on the right, the parts with stripes are resistors and the black items are diodes. On the right is a view of the end of the card, showing test points for use during production or repair.

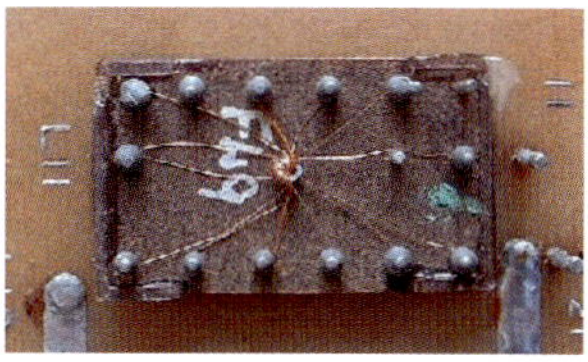

One of the grey boxes with the lid removed
(Courtesy of Andrew Wylie)
The box was about twenty-eight millimetres long.

The little doughnut with wires threaded into it is a magnetic "core" made out of ferrite. It can be magnetised so that the magnetic field is going clockwise or anticlockwise around the ring. If clockwise is binary "one" then anticlockwise will be binary "zero".

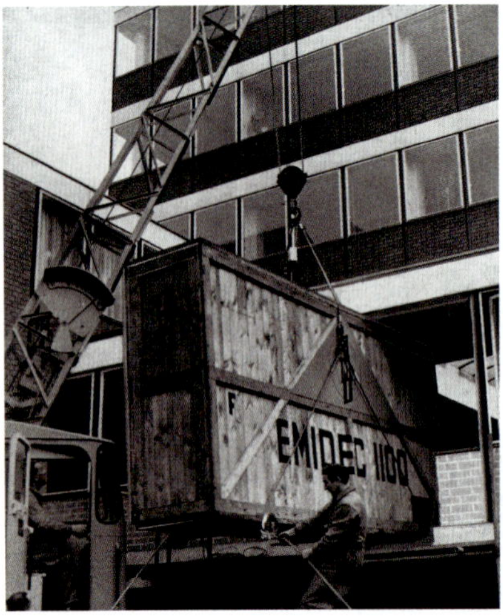

The main cabinet of an EMIDEC 1100

(Copyright EMI Music)

The computer is on a crane, about to be installed in EMI's head office to help to automate the business.

David Robinson remembers Godfrey and Bob Froggatt going on a trip to Paris to try to sell an EMIDEC 1100. Bob arrived at the airport wearing a suit and carrying his briefcase, but was rather surprised to see Godfrey in his sports jacket, with no briefcase or papers. Perhaps Godfrey felt that he did not need any props, or perhaps he assumed that Bob would be fully prepared.

In 1958, even the best computers were vastly inferior to what we have now. The time taken to add two numbers together was 140 microseconds, and multiplication took nine times longer. The EMIDEC 1100 was a fast computer in its day, but you would need to be patient if it was running a complicated program.

Years later, Godfrey was at his nephew Andrew's farm: *I remember when I got my first farm computer, to keep the pig records, while we still kept pigs. Godfrey's comment when he saw it was 'It's incredible, you know, a computer like that is far more powerful than the one which I made which would not fit in this room!'*

François Mémeteau was servicing and maintaining an EMIDEC computer at Pathe Marconi near Paris in France when he took the following photos. He says that, *every morning we had one hour of maintenance for which we stress-tested all voltages by 50% to find anything that was marginal.*

Godfrey was called "H" at work for many years. Bill Ingham says, *One episode in the computer period illustrates the way in which H inspired great loyalty in his colleagues. Bob Froggatt told me how H used to redesign a bit of the hardware and how his staff used to wait until H was away to put the system back as it was! I thought this was a joke but Bob said in all seriousness that it was true.* This loyalty was inspired by the fact that working with Godfrey was enjoyable. He was a pleasant person, and he found exciting new projects. The loyalty easily overcame the irritation of him getting too involved in details that he could have delegated.

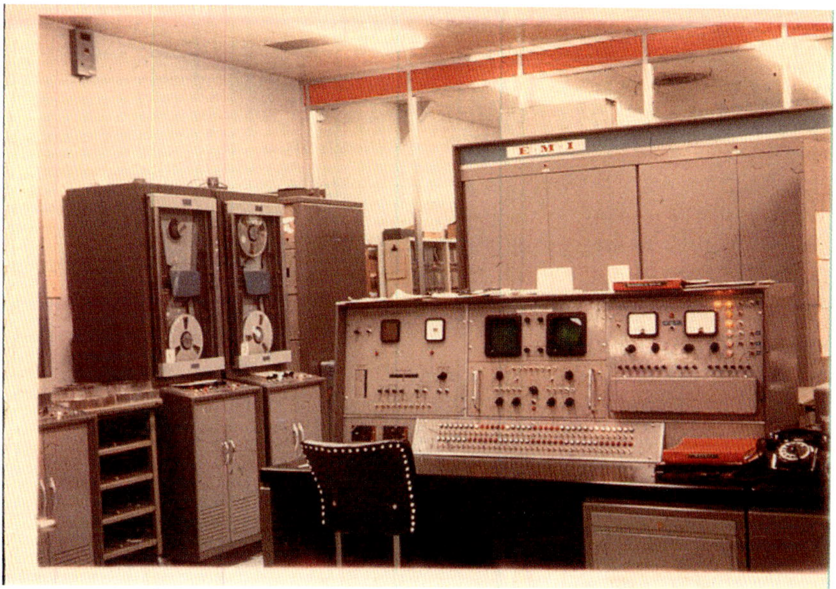

The EMIDEC control panel and two tape decks

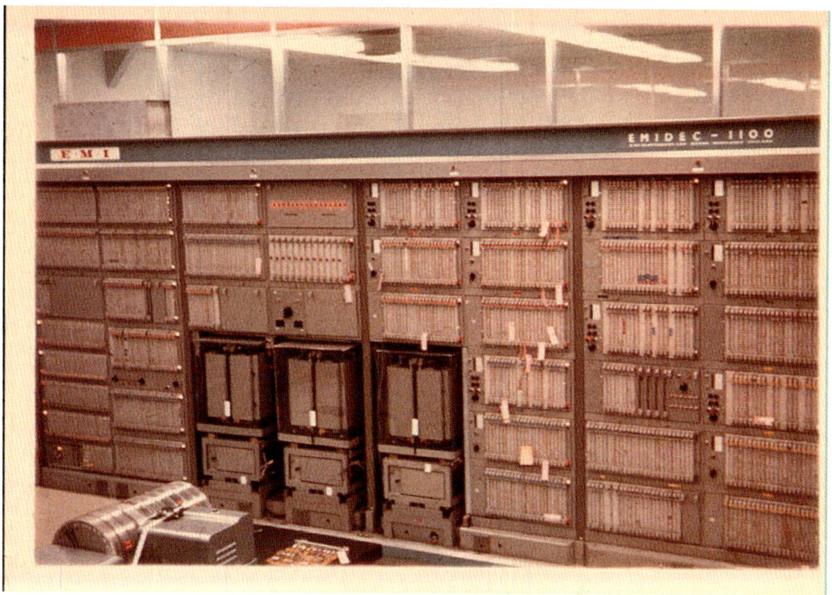

The main cabinet of an EMIDEC 1100 with the doors removed

(Both photos courtesy of François Mémeteau)

About a thousand circuit cards are visible. Three magnetic drums are in the lower half of the picture. On the left of the drums is the processor. On the right are interfaces to tape decks and printers.

Malcolm Fidge worked as an apprentice on the EMIDEC 1100 machine, and remembers Godfrey. *I was based at the Dawley works and served on the Test engineering side of things. My particular area was the peripheral equipment in particular the Elliot Card reader and the Ferranti Paper Tape reader. I worked with Mr Hounsfield on a mock up of the 1100 machine that was used at the first computer exhibition at Olympia in 1959. We had a card reader feeding a buffer store and then a Powers Samas Printer reading from the buffer. The rest of the computer frame was filled with empty panels. Once we got the machine installed on the stand, Mr Hounsfield insisted on running some tests and the two of us worked together into the early hours before Mr H drove me to my home in North Kensington in his Standard Vanguard car. On another day several of us were having lunch in the staff canteen in Hayes and he literally drew a circuit diagram out on the back of a cigarette packet. He often said 'If I was you I'd be inclined to do this or that' to give us a sense of the direction in which to proceed rather than a definite instruction. I remember another apprentice who when he heard Hounsfield say that would lean to one side in a humorous way! ... There was a great sense of excitement at being at the cutting edge of things.*

One of the letters that congratulated Godfrey on the Nobel Prize in 1979 came from John C. Howard, who worked in EMI's drawing office on the EMIDEC 1100 circuit cards. He recalled, *the day that you begged a lift home in my A40 Somerset. We had hardly got over Dawley Bridge when you banged on the dashboard and demanded that we stop. Enquiring whether you were ill, you replied 'I've just remembered – I came on my bike this morning!'*

A similar story comes from Dennis Hacking who heard it from Sam Yates, sadly now deceased. *When the tea-trolley arrived at the door of the lab for the mid-morning break, my friend Sam was waiting in the queue behind Godfrey. The tea-lady said 'I am sorry, Mr Hounsfield, but I cannot let you have anything more from the trolley until you have settled your account'. Godfrey rifled though his pockets, unearthing many unopened brown pay envelopes (which only contained pay-slips), but failing to find any cash. Eventually he had to turn to my friend and borrow some cash from him. It is not clear whether he ever paid back the loan!*

The EMIDEC 1100 was a large and successful computer in the UK market, but EMI faced difficult headwinds. The computer industry was entering a period of globalisation in which the biggest manufacturers prospered, while smaller manufacturers merged or closed down. In the UK, IBM sold twenty-one of its type-1401 computers in 1961, so it was leading the field there, but it was its global sales figures that really frightened the UK manufacturers. By the end of 1962 IBM had sold four thousand of these computers worldwide, so it had a far greater ability to fund future developments than any UK company. EMI sold its EMIDEC business to ICT and over the next six years there were further mergers.

By 1968 the business was called ICL and it was the only mainframe computer manufacturer in the UK. It faced global competition, with IBM still in the dominant position.

When EMI's computer business transferred to ICT, it was a transfer of only the manufacturing and servicing of the EMIDEC computers. EMI continued to develop and manufacture various computer-related items that could be sold separately, such as computer memories. About one hundred EMI staff transferred to work for ICT. Godfrey stayed with EMI, and he transferred to Central Research Laboratories, also known as CRL, which was in another building on EMI's Hayes site.

The IVC made a block booking at the "California in England" holiday camp, which was by Longmoor Lake in Finchampstead, about thirty miles from London.

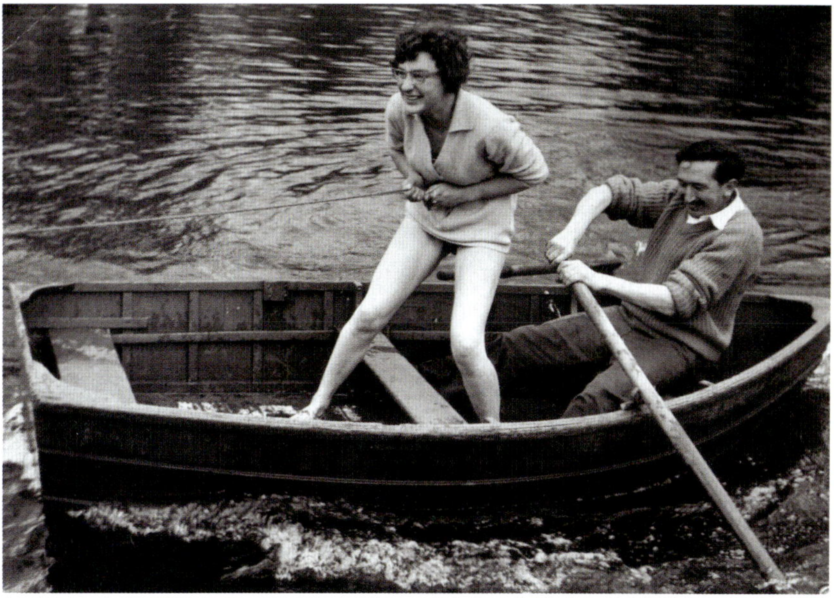

Boating, May 1961
(Copyright uncertain, possibly Inez Pugh)

Joanna Irvin recalls, *We were in a tug-of-war in a fun regatta, doing daft things. Another boat was rowing the other way, which is why I am holding a rope. We were in fits of laughter. It was a cold day in May, so I wore a sweater over my swimsuit – I thought I'd fall into the water. I saw Godfrey a few years before he died and showed him this photo, and he smiled and said 'yes, I've got a copy too.'*

I met him soon after I joined IVC in 1957. He came to the painting group – he was very talented - he didn't draw much, but when he did it was good. Sometimes we drove to the countryside but if we met in London in the evening he usually arrived too late for us to see anything he drew.

I used to invite him to parties because he would talk to everybody, although normally he was rather shy. If I didn't have a boyfriend and was going to a dance he was happy to come along, have several dances and then give me a lift home in his car.

A journey in Godfrey's car could bring unexpected surprises. Mac Gollifer remembers a Ramblers outing with Godfrey, in which he had to stop frequently to refill his car radiator. Godfrey told a story about running one of his cars without any water in the radiator, simply turning off the engine at traffic lights so that it did not overheat. He told John Ryan about refilling his radiator and then finding all the water running out of the exhaust pipe!

Godfrey's niece Lynda Hounsfield remembers his visits to the farm around this time: *he used to come up all the time at Christmas and for any breaks. I remember him arriving at Christmas and it was always touch and go, because sometimes he would ring up and say 'I am going to be a bit late because I am in Newcastle!' 'What are you doing in Newcastle Goffa?' 'Well I went to sleep and didn't get off the train!' When he visited we used to find everything that had gone wrong, because he used to love it if we had something for him to mend. Sometimes it was the clock, sometimes it was something on the car, sometimes it was something in the kitchen. He would get straight on with it. We would all think he was absolutely superman, because he always made it work. One year he brought only the underpants that he was wearing and was too embarrassed to tell anybody. He washed them out every night, until mother found them and whisked him off down to Newark to buy some new ones!*

If you hummed anything to uncle Godfrey, you only had to hum a couple of bars, and all of a sudden he was playing it on the piano with all the accompaniment, as though it was a master-piece: absolutely unbelievable. I have never seen anyone do it by ear, and be able to translate it straight onto the keys. When he wrote his own music, he wrote it upright, so the keys go across the front of the piano: that was his brain, seeing it like that.

Godfrey was on an outing with some friends when his Jaguar car got stuck in a ford. He told his nephew Andrew that eventually he had to persuade a rather angry farmer to tow him out.

Godfrey may have got stuck in a ford more than once; Heather Rowe recalls it happening in 1964 with no farmer: *Godfrey was in his large Jaguar with me, Harold Scarlett (the Chair of the IVC Churches and Castles group) and his wife-to-be, Cecily. Godfrey blithely ignored a 'Ford' sign ahead on a country road and merrily attempted to drive through only to stall in mid-water. He took off his shoes and socks, rolled up his trousers, dived under the bonnet, produced – as I recall – a piece of string, and got it going again. Harold was furious at this delay to the schedule and, similarly barefooted, paddled out and up the hill to the next Church.*

He was popular in the Travel group as he possessed a projector (not everyone did then) and was happy to offer it round. I recall him delivering

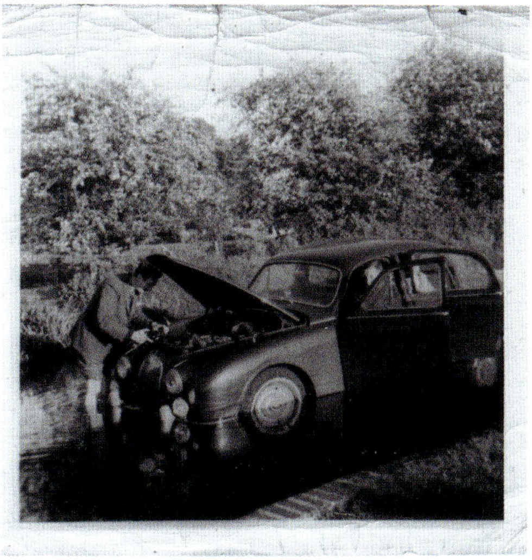

Stuck in the ford
(Copyright ownership is unknown)
Godfrey has his trousers rolled up above his knees, but is still wearing his jacket and tie.

it once to our flat in Marylebone and not bothering with the one-way entry into the Mews which caught the eye of a bobby. Godfrey was quite unconcerned.

Amy Myers remembers an incident a few years later, *I first met him in 1966 or 1967 at an IVC Churches and Castles weekend, in which 20 or 30 of us stayed in a hotel or country house and went sightseeing during the day. This was in, I think, Suffolk and Norfolk. I thought what an interesting and lively person he looked. I wasn't wrong. With two or three others, I was a passenger in Godfrey's Jaguar – not a new one, probably a fifties' model and an automatic. On the way back to where we were staying, Godfrey spotted a sign which said something like 'Ford – Deep water' and decided it was just the place to see how his Jaguar would like it. It didn't. It stopped in the middle as can be seen in the photo. Godfrey (and I think Harold Scarlett) nobly remained to tinker with the engine while we girls paddled our way out. We were in the middle of the countryside with only one house (and no phones) in sight. Eventually the car had to be towed out by a local farmer. Set down in cold print, this sounds a fairly dull episode – but it wasn't. It was fun, because Godfrey was there!*

My last vivid memory of Godfrey was in the seventies when my husband and I went to a mutual friend's New Year party. She lived in a high-rise block near Baker Street, and as the evening wore on her flat became too small for exuberant dancing and we all spilled out into the corridor – I think at Godfrey's instigation. My memory is of him wildly swinging his partners round in some kind of barn or country dance – the life and soul of the party.

Godfrey visited his brother Paul, whose daughter Ruth Harston remembers it very clearly. *He came to see us in Shropshire. He turned up in a great big Jaguar car. I was seventeen and I had just passed my driving test, and I proudly told him about this. Without a thought he just offered me the keys and said 'Would you like to go for a run in my Jaguar?' My father was absolutely horrified by this idea, and he said 'No, definitely not.' I think my father could see me wrecking Godfrey's car! But Godfrey didn't worry about the fact that I had only just passed my test.*

When we visited my grandparents in Sutton on Trent, grandmother often said that one day Godfrey would do great things. My parents thought that this was a great joke, and they would laugh about it in the car on the way home! They were very surprised, but pleased, when she turned out to be right.

Iris Glass met Godfrey via the IVC. *He loved to play the piano. His party piece was 'Go it ancient B's'. He had perfect pitch and he could play anything in any key. Late in life he realised that he could name the key which any piece of music was being played in, and he was surprised that he could do this. He could not read music: he objected to the way it was written. On his piano was a piece of paper on which he was trying to develop a better alternative! He had dreadful spelling, and he wanted to revise English spelling.*

He was not often angry, and he was not one to swear. We went to a meeting in a pub where there was only one other person, a new member, so I tried to make him welcome, but Godfrey didn't join in. There were times when he didn't quite seem able to join in, or possibly he didn't see a need to join in. Perhaps he had a bit of a blind spot in some social situations, but he was a charming man.

Geoff Lewis and Pat Scholes (now Lewis) organised an IVC skiing trip to Cervinia in Italy, taking about twenty people including Godfrey.

Pat Lewis remembers Godfrey describing *the time when his elderly Jaguar broke down at the traffic lights. He leapt out of the car and offered it to a passer-by, who accepted, for £5.*

He joined in rambles and in the painting group, doing watercolours. The group went on sketching expeditions around London in the evenings and further afield at weekends. Godfrey gave welcome lifts in the unreliable Jag!

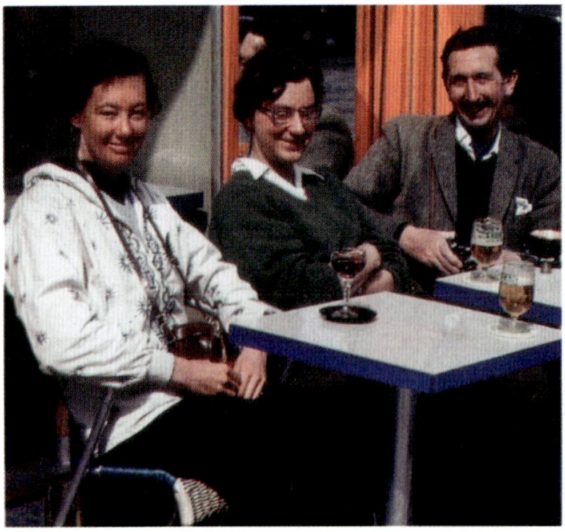

In Paris about 1963, returning from Italy
(Courtesy of Geoff Lewis)
Pat Scholes (now Lewis), Joanna Irvin, and Godfrey.

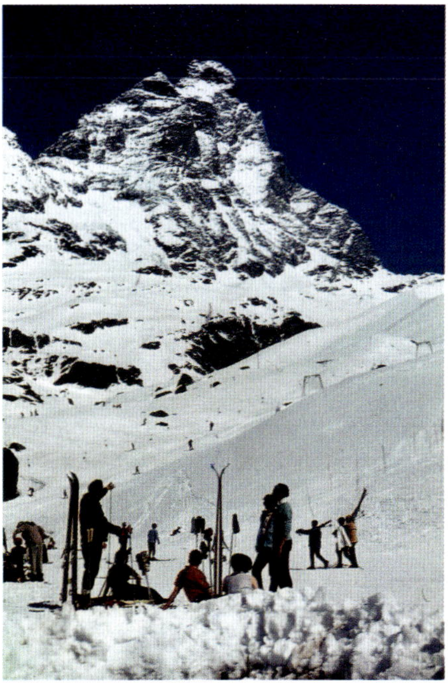

Godfrey (on the left) and the Matterhorn
(Courtesy of Geoff Lewis)

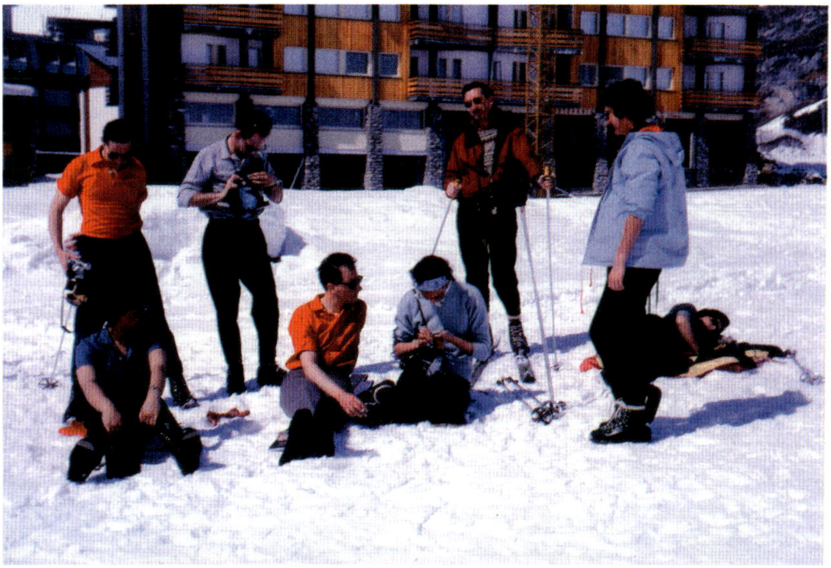

At the hotel with friends
(Courtesy of Joanna Irvin)
Standing, left to right: Richard Swain, Geoff Lewis, Godfrey, and Inez Pugh. Seated in the centre: Alan Richardson and Pat Lewis.

In September 1962 Keith Jones moved into the same lodging house as Godfrey in Isleworth: *I was immediately impressed by his thought for other people and his gentle manner. Nothing was ever too much trouble and nothing ever seemed to bother him. His car (a pale blue Standard*

10 or 12) was never washed or so it looked. Godfrey went out to drive himself to work. He was never in a hurry, but was back a few minutes later saying to those still at breakfast 'The car won't start'. An Australian, who was an aero-engine engineer at Heathrow for Quantas, went out to see if he could help. 'Open the bonnet'. 'How?' was Godfrey's reply. He had never checked his oil or water levels and said that he had only ever put petrol into the tank.

He had to move from one building to another at EMI while he was working on the first transistorised computers. He got a roll of newspaper, no I think that it was wallpaper, and slid it underneath the equipment which he had spread out all over his bench. He rolled it all up and then unrolled it at the other end. Typical improvisation!

Godfrey was now working in CRL on a project to design a new type of computer memory, which at that time was usually called a "data store" or simply a "store". EMI had several store projects: these were called HS if they were aiming at high-speed and LS if the target was to make a large store.

John Ryan, who worked with Godfrey on CT scanning from 1973, joined EMI in the 1960s. He first worked on the HS1 store, which was being built and sold by the Computer Components division. John says, *I joined Computer Components at the end of my graduate apprenticeship. It was a residue of EMI's computing division, and some EMIDEC prototypes were still there. This was when I first heard Godfrey's name. He was held in some respect even then. The market was too small and Computer Components was eventually closed. CRL continued work on the prototype HS2 store project and wanted to retain our expertise. Skills in digital electronics and integrated circuits were in short supply.*

Meanwhile, Godfrey worked on his large thin-film store. A patent in 1961 shows that he was working on this before the EMIDEC business was sold to ICT. The production route for that store would be the Computer Components business which remained with EMI, which may explain why Godfrey stayed with the company.

The store was like a sandwich. The "bread" was two large sheets of copper. Grooves were cut into the copper and long straight wires were laid into them. The top half of the next diagram shows X and Y wires crossing, and there were several hundred wires in each direction. One bit of data was stored at each place where two wires crossed.

The copper sheets were plated with nickel-iron, which was the magnetic 'thin film' in which data was stored. Pressing the sandwich together made a magnetic loop around each place where wires crossed. This loop acted like the core in a magnetic core store. This technique does not need difficult hand-wiring, so it should cost less than a magnetic core store.

The target was for a store of twenty-five million bits, an increase of seven hundred times from the memory in the EMIDEC 1100. Godfrey had an ambitious target! His team included Patrick "Pat" Brown and Peter

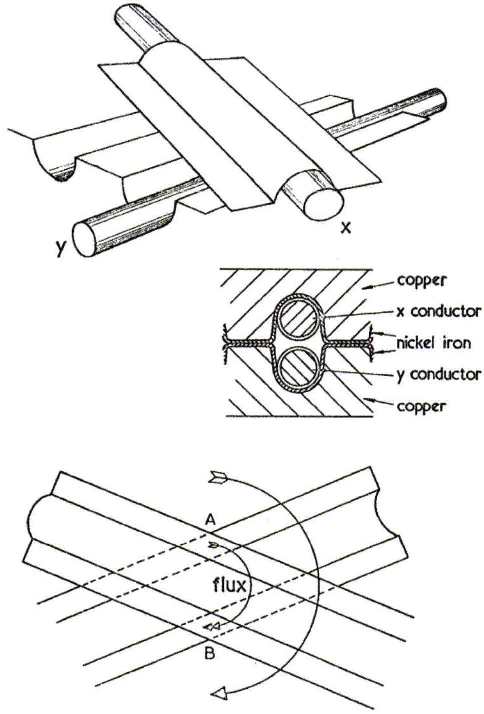

Diagram from Godfrey's April 1968 report "A large thin film store"
(Copyright EMI Music)

Langstone who were co-inventors with Godfrey of patents for this store. Peter also worked on the CT scanner.

Pat Brown recalls that *One of our most persistent problems was the growth of 'trees' in the plated layer of Nickel-Iron. These were few and far between but, in such a large area, just one or two could interfere with the mating of the plates or the placing of wire in a groove. Nevertheless we fabricated enough plates for the Magic Roundabout to be loaded for the winding process. I wonder if there is a picture of this machine anywhere?*

Sadly, there is no known photo of the Magic Roundabout, which automatically put the wires in position, and whose name came from a children's television programme of that era. The trees that Pat describes were unwanted structures in the plated layer, named after their shape. The trees were small ridges on the surface of the plated layer, whereas Godfrey and Pat wanted that surface to be as flat as possible. Pat continues, *The deburring of the grooves in the copper plates was accomplished by a polishing pad and wheel and crank mechanism. Very basic. I do not remember any attempt at electropolishing.*

I recollect driving with Godfrey in his Jaguar up the M1 to an electroplating supplier in Birmingham. We had just passed a service area when I drew his attention to his glowing ignition light. After a hurried halt and conference, he decided to reverse all the way back down the exit road to the garage! This we did without mishap and were fitted with a new belt. I was much relieved at this successful outcome.

Godfrey liked jazz, and he took me to the Runnymede Hotel to see some band which he thought were quite good. All I remember is that we both enjoyed the music, and that the bass player was wearing Wellington boots! Godfrey did like his jazz.

Progress reports were written each month, but were not filed or kept indefinitely. A few survived by accident. The March 1963 report says that Godfrey was starting work on the LS store, and contains the last surviving mention of his gate-array concept. The August 1967 report says that the store was working but that the drive circuits still needed some improvement.

Don Tyzack says that the large thin-film store project was stopped because it ran out of money, and because Hong Kong was producing low-cost core stores. This was some time after July 1967 and before the first conversation Godfrey had about CT with Stephen Bates in November 1967. The report on the large store that he wrote in April 1968 seems to have been a final attempt to find a new source of funding, which failed.

The HS2 store project faced similar difficulties, as John Ryan recalls, *ICT soon became ICL by merging with English Electric and we then only had one potential customer. We subsequently lost the order to a US company that did not even have a prototype and after two years failed to deliver. At about the same time Malvern cut off the funds for the HS3 store, because the future was seen to be in semiconductor memories.*

Ian Kimber joined Godfrey's large store project a few months before it closed: *I had been working* [before joining EMI] *in a well funded research laboratory with the latest equipment. It was precisely regimented. If you weren't sitting at your desk, pen poised ready to work, when the bell rang at 08:30 you were subject to reprimand and if you weren't careful you could risk being trampled to death in the rush when the bell rang for the end of the day. You were considered to be mad if you stayed behind to finish off what you were doing. CRL was none of these things. People seemed to arrive and leave as they pleased, worked enthusiastically, and the equipment seemed mostly from war surplus shops. Considerable effort was devoted to inventing ways to do experiments with what was available but that enabled greater insights and often threw up design ideas.*

Godfrey was always late for work but he more than compensated for that by working late in the evenings. He suffered from frequent 'migraine' headaches and had good days and bad days. On good days on the way back from lunch we would have races up the stairs to the fifth floor where our labs and offices were situated.

This was a time of extremely hierarchical lunching facilities. There was a vast self service canteen for the factory workers, a smaller self service canteen for weekly-paid staff, and a waitress service restaurant for the monthly-paid staff. In the head office there was a lunch room for section heads and major project leaders (including H). Godfrey chose to use none of these but went to a 'greasy spoon' restaurant called Brills where we would continue to discuss the project and many other ideas over lunch.

Commercial integrated circuits were being developed and the computer manufacturers could see things going solid state for main memories even though tapes and disks would last much longer! After some months the project was closed down and I was very worried being the new kid on the block. (With hindsight he did not need to be worried: he stayed with EMI for many years.)

So Godfrey needed a new project, and his search resulted in CT scanners, as described in the next chapters. But first, it is worth describing how EMI came to be involved in electronics as well as music, because this was an important part of the context in which the scanner ideas germinated.

Two music companies, Columbia and The Gramophone Company, merged to become EMI in 1931. Until 1924, most music was recorded acoustically: the singer stood in front of an acoustic horn which drove the recording stylus directly, without any electronic amplification. EMI's predecessor Columbia was irritated by having to pay royalties on the "Westrex" patent for recording music which was held by the Western Electric part of AT&T. That patent covered the new electrical recording method. Columbia paid a royalty of around five per cent of the price of the records that used this method of recording.

Isaac Shoenberg recruited Alan Blumlein who quickly solved the patent problem by finding a better alternative, which was not protected by the patent. In the next thirteen years these two remarkable men sowed the seeds that gave EMI businesses in television, studio equipment, radar, and defence electronics. Sadly their partnership ended when Blumlein died in a plane crash in 1942. The loss to the war effort was so serious that Winston Churchill forbade any announcement in the newspapers.

Alan Blumlein filed an exceptionally large number of patents while he worked for EMI, including the stereo sound system used on vinyl long-player music recordings. He invented many circuit techniques, and almost everyone who owns a radio or a mobile phone is using his "long-tailed pair", which amplifies the difference between two input voltages.

Shoenberg and Blumlein began work on television in 1931. They wanted an electronic system, to give higher definition and less flicker than Baird's mechanical television system, but this needed a vast amount of preparatory work on camera tubes, display tubes for domestic televisions, and many new electronic circuit techniques. By March 1936 they had these in prototype form, and they produced a television picture with 253 lines. The government asked for bids to build a full broadcasting system with six cameras by November 1936. It was a big step to go from prototype to full operation in such a short time, but EMI's bid went even further and offered a 405-line system. This was built in competition with a parallel project by Baird and the EMI solution was the winner. This courageous leap set the television standard for the UK until 1964.

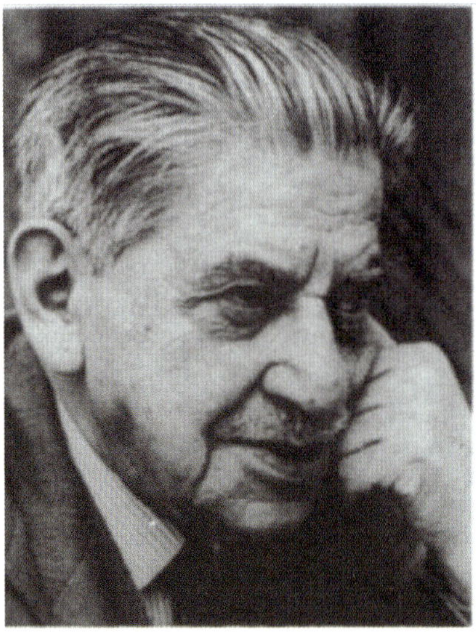
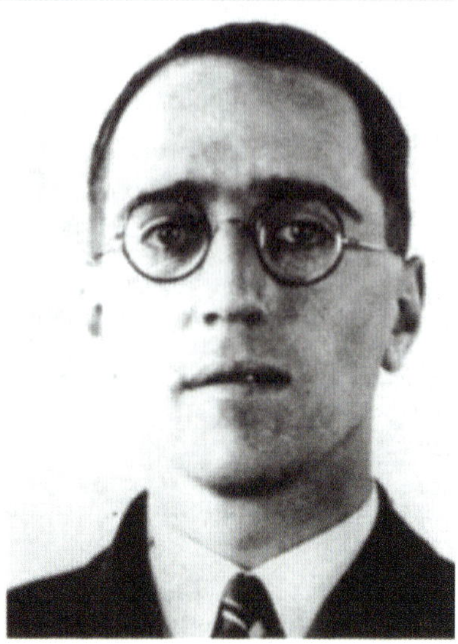

Sir Isaac Shoenberg and Alan Blumlein
(Copyright EMI Music)

All television work was put on hold when the war started in 1939. EMI had not previously worked on defence projects, but the secret work on radar needed similar receivers and display screens to television, radar transmitters were similar to television transmitters, and EMI's test equipment for television was equally useful for radar. In October 1940 it delivered the world's first effective radar for fighter aircraft. Blumlein died on 12 June 1942 during flight tests for another airborne radar, the H2S, which ultimately helped to win the battle of the Atlantic by finding the U-boats. (The H2S radar would have been included in the courses that Godfrey taught at RAF Cranwell.) EMI also built the proximity fuses that helped to destroy two-thirds of the V-1 flying bombs.

Alan Blumlein was one of the greatest engineers, and his director, Isaac Shoenberg, had the courage to back him. Together they had expanded EMI from being purely a music company to being one of the best electronics companies in the world, active in new radar and television industries. Who knows what more they would have achieved if Blumlein had survived the war?

After the war ended in 1945, the UK economy was in a dreadful state. The war had inflicted great damage to people, homes, and factories. The country was deep in debt, and it was difficult to import goods or to travel overseas because of a lack of foreign exchange. Food rationing was introduced during the war, but it continued for **nine** years after the war ended. Sometimes labour relations were poor. Trade unions were blamed for inefficient working practices and unnecessary strikes. Companies were accused of poor management and under-investment. Millions of people were trying to adapt from war to peacetime. The 1948 Olympic Games were held in London but there was no money to build new facilities. The athletes had to stay in army camps and college dormitories and bring their own food!

As far as EMI was concerned, defence electronics projects were still needed, but they were often more incremental than the radical innovations during the war. The procurement processes were arguably less beneficial for both sides in "cost plus ten per cent" contracts, in which the suppliers could make easy but undramatic profits simply by spending time on a project. Bill Ingham joined EMI's CRL in 1946. His recollection is that *EMI was of course very different in those days. I joined the audio department and worked on the Outside Broadcast van for the Olympics but was lucky enough to be given a project to devise an information interchange system which used digital logic, and then worked on circuits for some of the very first transistors.*

There were several massive cost cutting exercises. Joseph Lockwood said things were so desperate when he took over that he was unsure whether he would be able to pay the wages.

EMI went into computers in much the way it had operated in defence, using its technical know-how and winning contracts, e.g. from the NRDC [National Research Development Corporation]*, so that its investment was small.*

Sir Joseph Lockwood was chairman of EMI from 1954 to 1974, and chief executive for the first fifteen years of that. There were coincidental links between Sir Joseph and Godfrey: their brothers farmed about five miles apart and they both attended the same school, although their time at Magnus school did not overlap. Sir Joseph was on the NRDC advisory board for computing from 1951, so they were both interested in the early years of computers. But it was the EMIDEC, not the coincidences, that was the first reason for Sir Joseph to talk to Godfrey about his work.

Sir Joseph was interested in research, although he did not specifically sponsor Godfrey's 3D X-ray project. He was an industrialist with a strong vision: Ray Gilson recalled him saying, when someone talked about studying the market, *This is EMI. We don't follow markets, we create them!* William Cavendish, who assisted Sir Joseph, notes that he set up a research facility at his previous company, Henry Simon Ltd., and that he visited CRL whenever visiting Hayes, and saw Godfrey's early CT scans of a pig carcase as well as the research for the music business.

In his history of EMI in the book "From Making to Music", S. A. Pandit says, *Sir Joseph Lockwood was a dominant figure in the post war history of EMI. [...] After years of moribund financial results, between 1954 and 1960 pre-tax profits grew at 30 percent per annum. [...] He was the first board member to see the potential for popular music and to make a point of taking an interest in it.*

While Godfrey was developing his prototype CT scanner, EMI had a very diverse collection of businesses. It recorded and sold music in markets all over the world. It owned Elstree Film Studios, the ABC Cinemas that were present in most towns in England, Thames Television (a commercial broadcaster who competed with the BBC), and the Blackpool Tower seaside attraction. It made ten films during 1970 for release in cinemas, and was active in the theatre market in London. EMI made television cameras, television transmitter aerials, studio equipment, loudspeakers,

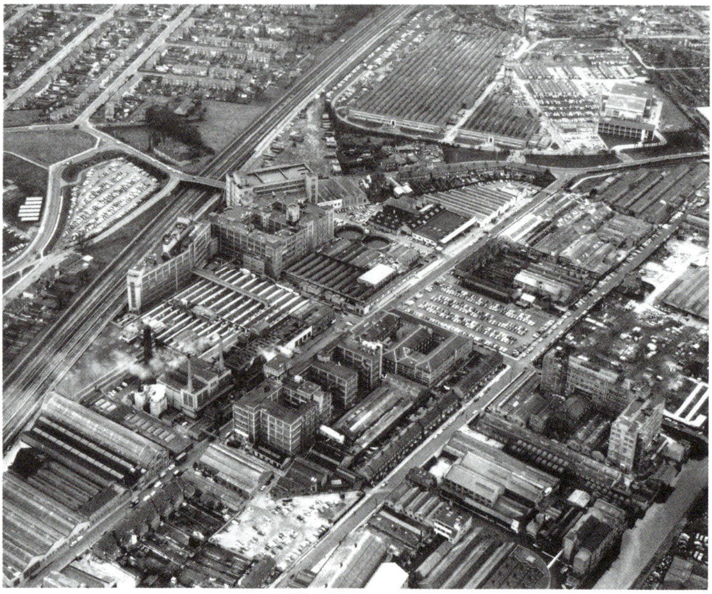

EMI's Hayes site
(Copyright EMI Music)
There is an annotated version below.

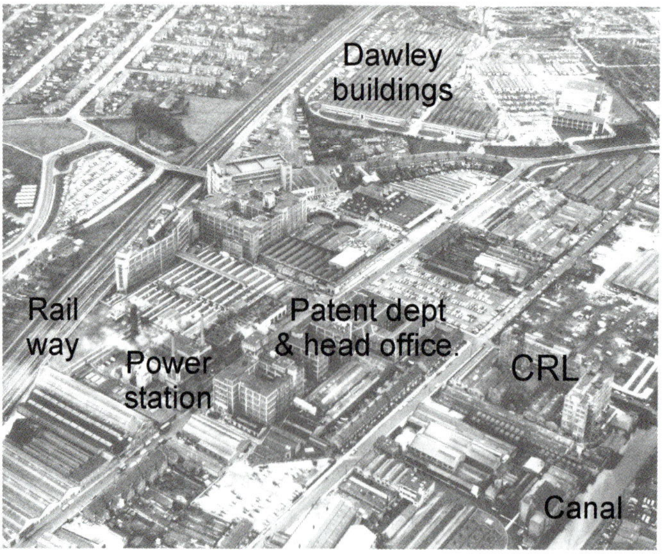

magnetic tape, tape recorders for military and commercial use, products to automate factories, oscilloscopes, flow sensors and photo-multipliers, thermal imagers, and radars for defence, commercial airports, and privately owned boats. It also made and installed fire alarm systems. It was a vast array of activities. EMI employed 28,000 people in the UK, and its main site in Hayes had its own power station to supply the factories.

The Dawley Road buildings where the EMIDEC 1100 was made are top centre. Smoke and steam come from the electric power station chimneys on the left of the photo. Godfrey invented CT in the L-shaped CRL building on the right of the photo next to the Grand Union canal.

The split of sales and profit for the year to 30 June 1970 was:

	Sales	**Profits**
Leisure, including records and tape	60%	66%
Entertainment, including film production and exhibition	14%	16%
Television	5%	4%
Electronics, radio, and television equipment	20%	13%
Other activities	1%	1%

The "electronics" business, which included Godfrey, delivered only twenty per cent of sales and thirteen per cent of profits. An accountant might think that the electronics activities should have been sold off, to focus efforts on the more profitable leisure and entertainment areas, but the 1970 annual report declared an intention to grow the electronics business and make it more profitable.

In the book "From Making to Music", S. A. Pandit says that EMI's board wanted to balance the business, with a diversified portfolio of activities across a range of markets. He argues that it is better to focus and that conglomerates are bad at managing businesses that are undergoing rapid changes in technology or markets. He uses memorable phrases, such as *a conglomerate is particularly prone to pointing fingers and not learning from events. [...] Perversely, risk taking is greatest when the issues are least understood, and is discouraged where it is most necessary.* It would be grossly inaccurate to apply these criticisms across all parts of EMI at all times. However, it is fair to say that EMI was a curate's egg, in that parts were good but others were less so.

When Godfrey Hounsfield joined EMI in 1949 it was among the leading companies in electronics, and it still had a positive attitude towards innovation. Shoenberg and Blumlein established a track record of bold research funded from within EMI, leading to strong patents and new industries. By the time Godfrey ceased computing work in 1967 the post-war changes (and the loss of Blumlein) had dented but not eliminated this legacy. Godfrey and the directors of the research labs, Len Broadway until

1969 and Bill Ingham thereafter, were well aware of that track record. It was still possible to make big innovations at EMI, but it was certainly not at all easy. The easy path was to make incremental developments in established markets where funding could be obtained from outside, rather than from within EMI. Godfrey preferred to be more radical.

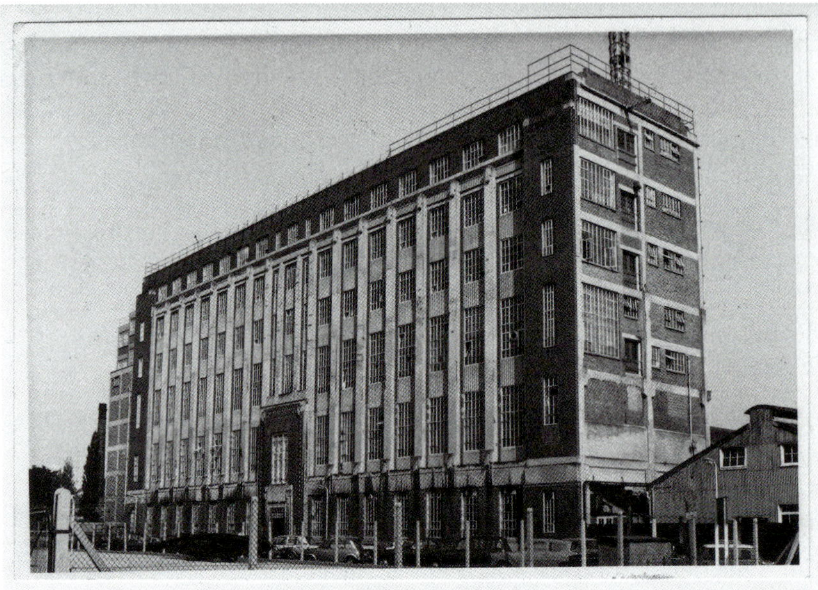

EMI Cental Research Labs; CRL
(Copyright EMI Music)
This is where electronically scanned television and stereo music recording were invented in 1931–36. It was the home of vital radar work from 1939 onwards. It was where Godfrey pioneered CT scanning. It usually housed about 250 researchers.

Chapter 5
Early struggles to develop and test ideas

Groundwork on image reconstruction, and first meetings with the DHSS

Godfrey's autobiography describes 1962–76 as follows: *When this* [work on the EMIDEC 1100 computer] *finished I transferred to EMI Central Research Laboratories, also at Hayes. My first project there was hardly covered in glory: I set out to design a one-million word immediate access thin-film computer store. The problem was that after a time it was evident that this would not be commercially viable. The project was therefore abandoned and, rather than being immediately assigned to another task I was given the opportunity to go away quietly and think of other areas of research which I thought might be fruitful. One of the suggestions I put forward was connected with automatic pattern recognition and it was while exploring various aspects of pattern recognition and their potential, in 1967, that the idea occurred to me which was eventually to become the EMI-Scanner and the technique of computed tomography.*

The steps in my work between this initial idea and its realisation in the first clinical brain-scanner have already been well documented. As might be expected, the programme involved many frustrations, occasional awareness of achievement when particular technical hurdles were overcome, and some amusing incidents, not least the experiences of travelling across London by public transport carrying bullock's brains for use in evaluation of an experimental scanner rig in the Laboratories.

After the initial experimental work, the designing and building of four original clinical prototypes and the development of five progressively more sophisticated prototypes of brain and whole body scanner (three of which went into production) kept me fully occupied until 1976.

Godfrey did not easily abandon his computer store project. He thought that it could still be commercially viable, and he did not immediately have a better project to work on. The computer store was not quite finished, and he worked very long hours to complete it. This was in spite of the facts that he was not being paid for the extra hours, and he had also been told to stop the project because the money had run out. He even had a camp bed in his lab. Persistence and determination were hallmarks of his character. It would have been understandable if he had been worried about not knowing what work he would be doing next. He had spent the last eleven years working on computers and his employer had lost interest in that field. He was forty-eight years old and did not yet own a house. What was he going to do next?

Godfrey was not the only person whose project faced an uncertain future. Several other projects had run out of money and did not seem to have a viable future, so the overall financial position of CRL was not good. At the same time, EMI was making its financial controls more rigorous. The next few years saw a reduction of about twenty-five per cent in the number of research staff, some of whom were redeployed into other parts of EMI, and some of whom left the company. Ian Kimber who had worked on Godfrey's computer store says, *I was then moved to work in the high speed military store area. Peter Langstone was moved out to work at Springfield Road and Godfrey was on his own.* Peter Langstone did not like being transferred to Springfield Road, where he worked for EMI's defence electronics business.

Roger Voles had an interesting conversation during a walk with Godfrey sometime in the 1960s: *the conversation turned to the question of whether there was any way of finding any undiscovered chambers in the pyramids. At this distance in time, I forget who said exactly what that day, but it went something like this. Suppose that certain rays from the sun could penetrate deeply into the pyramid. [...] If we put a detector outside the pyramid on the far side from the sun and moved the detector, day-by-day, across the two shadow areas as the sun rose and set, the whole volume of the pyramid could be explored for undiscovered chambers. The intersection of two lines of detection would give the position of the chamber. Godfrey and I never spoke about this discussion again. However, when he was chatting with my wife after a lecture and dinner at the IEE in 1993, Godfrey reflected that it had all started when he and I had been speculating on a ramble one day.*

In a video conversation with his friend and former colleague Bill Ingham, Godfrey said that he started working on seeing inside a "box" purely as a puzzle, before he thought of the medical X-ray application: *I was walking with Roger Voles at the time. When the box idea came up I remember asking him the question why can't we do that?* The idea stuck, "niggling" in Godfrey's mind for months after this walk, as he says at another point in the same conversation: *if I had a number of readings taken through a box from various angles, could I find out what was in the box? It was a puzzle that kept on niggling at me. Just for fun I worked it out.* After a short pause, with a shy smile, he continued, *It turned into something worthwhile in the end.* What an understatement!

Roger and Godfrey were dreaming up ways to find big targets like chambers inside a pyramid, using a form of solar radiation that may not exist. It was a game: it may seem strange to non-technical people, but quite natural to scientists and engineers. We do not know if they were aware that the idea of finding chambers in pyramids had been suggested by Luis Alvarez in 1965. His expedition searched the second pyramid of Giza from the spring of 1967, and reports of it were in the press at that time. Alvarez used bubble chambers to detect muons, which are created in the upper atmosphere by cosmic rays, which arrive from outside the solar system. He recorded the paths of more than a million of these that had penetrated through the pyramid into the Belzoni chamber. His plan was to move the detector around the inside of the chamber and triangulate to find the location of any unknown chambers. He proved that there were no undiscovered chambers in the area he searched, and his test stopped in late 1969.

Godfrey leapt on to consider a much harder problem: he wanted an accurate solution that would work regardless of the contents of the box. He was no longer starting from the knowledge that the box contained only stone and air, and his problem could not be solved by triangulation. The conversation with Roger had made him aware that working out the exact contents of a box was an interesting and, as yet, unsolved problem. This was not a Eureka moment: after this ramble Godfrey was at a stage that a patent agent would dismiss as "free beer". You cannot write a patent that simply says, *I would like to produce free beer, or at least cheaper beer*. You can only write a patent that says, *I have a method of producing cheaper beer, and here is a full description of how to do it*. The cogs in Godfrey's brain had started to turn, but the problem was still niggling – it was under investigation, rather than solved.

Godfrey seems to have quickly forgotten all about the pyramid. His target was to get accurate knowledge of everything in the box, not simply to detect the presence or absence of chambers. He was interested in the puzzle, not the pyramid.

In a speech to pupils at his former school, Godfrey said that his ideas came gradually, and people were often disappointed that he could not tell them about a Eureka moment. Perhaps there is a natural tendency to dream that *it could have happened to me: if only I had the idea of inventing the electric light-bulb ...,* but it remains a dream. Thomas Edison (a prolific inventor who developed the first commercially useful light bulbs) said that *genius is one percent inspiration, ninety-nine percent perspiration.* Dreamers run out of steam, but the dogged determination of people like Hounsfield or Edison drives them through the long and difficult process of turning a fleeting thought into a whole new industry.

There were several significant changes during the summer months of 1967 that conspired to give Godfrey the time to look again at this "niggle". The director of CRL (Len Broadway) was assisted by Don Tyzack, who already knew Godfrey from working with him on radar in the 1950s. Part of Don's role in 1967 was to help to keep the research projects on the right lines financially. Don describes Godfrey's dogged persistence on the over-spent large store project: *Len and I discussed our problem. We had already told Godfrey to stop the computer job but the costs kept going up. He clearly needed another interest.*

The next step is described by Bill Ingham in his unpublished document "The Scanner Research in the Central Research Laboratories of EMI", copyright of which is held by the Royal Society. Bill wrote most of this during the 1980s, but it is based on his detailed contemporary files: *As is well known, Godfrey Hounsfield's remarkable discovery arose out of an involvement in research on pattern recognition. What in fact happened was that Len Broadway, then the Director of the Central Research Labs, called me in confidence to say that the work on computer stores in CRL was to be terminated and that he was considering what to ask Godfrey to do next. I had established the Cognitive Systems Research Group in EMI Electronics, working on pattern recognition research, and Broadway wondered whether I had any suggestions for future work either in my own field of pattern recognition or any other area of research for EMI Electronics.*

I suggested work on the basic problem of recognizing printed characters or shapes, and Broadway then asked whether I would be happy for Godfrey to work in this field and have some sort of liaison with my group. I told him that I would be delighted: Godfrey knew many of the people in the group from the time when he was in EMI Electronics himself, and I thought that such a link would be very valuable. However I said that Godfrey was such a creative person that it might be a good idea, at the start, for him to begin to think about the problem on his own, without the influence of existing theories and ideas, as I was sure that he would come up with a fresh approach. I little knew how true this would turn out to be!

Bill is right, and Ian Green makes a similar point: *Godfrey used Michael Faraday's method of first working out the best way of doing something from first principles, and only then looking to see what others had done. Otherwise prior art prejudices the mind and inhibits original thought.*

Don Tyzack needed to stop Godfrey from working on computer stores and make him work on something more relevant to EMI, such as pattern recognition. *He had not taken any holiday for a year or two and looked a bit pale so we sent him on six weeks holiday break, and told the policeman on our gate not to let him in if he came to work. He went to stay on his brother's farm.*

Godfrey departed with the suggestion from Bill Ingham and Len Broadway about pattern recognition, and it seems to have re-awoken his interest in "the box idea", which had lain dormant (perhaps for a year or two), and he now looked at it in a new light.

Len Broadway describes an enforced holiday, possibly the same one, although his recollection was slightly different. In a letter to Charles Süsskind (whose history of the invention of CT can be found in the bibliography in Appendix 2), Len said that *I found that he was overdoing things and I instructed him to take a holiday. This he refused to do, but I said I would instruct the commissionaire to refuse him admission to the laboratories for a week, and so he capitulated. He came back refreshed after walking on the Yorkshire moors, and work proceeded with renewed vigour.*

Broadway places this enforced holiday during the development of the CT scanner, but it seems likely that Don Tyzack's account is more accurate, because he was more closely involved. (As a minor sidelight, the six-week holiday helped the accountants: while Godfrey was away his time was booked as holiday, and so was not booked to his overspent project.) Len Broadway is certainly correct about Godfrey walking while on holiday: he was a keen rambler.

Godfrey's nephew, Andrew Hounsfield, says that at about this time Godfrey met a doctor while on holiday in Malta and discussed the drawbacks of conventional X-rays with him. Six weeks would be long enough to include a trip to Malta, walking on the moors, and some time with his family, or perhaps the holiday in Malta was the following year. Godfrey would talk about his work to anyone who would listen. He used these conversations to test whether or not the other person could see a flaw in ideas, which Godfrey had already thought of, or simply to talk about the topic that was uppermost in his mind.

Nobody kept detailed records of these early events in the development of CT scanning, but we can estimate the dates to within a few weeks. The estimated date of Len Broadway's confidential phone call to Bill Ingham is July 1967, and the best estimate of the date of Godfrey's enforced holiday, and the development of his ideas about CT scanning, is September and October 1967. Godfrey's development work on his computer store probably ceased in August 1967, although his efforts to sell the idea to other companies continued until May 1968.

This story of how Godfrey's ideas for CT germinated is interesting but incomplete. He had his most important ideas about the scanner in 1967–68, but it was not until 1972 that his breakthrough was published, so five years elapsed before any press reporters started to ask how the ideas developed. However, by 1972 Godfrey probably had only a patchy recollection, and he was also too busy to answer such questions.

Don Tyzack picks up the story again after the holiday, at the point where Godfrey's ideas were fairly well-developed: *Six weeks later he returned to work and came and sat in my office for a chat. 'You know Don,' he said, 'I've been thinking of an interesting idea. Suppose you took a single page of a book and imagined that it was possible to shine a very bright light through the edge. Then you collected the light that came out from each position across the bottom of the page. And suppose you did the same thing along the side from one side to the other, and then from the brightness values that came though the edge of the page, given enough information, you could calculate what was written on the page!'*

One step towards the scanner was the idea of looking through the 3D object from all angles – the full 180 degrees. Another step was realising that the task could be simplified using the concept of slices. Godfrey described this as being like putting the object through a bacon slicer, with each picture being a 2D "slice" from the 3D volume. Each image could be calculated from a set of rays along different paths. All of these rays could, if he wished, be in the same plane as the slice, as shown in the diagram on the following page. Godfrey had simplified the challenge by

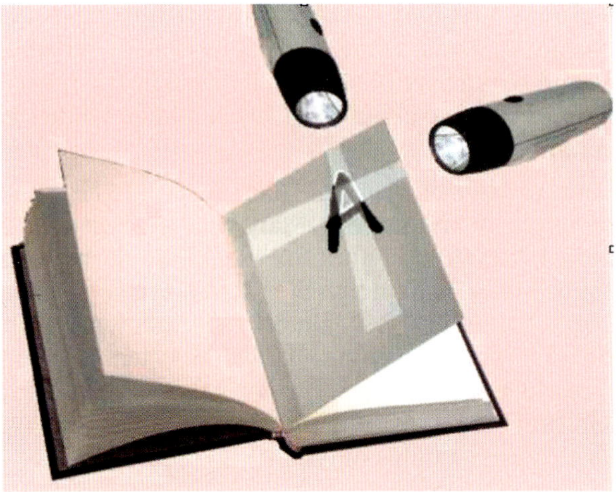

Reading a book
(Diagram courtesy of Don Tyzack)

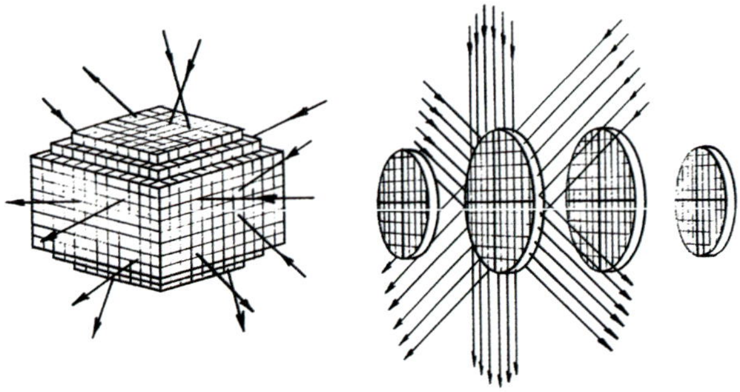

It is easier to scan a volume one slice at a time, with all of the beams being in the same plane as the slice, as shown on the right-hand side of the diagram, rather than if the beams intersect the plane of the slice at an oblique angle, as in the left-hand side of the diagram.

How to scan a volume
(Copyright EMI Music)

dealing with one slice at a time. He could view the complete volume as a series of these slices. If it worked, he could see all of the details of what was written inside a book by looking at the shadows. He could read every page in the book without opening it.

In developing this idea Godfrey had gone beyond the pattern recognition projects that the operating divisions of EMI were interested in, such as recognising addresses on envelopes or missiles in the sky. He was still talking about recognising printed text, but perhaps even as early as November 1967 he was already diverging from the company's existing business areas.

Reconstructing the image for each slice was still a major challenge. In later years, Godfrey said that he was "very lucky" to have found a shortcut that avoided a labyrinth of mathematics. He found a practical engineering approach, which homes in on the right answer remarkably quickly.

When Godfrey returned from holiday he wanted to test his ideas. The central idea was that if you looked through an object from many different angles you could calculate a map of what was inside it, giving exact values for every point. It is exactly the same idea, regardless of whether you use it for reconstructing a CT scan to give a "slice" through the human body, or as an unusually complicated way of reading a book, as Godfrey had described to Don Tyzack. Godfrey wanted to try this idea out on a computer, so he started asking around CRL looking for the best way to get time on a computer. This led to him meeting Stephen Bates in November 1967, as Stephen recalls, *I had joined the Research Laboratories of EMI (I shall refer to it as Central Research Laboratories or CRL, as it became later) in January 1967 and was part of a computer group in the High Power Klystron department. The group was engaged in the analysis of electron beam paths in microwave devices using both analogue and digital computers. We had been using computers that we bought time on, but had recently installed a link to a remote time-sharing computer that gave us in-house access to a computer for the first time in the Lab's history.* [The computers were expensive and they needed teams of operators and maintenance staff, and they usually needed air-conditioning. So it made sense to buy time on a computer if you needed to use it only on a temporary basis.] *John Hatton, my immediate boss, was keen to extend computing to other applications beyond klystrons. This and the fact that there was no way that one department could meet the funding requirements of the time-sharing link meant that we made it available to others in the Company. I was the contact point for any who wanted to use the facilities and we were, in effect, running a mini business selling computer assistance to other departments.*

The time-sharing link gave us access to a computer that by today's standards was of extremely limited performance and capacity but the ability to obtain instant results within the Labs was an enormous benefit. The instant access and the fact that it was programmed in BASIC (a much limited version of the language still in use today) considerably speeded up the development of software.

Computers at that time were evolving rapidly but were of limited power and incredibly expensive, although plans were being made to install a large mainframe computer, an ICL 1905, in the defence electronics part of EMI located on the same Hayes site as CRL.

I first became aware of Computerised Tomography in November 1967 when my boss came to see me and told me that he had agreed to give someone a small amount of time on the link. He said that this person was Hounsfield (later Sir Godfrey Hounsfield) known as 'H' and that he had a 'crazy idea'. He said that H (I shall refer to him as Godfrey from now on) knew how to programme the computer and that I was just to show him how the terminal worked and let him get on with it. I was not to waste any time with him as he had no research money.

Godfrey came to see me later that day and described his idea to me. It soon became apparent that although he had a good idea of the operations he wanted carried out that he did not have the first idea as to how to programme the link to achieve them. His idea however was so intriguing that I was soon persuaded (despite my instructions) to carry out the programming for him.

Godfrey described his idea using a simple 3×3 matrix of numbers. He first placed a set of numbers in the matrix to represent the cross section that would be reconstructed then added up the horizontal, vertical and diagonal columns and rows to give 'edge readings'. Then starting with a clear matrix new edge readings were again calculated for each angle in turn and compared with the original edge readings and an 'error' calculated by subtracting the new readings from the originals. These errors were then proportionally added back into the matrix along the appropriate column or row so that the summation of that row or column now agreed with the original. This simple example quickly converged to give a resulting matrix in good agreement with the original after only two or so iterations through the angles. Godfrey described this as being able to look inside a box without opening it and likened it to solving simultaneous equations.

I remember being fascinated by Godfrey's description of this simple but effective example and it was the start of a subject that was to dominate the next fifteen years of my working life.

Godfrey wanted to extend his simple example to prove that it still held good for a larger sized matrix and seek funding for further work. We went on to an 8×8 matrix. This larger sized matrix proved successful and Godfrey was able to obtain funds for a feasibility study.

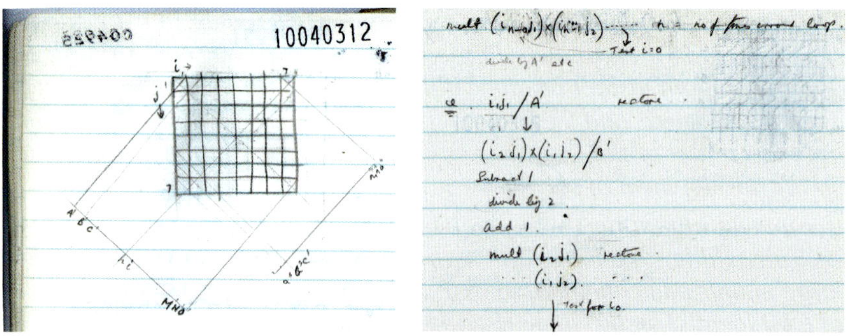

Extracts from Godfrey's daybook
(Copyright EMI Music)
Left: diagram of an 8×8 matrix. Right: calculation sequence.

Again, there is no record of the exact date, but this 8×8 matrix was produced around December 1967. As Stephen says, the readings were simulated by a computer program to avoid the expense of using real X-rays at this stage and, *in typically Godfrey fashion he kept coming back for 'one more experiment' after another, including some early tests on noise. I remember Godfrey having grave doubts about my use of the computer's random number generator and doing tests to convince him it was truly random. The costs (for the time on the computer and for my time) would have been 'lost' on other projects as Godfrey had only been given permission for one run on the computer.*

In his filmed recollections with Bill Ingham, Godfrey says, *it was easier to reconstruct a slice than a volume and I started working out mathematically how I could do this. There was very little in mind at this point of X-rays used in medicine, it was just a good exercise to think about. I took a matrix of numbers, put a square with a hole in the middle putting the numbers, a series of ones for the square and dots for the rest of it, the numbers were around a thousand as we were looking for accuracy in reconstruction at the end, so we put big numbers in. We scanned this data into a computer programme and we got the values of the addition of the absorptions through these numbers and reconstructed the picture in another programme and got it back and I was surprised how well it worked. I could actually reconstruct the square with the hole in the middle accurate to about six digits, one part in a million. Which meant, at least mathematically, that it was sound, although I didn't expect that X-rays would be accurate to one part in a million. Eventually it was necessary to get very accurate results because we could get accuracy of five parts in a thousand.*

Godfrey had proved that his method of reconstruction worked. By now he was describing it as a way of taking 3D X-rays, but nobody knew if it was going to be useful medically or if it would be viable commercially, and his project still had no money.

Don Tyzack says, *Godfrey came up with the application that we all know about today. Len Broadway's first reaction was that EMI had absolutely no interest in the medical market so there would be no group company money to fund it. At that time our Central Research Laboratory was supported mostly by projects done for subsidiary companies and funded by those companies. However, fortunately, there was a small percentage group levy on all the operating companies. This levy was spent at the discretion of the Director and monitored on a quarterly basis by the main EMI Board. We kicked this new project idea of Godfrey's around for a while and eventually Len Broadway said, 'I'll tell you what I'll do. You two go up to the Department of Health head office in London with Godfrey's idea. If you can persuade them that the idea is good enough to give you any money for research I will authorize you to open a project on company funds.*

Godfrey now needed to check whether or not his ideas could be patented. Patents are granted only for new ideas that have not previously been discussed in public. Godfrey and Don could talk in private with the DHSS using a confidentiality agreement, but it was best to apply for a patent before holding the meeting.

Godfrey already knew Allan Logan, a patent agent at EMI, and Allan worked with him on this patent. EMI's patenting process asked the inventor to write a "PQ" or Patent Query to describe the invention in ordinary language. On about 6 June 1968, Godfrey's PQ 10,166 was passed to Allan in a building a hundred yards away from CRL. Allan's job was to judge which aspects could be patented and to express them in the legally exact wording of a patent application. This application described how to image a slice from a volume using efficient collimated detectors and the use of logarithms to minimise the number of multiplications. It described how CT pictures produce more levels of grey than the human eye can see, so doctors need to select which density range they want to focus the display onto.

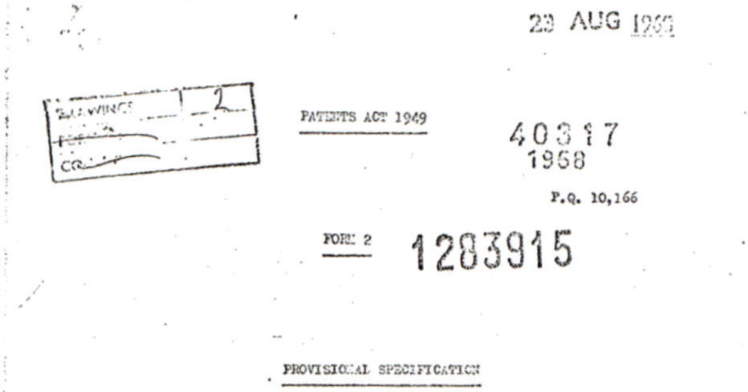
PATENTS ACT 1949

40317
1968

P.Q. 10,166

FORM 2 1283915

PROVISIONAL SPECIFICATION

Part of Godfrey's 1968 patent application
(Copyright EMI Music)

On 23 August 1968, Allan sent the patent application to the UK Patent Office. This was "provisional", meaning that it could be amended over the next year. Godfrey was protected by this patent application when he first met the Department of Health.

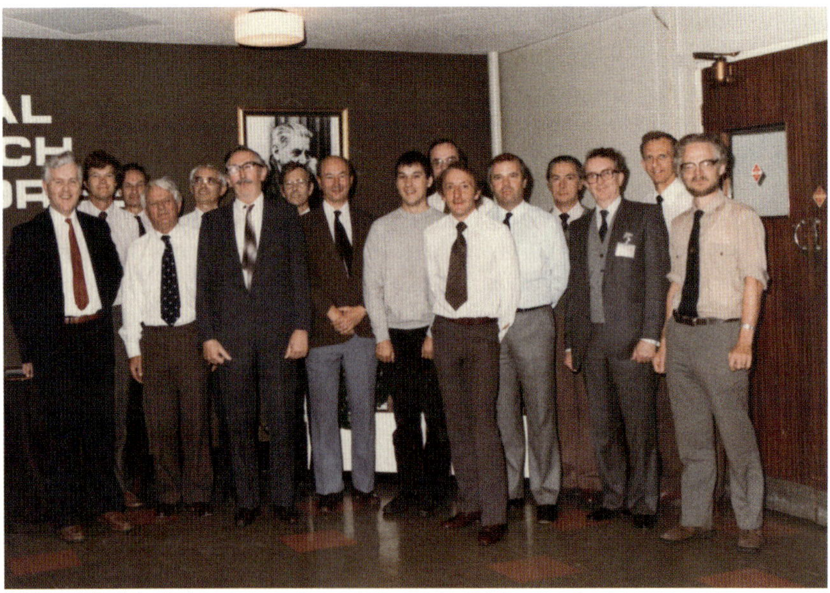

Godfrey's retirement, CRL, 1984. Allan Logan is third from the right
(Copyright EMI Music)
Other names are Alan Blay, Brian Lill, Colin Oliver, Bob Froggatt, Ian Fairbairn, Godfrey, Roger Waterworth, Jim Lodge, Neil Meek, Richard Waltham, Tony Williams, John Ryan, Arthur Harvey, Allan Logan, Mac Gollifer, and Peter Langstone.

The only available photo of Allan Logan is from Godfrey's retirement (twelve years after this point in the story), but Logan played a very important role, so it seems to belong here. Allan Logan is wearing a visitor badge, so perhaps he retired before Godfrey.

Robbie Marsh, who worked with Allan Logan on Godfrey's later patents, recalls: *I still miss Allan; he had a great influence on my career and was a true gentleman. If ever there was such a thing as a natural born patent agent, it was Allan! As regards Godfrey, I remember him as being always kindly and helpful, but genuinely somewhat confused about the whole patent thing! He was prone to produce ideas, literally, on the back of an envelope and then be utterly surprised when a draft specification turned up describing the ideas at length and with attempts by Ian Fleming or me – or sometimes both of us – to embody them in something that looked practical! It was a similar story if we had to consider patents belonging to other people, for example as potential prior art. Because he had such a clear picture in his mind of his own ideas, he could rarely see the relevance of other people's! I think the whole thing frustrated him, and he saw it as a distraction from the real work he was doing, but he was too much of a gentleman ever to complain about the intrusion.*

During this period, Godfrey went to see Peter Murden: *I cannot recall the specific date, but Godfrey sought me out sometime in 1967 or 1968, when I was heading a team in EMI Electronics working on a Ministry of Defence contract attempting to achieve computerised pattern recognition, using photographs of five types of blood cells as an initial task. Since this was funded, Godfrey wished to know if there was any chance of diverting any finance to help him progress with his attempts to prove the concept of the scanner. He was meeting great difficulty in persuading his management to provide him with finance directly.* They also discussed the computer power needed for CT scans, but Peter recalls that it did not seem feasible at that time. His team had been paying several hundred pounds per hour to IBM for the use of an IBM 7090 computer. That was a lot of money when a new car could be bought for £700, so Godfrey faced big challenges both in getting funding and in carrying out the computing at an acceptable cost.

A vital part in the story was played by the UK Department of Health and Social Security (DHSS). Godfrey first met Cliff Gregory, who was head of the Scientific and Technical Services Branch of the Department of Health, around the end of July 1968. Godfrey showed him the simulation and proposed the idea of X-ray CT scanning. Cliff Gregory listened, understood, and said that Godfrey's idea sounded good.

It would have been very easy for Cliff Gregory to reject this idea, because he was subjected to a regular stream of hopeful inventors and hardly any of them were worth backing. Godfrey was proposing to make a CT scanner (or as he called it then, a 3D X-ray machine), and he also proposed to use pattern recognition for automated diagnosis in mass-screening applications.

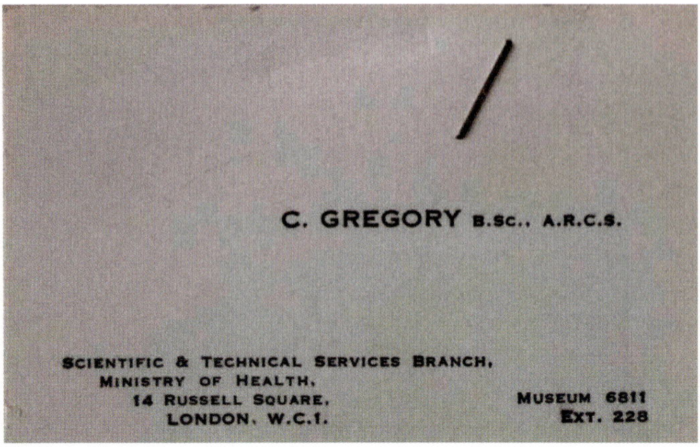

Business card (c. 1968) found in Bill Ingham's X-ray file No. 1

Cliff Gregory understood what Godfrey was proposing, and could see the benefits of such a machine. This reflects great credit on Gregory, because Godfrey spoke to many other medical people in the next three years who were deeply doubtful about the proposal.

William Oldendorf faced similar discouragement after patenting a machine to produce cross-sectional X-rays in 1963. He approached the major X-ray manufacturers but they rejected his idea, and one replied, *even if it could be made to work as you suggest, we cannot imagine a significant market for such an expensive apparatus which would do nothing but make a radiographic cross-section of the head.* (Quotation from Steve Webb's book "From the watching of shadows".) History shows that this person was spectacularly wrong, but at the time this view was so widespread as to be almost universal. Godfrey's proposal was for an even more expensive apparatus – Oldendorf's technique did not use a computer.

In hindsight, Oldendorf's method needed to use a high dose of radiation to get a useful picture. But the major manufacturers rejected it because they saw no need for it, not because it made inefficient use of the information from the X-ray beams.

Returning to 1968, it is remarkable that Cliff Gregory understood both that a "radiographic cross section" could be useful, and that Godfrey's technique was a very efficient way of using the information from the X-ray beam. Godfrey had persuaded Stephen Bates to write the computer program and now he had persuaded the DHSS that the proposal was worthwhile.

Something must have made Godfrey stand out from the crowd of other inventors: perhaps he mentioned designing a successful computer, or perhaps his understated but quietly confident manner was convincing. He said, *I went to the DHSS waving this piece of paper saying I could reconstruct a picture, a slice through the body, with great accuracy provided that I have enough photons to do it. They were very helpful....*

Godfrey returned from that meeting and wrote a project proposal dated 13 August 1968 seeking funding from EMI only, with no contribution from the DHSS. That proposal did not yield any funds, because Len Broadway would proceed only if the DHSS showed confidence by contributing to the funding. This triggered another meeting (on about 1 October) at which Godfrey and Don Tyzack met Cliff Gregory, as Don describes: *up we went by train from Hayes where we were based. The London office of DHSS in those days – 1968 – was a bit tatty. I remember it a bit like a kitchen table with lots of samples of equipment littered around. I think there were some new designs of stretchers in the corner. Godfrey did a great presentation but all by word of mouth, no props, and I did my bit. Somehow or other the discussion gravitated down around a sum of £2,500. I don't really remember the negotiations to that figure but I do remember the DHSS officer saying they would have to forego a hell of a lot of bandages and things like stretchers for that! We came back to Hayes not realizing that we had made such a momentous achievement. Next day Len Broadway called me in, 'Well? Get anywhere?' '£2,500', I said. There was a silence, and then, 'Oh well I did say I'd authorize it if you got any money I suppose!' So that was it. We opened a works order and for a few weeks Godfrey worked alone and then with a young assistant. Some months afterwards I was going home late one night and noticed Godfrey's lights on near 8pm. So I went up to his lab to try to persuade him to go home and take a rest. On the bench was a Perspex box full of formaldehyde. 'What's that in there Godfrey?' 'Oh it's just a human brain.' 'And what's the lump in it?' 'Oh that's a tumour!' It was all so casual.* (Godfrey scanned the pickled brain in the autumn of 1969.)

A widespread myth suggests that it was easy for Godfrey to get funding for his work. It seems important to give an accurate view of the funding of this vital phase, because it had such a strong influence on how he worked. It has been said that EMI and the DHSS each contributed half of the cost of the development of CT, but the documents show that this is not quite correct. Godfrey had no funding for CT from November 1967 to 30 June 1968 when EMI's financial year ended. His time must have been booked to some heading such as "general physics" or the even more embarrassing "waiting time". Booking many months to such headings would be a blot on his personnel records, because his work was not earning money for CRL. Until July 1968 Godfrey carried out unfunded work on 3D X-rays, and CRL began exploring other new projects such as a digital display unit (a very early computer screen) and a printed circuit motor. In the new financial year from 1 July 1968, a project called New Product Investigation reported on these embryonic activities, but they each still needed to get authorisation as independent projects. CRL was shrinking owing to lack of funds, and we already know that Len Broadway would not allocate any of the small amount of available EMI funds to 3D X-ray unless there was external funding as well. So much for the myth that EMI was funding "blue-sky" speculative research on the back of vast profits from pop music. The reality was that Godfrey was under intense pressure on funding.

Another point that should be mentioned is that although Allan Cormack and Godfrey Hounsfield shared the 1979 Nobel Prize, they worked independently, with no links. Allan Cormack said, *Hounsfield's algorithm bore no relation to any of mine.*

Godfrey wrote a project proposal dated 7 October 1968 following the meeting at which he and Don Tyzack persuaded Cliff Gregory of the DHSS to offer £2,500 of funding. The differences between the two proposals indicate progress in the intervening period. The 13 August proposal ends with the extract shown below.

> Enquiries at the Scientific and Technical Services Branch of the Ministry of Health have revealed that they have given financial backing to feasibility studies of this nature on previous occasions, and it appears likely that similar backing would be given to this project. Since the Ministry will be preparing their estimate for the next financial year in September, it is necessary for a preliminary technical report to reach them as soon as possible for assessment. It is accordingly essential that this preliminary work should start immediately.
>
> B.653
>
> G.N. Hounsfield.
>
> 08314/R/GNH/EMW.
> 13.8.68.

Extract from 13 August 1968 proposal
(Copyright EMI Music)

The 13 August 1968 proposal was for a gamma-ray prototype. It used the pages-in-a-book analogy described by Don Tyzack earlier in this chapter. It explains how to examine a slice with a narrow beam using an efficient detector. Medical uses include early detection of tumours and mass screening combined with pattern recognition. The proposal forecasts a resolution of one millimetre, and it estimates the UK market as 20–150 scanners.

The 13 August proposal requests EMI to fund the remainder of the financial year, until the end of June 1969, without any money from the DHSS. It seeks funding for three people on average, at a total cost of £20,000, including £5,000 to make a scanning gantry and £1,000 for a magnetic tape deck. This was not approved, and Godfrey proceeded with a budget that was a quarter of this. So he had to pare back the expenditure drastically, and he used any available free equipment. As Stephen Bates says, *Throughout this early phase of CT lack of funding was always a major issue. I was never sure at the time of the reasons for this but I have never, before or since, been involved in any project that took so many short cuts or utilised so many items of seemingly unsuitable pieces of equipment. One look at the lathe-bed* [in the next chapter] *shows the level of improvisation that was used by Godfrey. Many of the tests carried out on the computing were always in danger of being compromised by the need to minimise the costs involved.*

The proposal of 7 October 1968 is remarkable because it shows that at this early stage Godfrey foresaw most of the next 40 years of CT. The full document is reproduced in Chapter 12. For those with a detailed interest in CT, it shows a clear view of the benefits of CT: efficient use of dosage, better than one per cent sensitivity, and no confusion from shadows of other objects. It describes why the highly accurate images will need "window" controls because the human eye can not see all of the detail. A gamma-ray source has the ideal spectrum, but X-rays will be useful later and beam-hardening is tractable. Compton scatter will be no problem in a well-collimated test-rig, and it can be tackled when it becomes more of an issue in future. The proposal envisages future multislice machines with banks of detectors and rapid scan times. The main differences from the 13 August proposal are:

- There is increased emphasis on X-rays, although gamma-rays will be used for early tests. The advantages of the new method are more clearly and convincingly expressed.
- A new section proves that CT gives more information than a tomogram for the same dose. Perhaps Gregory or Broadway had asked for this. Conventional tomography moves the X-ray tube and the film in opposite directions, which leaves one plane in the patient in focus but blurs out the rest. It has similar aims to CT, but it is less efficient and less accurate.
- A new section on Technical Considerations shows greater understanding of producing and detecting X-rays and the effects of scatter. During a patent litigation interview, Godfrey said that at about this date a "junior who was a trainee" studied X-rays for him. Possibly this was a vacation student, who was free of charge (being paid by the training department).
- All of the detailed cost calculations have been cut out, and the funding request is cut to £10,000. The work plan is shortened to only eight sentences, seven of which contain the word "could", suggesting that Godfrey's confidence in reaching the objectives was reduced by having such a radical cut in budget. In practice, he faced an even steeper cut, to only £5,000.
- Existing components will be used to prove the principles, while accepting the consequent long scan times.

The 7 October proposal has Dr Frank Doyle of Hammersmith Hospital on the circulation list. So the evaluation of the proposal extended to people outside the Scientific and Technical Services Branch.

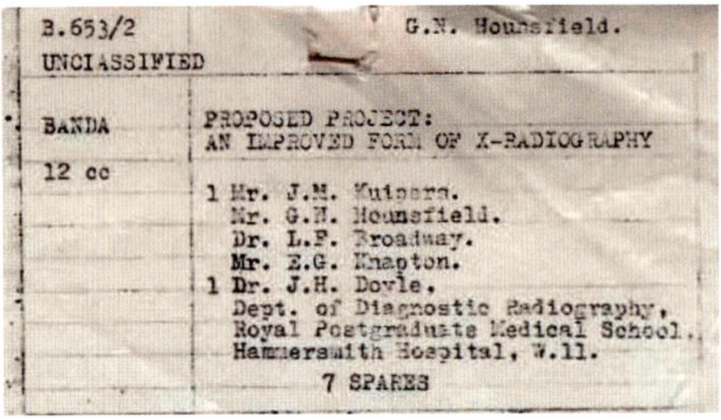

B.653/2 G.N. Hounsfield.
UNCLASSIFIED

BANDA PROPOSED PROJECT:
AN IMPROVED FORM OF X-RADIOGRAPHY

12 cc

1 Mr. J.M. Kuipers.
Mr. G.N. Hounsfield.
Dr. L.F. Broadway.
Mr. E.G. Knapton.
1 Dr. J.H. Doyle.
Dept. of Diagnostic Radiography,
Royal Postgraduate Medical School.,
Hammersmith Hospital, W.11.
7 SPARES

Distribution list for October 1968 project proposal
(Copyright EMI Music)
Dr F. H. Doyle ("J.H." is a typing error).

This links with comments by Frank Doyle quoted by James Bull:

> I was troubled about the use of heterogeneous x rays and the effect of the variation in absorption coefficients that this introduced; about the fact that it was not possible to achieve a completely parallel beam of X-rays by collimation; about the effects of scatter and a number of other things. Godfrey Hounsfield was a knight's move ahead of me at every turn. Any objection I raised he had already thought about and had satisfied himself by calculation that it was not a serious problem. To cut a long story short, I was able to report that I could not fault any of Godfrey Hounsfield's ideas and could find no flaw in anything he had said. His notion of computerised tomography was very much worth backing.

Dr Frank Doyle as quoted in Bull J. History of computed tomography. In "Radiology of the skull and brain: Technical aspects of computed tomography." Newton TH, Potts DG, editors. St Louis, MI: C.V. Mosby Co; 1981. pp. 3835–49
(Copyright Elsevier Ltd)

It is interesting that Frank Doyle says that Godfrey was *a knight's move ahead of me at every turn.* By the time he wrote this, Frank Doyle knew Godfrey well. The "knight's move" neatly hints at Godfrey's unconventional and intuitive explanations, and it echoes the fact that Godfrey often arrived at work in the morning with the results of his work at home the previous night. We can not be sure that Doyle intended both of these overtones, in addition to his fundamental point that Godfrey had a worthwhile and well-thought out proposal, but it seems likely that he did.

On 29 October 1968, a year after Godfrey's first ideas, Len Broadway gave him funding from EMI based on a verbal agreement from Cliff Gregory that the DHSS would also contribute. This funding was important: it allowed Godfrey to buy parts and to pay for services such as machining

Diagram of a fast scanner
(Copyright EMI Music)
Godfrey's far-sighted October 1968 project proposal anticipated most features of modern CT scanners. For example, the recent "slice war" goes back to this diagram. (It was a race to take more slices at once.)

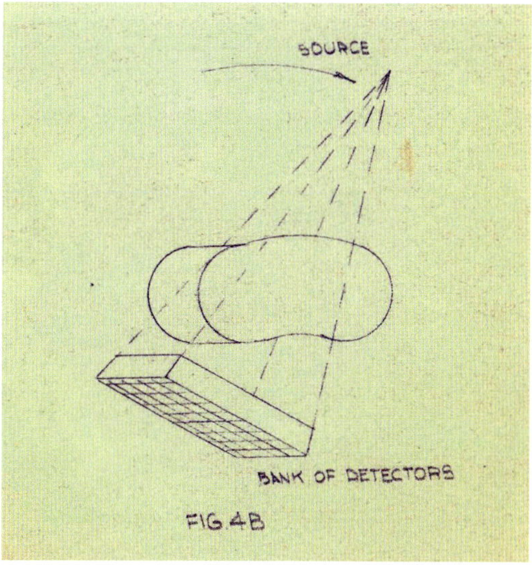

in the workshops of CRL. Now EMI (and Godfrey) were exposed to the risk that the DHSS might delay its decision or perhaps change its mind. Delays often occur in obtaining funding from government bodies while waiting for the proper approval processes to complete. Nothing survives to show whether or not EMI became nervous owing to this delay, but it probably made Godfrey very careful with the small budget for his work.

His first year of work on CT had taken him from general ideas about seeing inside a "box" to a specific target of medical X-rays that could measure tissue densities to within one per cent. He had developed his reconstruction method using simulated data and he had obtained verbal support from the DHSS. He had done a huge amount without any formal funding. Now that his project was funded by EMI he could start work on a practical demonstration.

He often led IVC rambles. His friend Roger Tripp says, *most of the people attending were younger than him, but he was comfortable with young people, and always interested in lively discussions.*

David Bosomworth knew Godfrey through the IVC from about 1964, and he recalls some stories from the 1980s as well as the photo from October 1968: *Although he must have been by no means poor, Godfrey had a modest taste in cars. He wanted a car to be big enough to be comfortable but was not interested in expensive cars which were designed to impress. The engineer in him ensured he chose an automatic transmission and I got the impression that what happened under the bonnet was of more interest to him than what was going on the road. But he enjoyed driving, always offered to drive, never counted the cost and was invariably courteous to other road users.*

I remember drifting around Lincolnshire and across the then new bridge into the East Riding visiting various places of interest in the company of our esteemed driver and three lovely ladies. I can only hope he heard

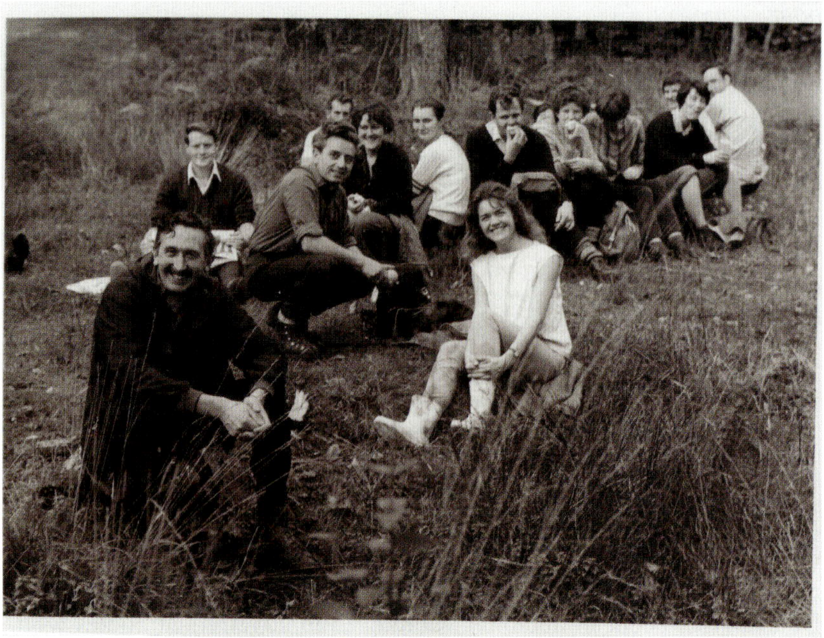

IVC outing, 20 October 1968
(Courtesy of David Bosomworth)

my instructions as a navigator above the excitement from the rear seats. (The Humber Bridge opened in July 1981.)

Eric Solomon met Godfrey through the IVC in the early 1970s. *On a house party at Halsway Manor in Somerset he devised a conjuring trick. 25 playing cards were laid out in a 5×5 array. I was sent out of the room, and the audience selected one of the cards. All the cards were then turned face downwards. When I returned to the room Godfrey would point to a card with a long stick, and say 'This?' I would reply 'Yes' or 'No'. No clues could be given in Godfrey's one-word query, and there was nothing on the backs of the cards which might give a clue. After successfully identifying the card half a dozen times the audience was completely mystified. The way the trick worked was that when pointing to the selected card he positioned the pointer on the back of the card in a way that matched the card's location in the array. For example, if the chosen card was in row two, column three, he would place the pointer approximately two fifths of the way down the card and three fifths of the way across it.*

Godfrey could be rather absent minded. He often visited to play croquet in Clissold Park, and one day left his jacket at the court. I had to climb into the park after dark to recover it. Thankfully it was still there. As a croquet opponent he was hopeless because he seemed to lack any competitive instinct. For Godfrey, winning did not enter the equation!

I must mention several ways that Godfrey's work has affected me. It struck me that deducing hidden detail could form the basis of an interesting board game. 'Black Box' was the result. This was first marketed by Waddingtons in 1974, and subsequently by other manufacturers. The web now has over 50 implementations of the game, and the Apple iPad and iPod Touch have 'Apps' for the game. But I did not, at the time, describe the inspiration for the game because I feared EMI would indict Godfrey for discussing his work with someone outside the company.

Finally, having suffered sudden weight loss, with suspected intestinal cancer, I was sent for a CT scan. I had aortic and iliac aneurisms, one in danger of rupturing with fatal consequences. As a result I had the procedure for an Endovascular Aneurism Repair. So, indirectly, Godfrey might have saved my life. There must be thousands who could echo this. Shortly before he died an American friend asked me to thank Godfrey for her CT scan which revealed an osteoma pressing on the brain.

Chapter 6
Miracles with very little money

The lathe-bed prototype and designing the Mk1 EMI-scanner

Bill Ingham describes Godfrey's early work on CT scanning as *miracles with very little money*. In October 1968 Godfrey's 3D X-ray project had funding and so he could begin building a prototype to test his ideas. He had only £5,000 instead of the £20,000 that he had asked for, so he had to be very careful with the funds. Instead of making a purpose-built prototype, he saved money by adapting the lathe that was left over from his large thin-film store project. The aim of the project was to prove *that the theory works in practice with currently available components*, by testing whether or not the scans were as accurate as he predicted. Using available components saved money, but it meant that the prototype scanner took a long time to take each scan.

34 COMPUTERISED 3D RADIOGRAPH

OBJECTIVE	TARGET DATE
PHASE 1	
Construction of a simple test jig in which an object is rotated in front of a fixed radioactive source, measurements taken and accuracy assessed. Also preliminary study of the computer program for picture reconstruction.	March 1969
PHASE 2	
Development of computer program and construction of a picture of a known test object by computer.	
PHASE 2 is not yet financially supported; it is hoped that this will be obtained from the Ministry of Health.	

Quarterly report, 31 October 1968
(Copyright EMI Music)

Godfrey's first test used gamma rays from a small radioactive source. If radiation (also known as a beam of photons) is generated by an X-ray tube it is called X-rays, but exactly the same photons coming from a radioactive source are known as gamma rays. Using gamma rays costs less than using an X-ray tube. The source contained americium, which emits a beam similar to a medical X-ray tube. The source and detector moved backwards and forwards, driven by the lead screw of the lathe. They passed on either side of a turntable, which rotated in one degree steps until a full 180 degrees had been covered. The object to be scanned was placed on the turntable. The measured data was punched onto paper tape and then fed into a mainframe computer. The americium source gave a much smaller number of photons per second than an X-ray tube, and so it took nine days to take a picture. It was a far cry from modern CT scanners in terms of speed.

Incidentally, the pitch of the lead screw in the lathe set the distance between the X-ray beams, and it was the reason why the picture was 80×80 points.

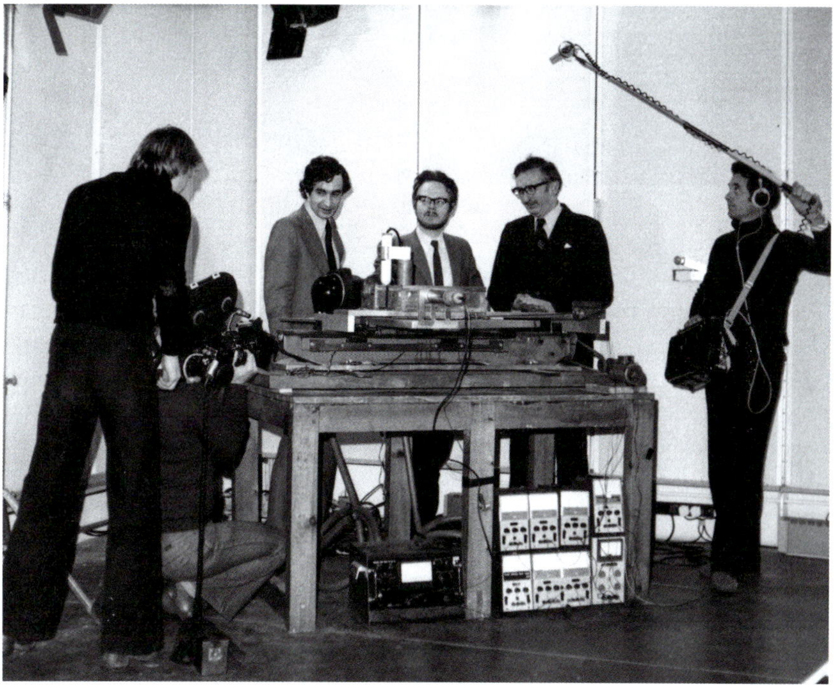

Filming the lathe bed
(Copyright EMI Music)

This photo was taken during the filming of EMI's "Scanner Story" in 1977. It shows the lathe bed mounted on a wooden bench. Left to right are Stephen Bates, Peter Langstone, and Godfrey. The lathe-bed prototype is currently on display in the library at the BIR.

In the following photo, the X-ray tube is at the top left, a pickled brain is in the centre, and the detector is at the bottom right. The detector is a sodium iodide crystal, which converts X-rays into visible light, followed by a photo-multiplier. The brain is in a box filled with formaldehyde

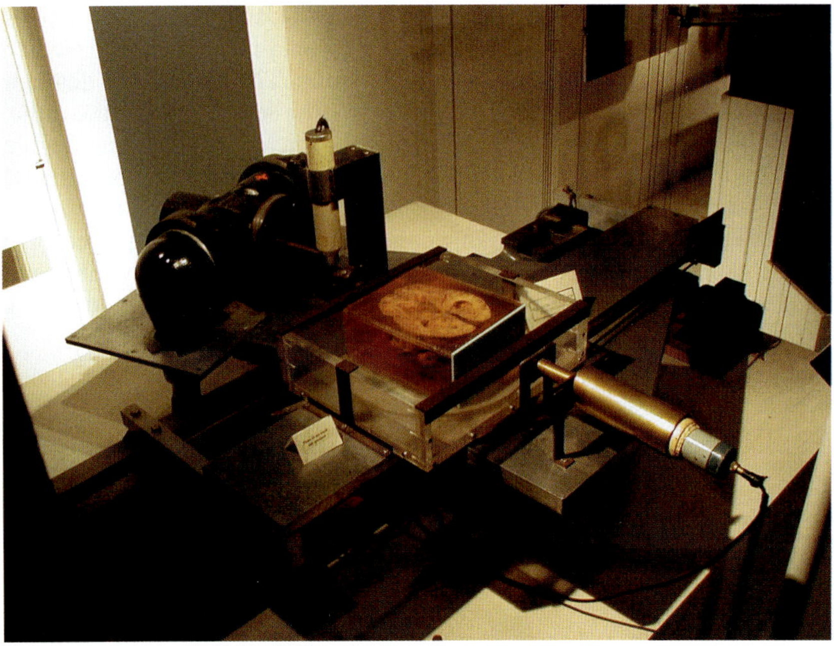

The lathe bed and pickled brain
(Courtesy of Peter Walters)

surrounded by a larger clear plastic box which can be filled with water. The water keeps the X-ray readings within a small range.

The X-ray tube and detector are driven from side to side across the plastic box, and then a turntable (with the brain on it) rotates by one degree. This process repeats until the turntable has rotated 180 degrees. The reason why Godfrey needed side to side movements and rotation is shown in the following diagram. The right-hand half of the diagram shows what Godfrey was aiming at. Each of the "scan 2" vertical lines through the patient's head is an X-ray beam that measures the absorption of the parts

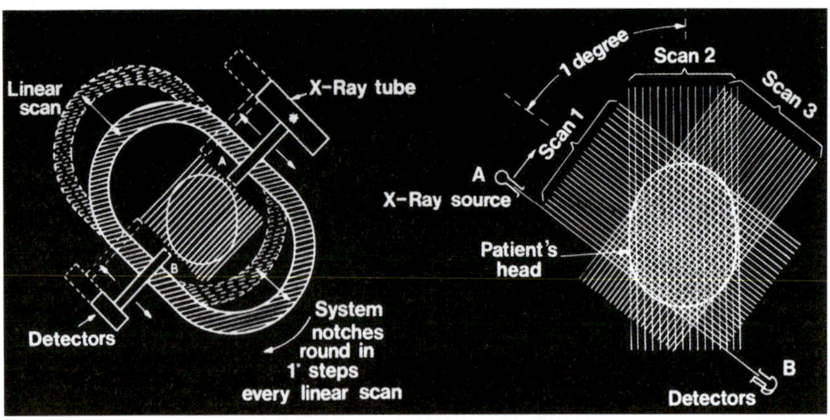

Method for scanning the brain
(Copyright EMI Music)

of the brain along that line. Those vertical lines are measured during the side to side movement of the scanner. Godfrey's brain scanner, and his lathe-bed prototype, repeated this side to side movement many times, with a one degree rotation after each one. This measures other paths such as "scan 3" in the diagram.

The left-hand half of the diagram shows that when scanning a living patient, the whole scanner rotates around the patient. In the lathe bed the pickled brain was rotated on the turntable, which is the easiest method when the brain is not attached to a living body.

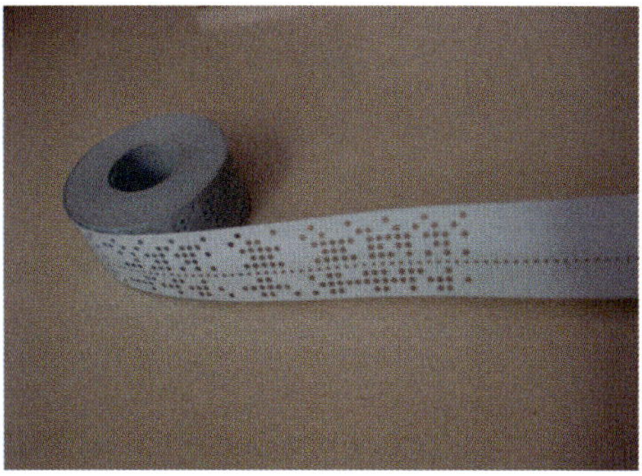

X-ray measurements from the lathe bed were stored on paper tape
(Photo courtesy of Richard Waltham; tape courtesy of Terry Froggatt)

The project had little money, so Godfrey borrowed a paper-tape punch to store the data. Measuring the absorption at 160 positions during each side to side scan and repeating that at 180 different angles gave 28,800 readings for each CT scan. This used about sixty metres of paper tape for each scan.

The reconstruction method was steadily improved from November 1967 onwards. Stephen Bates says that *the subsequent feasibility study extended the size of the matrix to the maximum that could be achieved using the time-sharing system due to its inherent memory limitations. I no longer have notes on this phase of work but I believe that the maximum*

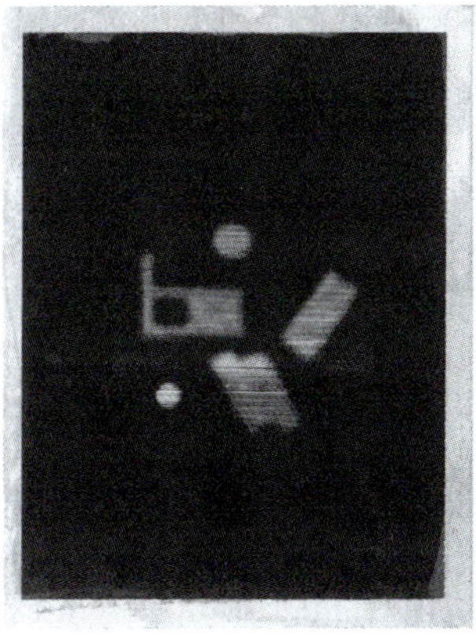

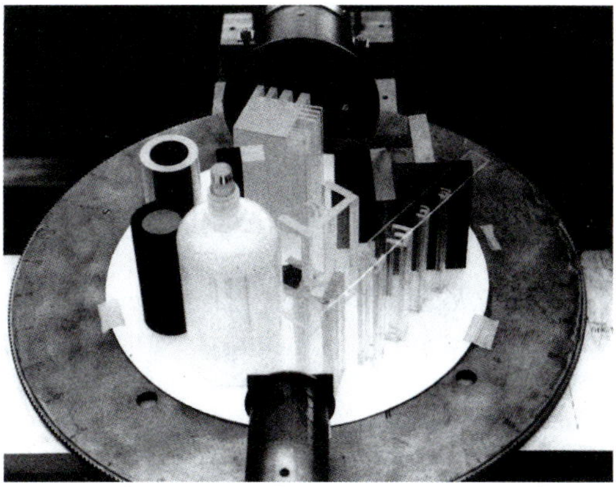

Gamma ray scan **Test objects on the rotating turntable**
(Both photos copyright EMI Music)
This scan shows objects in a different layout from those on the right.

size achieved was 32 by 32. Artificial random noise was added into the simulated edge readings in order to better represent a real situation with noise present on physical readings. All of this again suggested that Godfrey's idea was robust and capable of generating a practical system.

A gamma ray scan was taken in about February 1969.

There was no way of viewing the scan as a picture at this stage, so it was viewed as a printout of numbers. The photo on the previous page was taken several months later, after the DHSS had contributed towards the cost of constructing a viewer and buying an X-ray tube. The X-ray tube helped the lathe bed to more accurately model the proposed clinical scanner. It was low power to save money, and it shortened the time for taking a scan to nine hours.

Gordon Higson described the project from the DHSS viewpoint: *The Department of Health first became aware of CT scanning when Cliff Gregory was visited by Godfrey Hounsfield of EMI during 1968 and was introduced to Hounsfield's ideas for obtaining sectional pictures of the body by the use of a narrow beam of X-rays. He had in mind the location of tumours of about 1 mm in size and the use of his technique for mass screening and he came seeking a first view of the clinical potential of the technique. Gregory steered him away from the idea of mass screening and suggested that the application of the new technique to the location of abnormalities of the order of ½ cm size in the brain should be the first priority. In October 1968, EMI submitted a formal request to the Department for support of the costs involved in proving the feasibility of Hounsfield's ideas and examination of this was a job that was given to me when I joined DHSS.*

In January 1969, Gregory, myself and Dr Evan Lennon, a radiologist who was at that time on the staff of the Department, visited the EMI Laboratories at Hayes to discuss the scheme and see Hounsfield's equipment in action. At that time it consisted of a gamma-ray source and a Geiger tube detector, both fixed, and an old machine tool indexing table on which the specimen was mounted.

The equipment took about two days to examine a specimen and the first pictures were of various metal and plastic objects in a bowl of water. The feasibility study on which we eventually agreed was aimed at developing this equipment into a form in which biological specimens could be examined which involved changing to the use of an X-ray source in place of the mono-energetic gamma-ray source and the use of a CRT for picture display. We agreed a programme which was expected to take about six months with the relatively modest cost shared between EMI and DHSS. [Extracted from Higson G. Personal recollections. BIR Bulletin 1979;5(1).]

Evan Lennon's comment after visiting EMI in January 1969 was, *I remember being struck by the simplicity, not to mention crudity, of what was on view.* They asked Godfrey what a clinical scanner could do, and he wrote an estimation of a scan taking three minutes, and reconstruction in between eight and fifteen minutes on an ICL 1905 with high-speed tape decks.

The reconstruction program was moved to an ICL 1905 mainframe computer, and was extended to 80×80 pictures. The ICL 1905 computer was too large and expensive to be sold with each scanner. The plan was for EMI to provide a processing service, in which data from each scan was sent from the hospital (via telephone line modems) to be processed by EMI's computer.

It took about twenty minutes to reconstruct each scan on the ICL 1905 mainframe, and a printout of part of the program survives in EMI's archives. The program used the Fortran computer language, except where Stephen Bates used assembly language to make the most speed-critical parts run faster. The language is fast but the resulting code is certainly not easy to understand!

The description of how the program worked is handwritten. In those days, computer printers used only capital letters, and the use of the typing

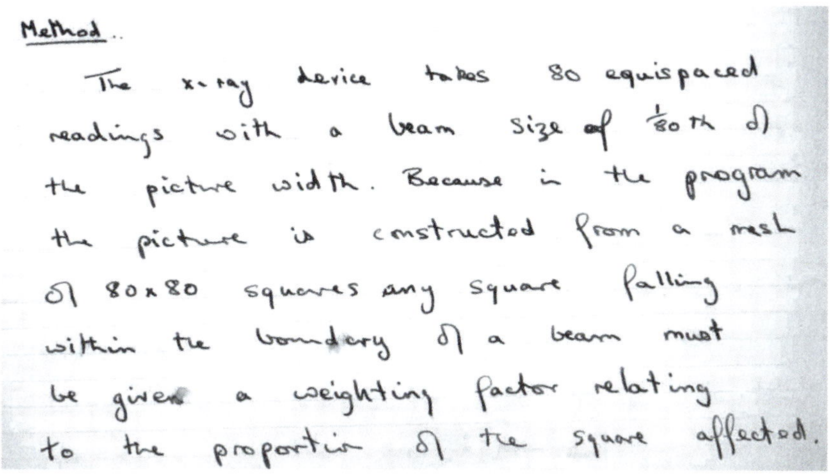
Method..

The x-ray device takes 80 equispaced readings with a beam size of 1/80th of the picture width. Because in the program the picture is constructed from a mesh of 80x80 squares any square falling within the boundary of a beam must be given a weighting factor relating to the proportion of the square affected.

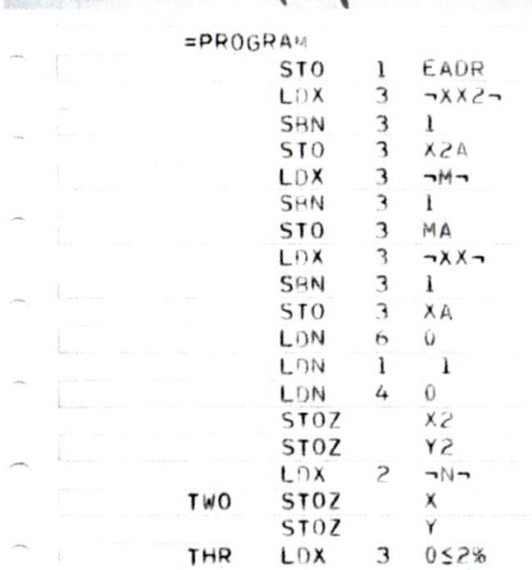
```
=PROGRAM
          STO    1   EADR
          LDX    3   ¬XX2¬
          SBN    3   1
          STO    3   X2A
          LDX    3   ¬M¬
          SBN    3   1
          STO    3   MA
          LDX    3   ¬XX¬
          SBN    3   1
          STO    3   XA
          LDN    6   0
          LDN    1    1
          LDN    4   0
          STOZ       X2
          STOZ       Y2
          LDX    2   ¬N¬
TWO       STOZ       X
          STOZ       Y
THR       LDX    3   0≤2%
```

Above: Part of the handwritten computer program description, early 1968
Left: Assembly code, 1969
(Both items copyright EMI Music)

pool would be charged to Godfrey's project. The description was written before Godfrey decided that he needed 160 reading points.

Godfrey and Stephen used an iterative method to reconstruct the CT scan. In this method, the only maths beyond the grasp of a sixteen year old at school is taking the logarithm of the detector readings. You start by guessing that the picture is all water. Then subtract the data at one angle from the projection of the guessed image, which gives you an error signal. You feedback a fraction of that error across the image. Then repeat all of that at another angle. It is an engineering approach, with minimal maths. To minimise overshoot you adjust the feedback fraction. To get fast convergence you take large steps such as thirty-seven degrees rather than one degree, and fill in the intermediate angles later.

Godfrey explained all of this using mental pictures. For example, his reason for using the large steps in angle was that it was like trying to flatten a ruck in a carpet. If you tried to do that at one-degree steps then you would just rotate the ruck, not flatten it out.

The method of interpolation was improved by modelling the X-ray beam as what Godfrey described as the "jacked up sine wave" in the diagram on the left below. This is an important part of getting a good-quality CT picture with low noise. (An engineer might say that this matches the frequency response of the reconstruction to the width of the X-ray beam.)

Another improvement was to correct the incoming X-ray readings for known imperfections, as shown in the diagram on the right below. The

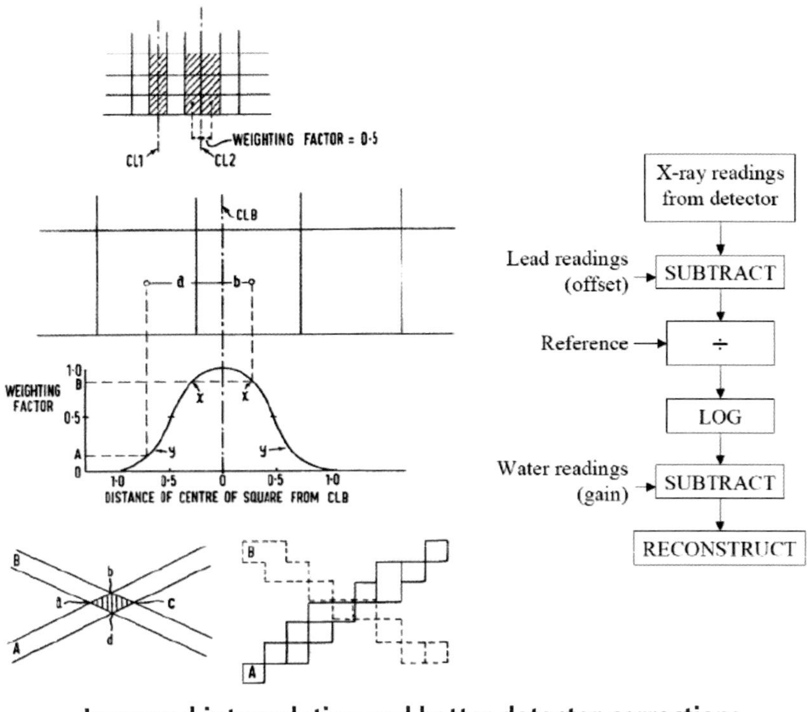

Improved interpolation and better detector corrections

detector readings could not go below zero, and in practice they were adjusted to be slightly above zero when no X-rays were arriving. This was corrected by taking an "offset" reading through a thick piece of lead outside the edge of the scanned object, and subtracting this from the readings through the patient. The gain of the detector was tested by taking a reading through the water bath outside the area of the scanned object. A reference detector corrected for variations in X-ray tube output. The previous diagram shows these improvements.

The three- or four-minute scan time restricted scans to organs that did not move when the patient breathed. Evan Lennon expected these to include scanning the brain and measuring bone density in the spine. He introduced Dr Frank Doyle, a specialist in bone density, to Godfrey. Doyle said, *I was asked to provide Godfrey Hounsfield with samples*

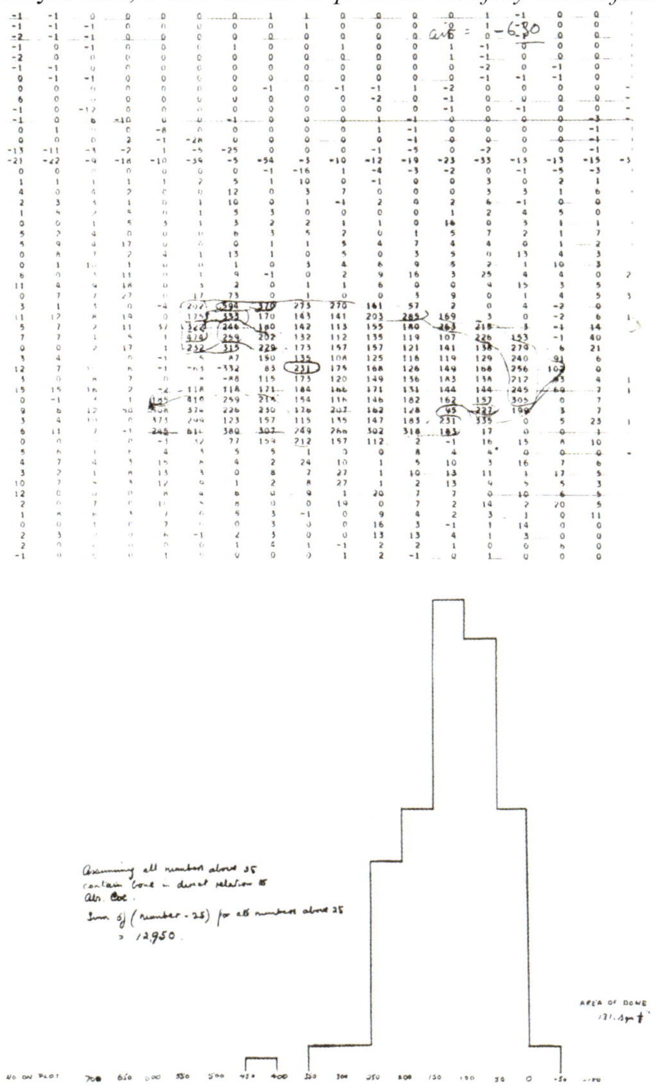

Scan of a bone sample
(Copyright EMI Music)

of bone for scanning with his technique. I was at that time personally involved with attempts at measuring the amount of bone in a vertebral body and had accumulated a large collection of third lumbar vertebrae from necropsies. I selected two vertebrae of different densities to send to him. Some weeks later we had a meeting at which he presented his results to me. He was clearly delighted that his method had come up with fascinating information about the amount and distribution of bone within the vertebral body. (Reproduced from Bull 1981)

The computer printout shows this picture as numbers, and Godfrey has drawn contours around regions of different density of bone. He also drew the histogram, and handwrote at the top "air = –630" to show the density scale.

In the spring of 1969, Godfrey saw Peter Langstone in the street at lunchtime, and asked how he was getting on. Peter was not enjoying his new role, and Godfrey asked whether Peter wanted to work with him again. Peter said yes, and always said that it was the best decision he ever made. His first task was to build a viewer so that the scans could be seen as pictures, rather than as numbers on a printout. The viewer was improvised at minimal cost. The screen was an oscilloscope, and the vertical movement was driven by an electric motor held in a retort stand. He used a paper-tape reader salvaged from an old machine tool, and it all ran far too slowly to see except by a Polaroid camera with a one-hour exposure time.

The same funding constraints applied to reconstructing the pictures, as Stephen Bates recalls, *Funding was incredibly tight and we debated carefully what experiments to conduct in the reconstruction. Each run on the computer cost the project money and Godfrey spent a lot of time trying to determine whether two or more experiments could be conducted at the same time, without confusing the results. Surprisingly few pictures were scanned (about 15) but they were processed several times as we experimented with different correction techniques.*

The results were outstanding and high accuracies were achieved. Godfrey's design and ceaseless attention to every detail had paid off. He had understood the principles of digitally sampling and processing noisy analogue signals to reconstruct a picture. He did this despite digital signal-processing being in its infancy at the time.

As a small detour from the main story, it is worth describing how Godfrey worked out how to sample the X-ray signals. He used first principles, partly because his formal education did not include any digital signal processing. Even non-specialists may find that this detour helps to show how genius sometimes relies on hard work rather than inspiration or mathematical ability.

To calculate how many different angles were needed, Godfrey pictured how a little ball of bone or metal would be scanned.

Godfrey drew diagrams of "jacked-up sine waves", which show the shape of the X-ray beam. The X-ray beams are never perfectly narrow: they

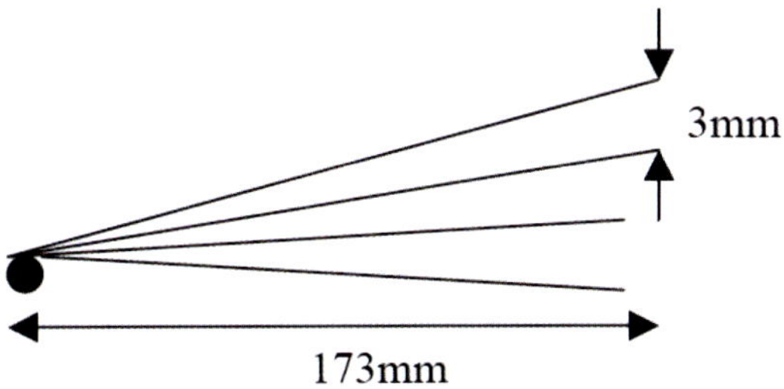

X-ray beams "see" the top edge of the black ball at several angles. For angles one degree apart, the beams spread by 3 mm at 173 mm from the ball.

always have some width, which limits how sharply focused the CT scan will be. He reasoned that these beams need to overlap sufficiently to produce a flat picture. By methodically adding up the beams by hand, he found that three-millimetre wide beams can only be allowed to diverge by three millimetres if you wish to be sure of having a flat picture. He called this "single-overlapped" sampling.

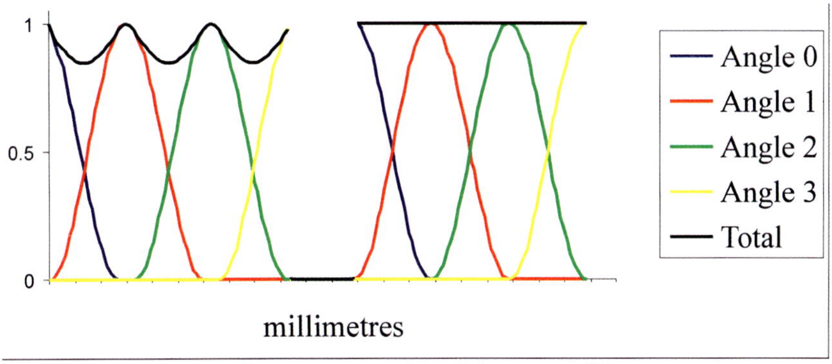

3 mm beams spaced at 3.3 mm and 3 mm

Left: too few angles, so the "total" black line is not flat. Right: just enough angles.

(In these two graphs, and in the graph below, the vertical axis is the X-ray flux using an arbitrary scale, and the horizontal axis is measured in millimetres.) If you let the beams separate by more than their width then you may get unwanted patterns in parts of the picture. These patterns usually appear far away from the sharp edges in the absorption that causes them, so they can be confusing as well as undesirable.

Godfrey used a similar diagram to work out how many times to sample the X-ray beam as it moved from side to side across the patient. In the diagram below, the X-ray beam is two millimetres wide if you measure across the bottom, and it is one millimetre wide if you measure between the points where it is fifty per cent of the full value, which is the usual way of measuring beam widths.

Godfrey worked out that the spacing shown in the "Double Overlap" diagram is the best way of sampling the X-ray beam as it passes across the patient. He did not use any complex maths: he simply used hard work. He did it without using a spreadsheet or a pocket calculator, because neither of those existed in 1969.

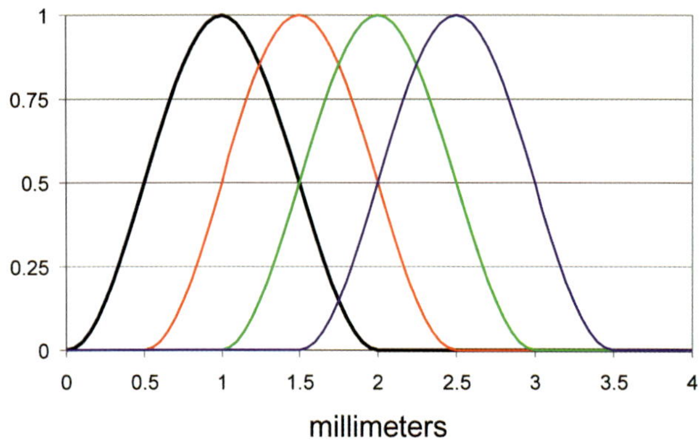

"Double overlap"
The black curve on the left is one of the X-ray beams. Three similar beams are drawn at equal spacing to the right.

He worked out how these beams would "see" an object such as a little ball of bone or metal that was smaller than the beam, say a tenth of a millimetre across. He added up the beams using pencil and paper, and then tried again using a different spacing of the beams. (From today's perspective it seems a very laborious process, but it gives a good insight into what is going on. It is an example of the definition of genius as the infinite capacity for taking pains.) Godfrey found that for a beam one millimetre wide, the best spacing between the samples was half a millimetre. Putting the samples further apart caused a loss of fidelity, but putting them closer together gave no further improvement.

Godfrey called this "double-overlapped" sampling, because it related to his "single-overlapped" method of working out how many different angles he needed to measure.

The same results can be obtained by signal processing theory, using maths that Godfrey had not studied. (For engineers only, taking the Fourier transform of the one-millimetre wide "jacked-up sine wave" shows that the information content falls to zero at two cycles per millimetre; thus the sampling theorem tells you to sample twice per millimetre. Godfrey was exactly right.)

What this little detour shows is that Godfrey used simple addition and hard work to calculate how many X-ray readings he needed to take. He did not use advanced mathematics: there was nothing that a schoolboy could not follow, although not every schoolboy would have wanted to spend long hours adding everything up by hand.

Returning to the main story, and specifically to Godfrey's problems with funding, Bill Ingham says, *The experimental work was done on an old lathe bed, first using inert test objects, then specimens obtained from an abattoir, and a preserved specimen of a human brain. All this was done on a tiny budget and Godfrey worked miracles with, at the start, one assistant.* (This assistant was Stephen Bates, who was available only part-time.)

Godfrey's funding problem from 1968 to 1972 was that the DHSS was not able to offer much money, and EMI was unwilling to allocate more funds than the DHSS, because EMI had no medical business. So Godfrey had to do everything on a shoestring budget. The easy path would have been to give up on 3D X-rays and find a different project with more realistic funding! He chose a harder path, as described in the following letter from David and Joan Clarke who he lodged with. The letter arrived in 1979 to congratulate him on the Nobel Prize, but it recalls how hard his life was in 1968–72.

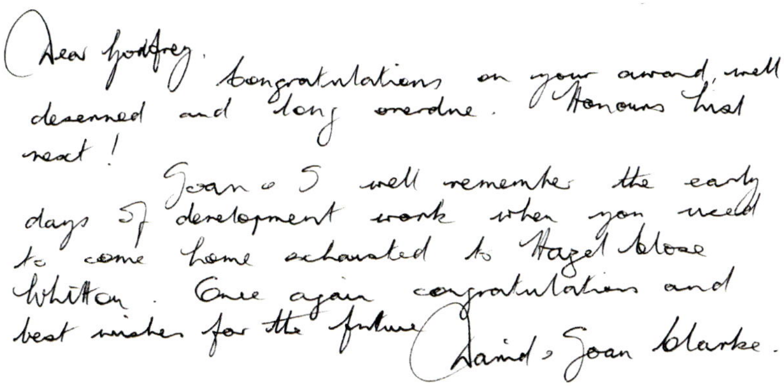
Dear Godfrey. Congratulations on your award, well deserved and long overdue. Honours list next!
Joan & I well remember the early days of development work when you used to come home exhausted to Hazel Close Whitton. Once again congratulations and best wishes for the future
David & Joan Clarke.

Letter from David and Joan Clarke
(Copyright David Clarke)

Congratulations on your award, well deserved & long overdue. Honours List next! Joan & I well remember the early days of development work when you used to come home exhausted to Hazel Close, Whitton. Once again congratulations & best wishes.

Godfrey always worked hard, but he was under extra pressure from lack of funds, as well as his usual dedication to his work.

An internal EMI memo shows the situation in May 1970. EMI allocated £5,000 in October 1968, and Godfrey overspent it by twenty-five per cent. The first funds from the DHSS arrived in December 1969, and the DHSS funded forty-one per cent of the project up to March 1970.

The 1968–69 cost includes nine months of work by Godfrey, a few months each by Peter Langstone and Stephen Bates, and a small amount for materials and computer time. The 1969–70 cost is higher because it includes the X-ray tube, and a full year of work by both Godfrey and Peter. The DHSS contribution of £12,419 is not a round number, probably because it includes part of the "picture service" under which the DHSS paid for some of the scans individually, as well as half of the cost of the X-ray tube and viewer.

EMI expected that its main income from CT would be from a processing service, rather than from the sale of the scanners. So Godfrey charged the DHSS a "picture service" fee from 1969 onwards to establish a precedent. The cost of this service for the first scans at Atkinson Morley Hospital was £10, including ferrying the magnetic tapes between the hospital and EMI in Hayes. This was projected to reduce to below £2.50

3D X-Ray

I can now give you what appears to be the true account of expenditures and recoveries of this project since the original P.D.C. authority dated 29th October, 1968. I have assumed this date to be the official commencement of the project. You will note that this information relates to expenditures up to the end of March 1970.

Financial year	P.D.C. authority (date given)	Actual expenditure	M.O.H. funding (month received)	Total project cost during year
1968/69	£5,000 (29th October 1968)	£ 6,283	Nil	£ 6,283
1969/70	Raised to £17,393 (3rd July 1969) leaving £11,110 for this year.	£11,713	£5,000 December 1969 £7,419 March 1970 = 12,419	£24,132
To end March 1970 Total	£17,393	£17,996	£12,419	£30,415

Memo from J. E. Dale to Bill Ingham 6 May 1970
(Copyright EMI Music)

if the total demand from all EMI-scanners increased to 400 pictures per day. Godfrey thought that it could ultimately reduce to £0.50. Today a CT scan of a region, such as the chest or brain, costs about £600 if paid privately, although that is for everything, not just for processing, and for a full volume not just one slice.

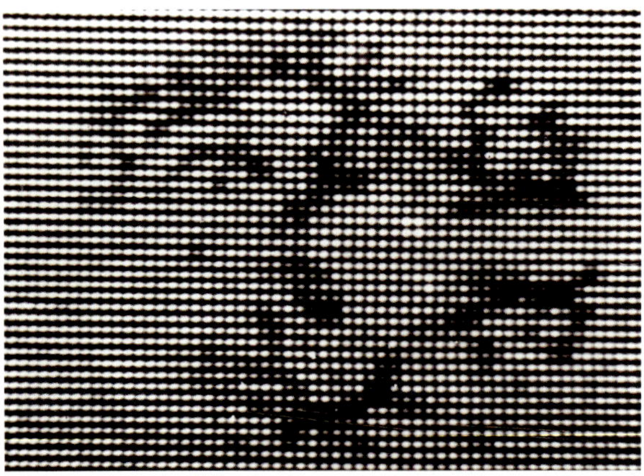

A scan of the pickled brain
(Copyright EMI Music)

The above photo was taken using the first version of the viewer. The lines and dots on the picture were removed when the viewer was improved. Evan Lennon said, *I take some joy in the fact that I was the first medical man to see this, and I recognised the suprasellar tumour which contained spots of calcium and that I realised that the picture differentiated white matter from grey.* (Reproduced from Bull 1981.)

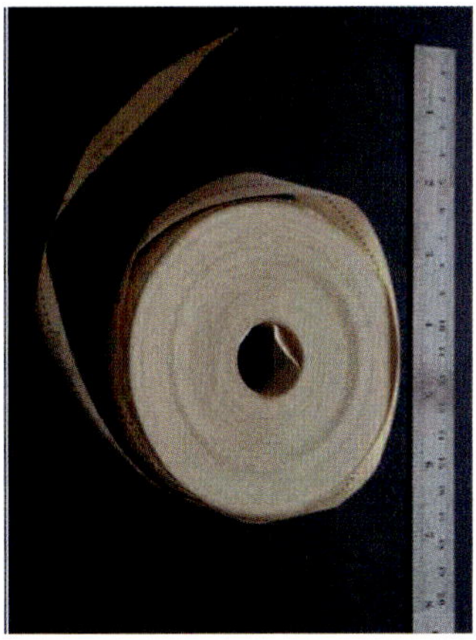

Punched tape of pickled brain, November 1969
(Courtesy of Stephen Bates)
This tape is labelled: X-ray picture no. 2, 5 November 1969, first iteration, brain.

Stephen Bates says, *the 1905 had an eight hole paper punch whereas Godfrey's reader was five hole. The tape width could be easily overcome on the 1905 but this resulted in holes being punched down the side of the tape leaving a somewhat serrated edge. Paper tapes snagged and tore in Godfrey's reader and so I entered the air-conditioned shrine that housed the 1905 armed with a wire link to short out the offending punch, much to the horror of the computer operators who were there to guard the treasure.*

To view the picture you had to wait for this tape, which was about ninety metres long, to be read by the viewer. The tape contained the full range of absorption values in the picture, whereas normally the doctor wanted to dramatically alter the contrast to see a narrower "window" of values. The doctor might have wanted fat to be black on the screen and a blood clot to be white, whereas their absorptions differ by less than fifteen per cent. To change that "window" or contrast setting took over an hour to rewind the tape and read it through the viewer again, or even longer if the tape broke!

Choosing the exposure settings for the camera was a very slow trial and error process until Godfrey hit upon the idea of mounting a small light bulb near the oscilloscope screen. The camera was set to expose the light correctly and then the picture brightness was adjusted to match the light bulb, resulting in a correct exposure. This explains the white dot below each of the four CT scans on the following page.

The two photos (below the CT scans) show the pig abdomen stuffed with offal, placed in a plastic bowl ready to be put into the lathe-bed scanner. The spine and the "pork chops" are at the bottom.

The stomach, liver, and pancreas were removed, and a bowl of water was put in their place. The letter E, made of Perspex, was about twelve per cent denser than the water. Godfrey planned to use three letters – E, M, and I – but they did not quite fit inside the bowl.

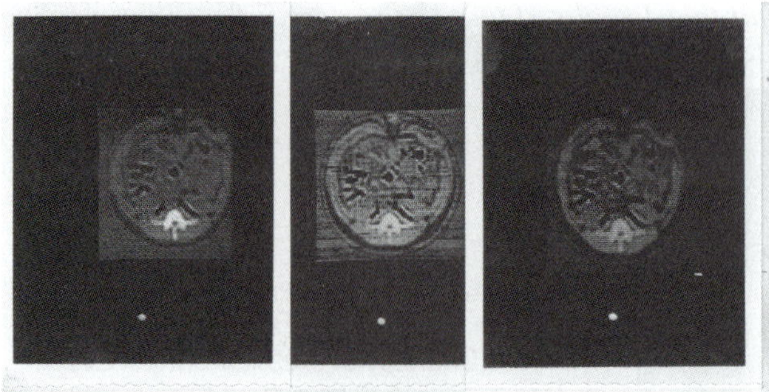

Early pig scans

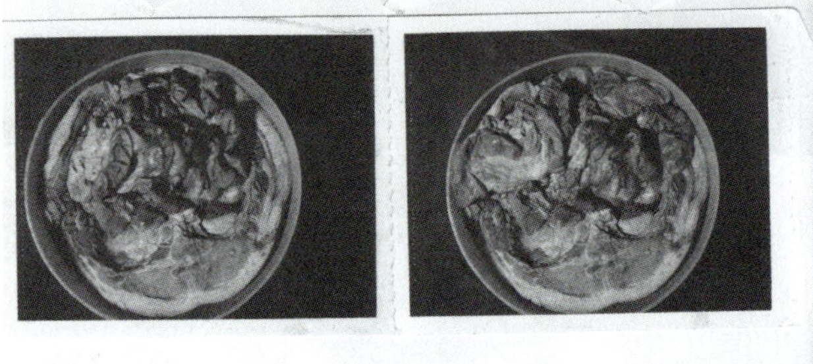

Photos of samples
(Copyright EMI Music)

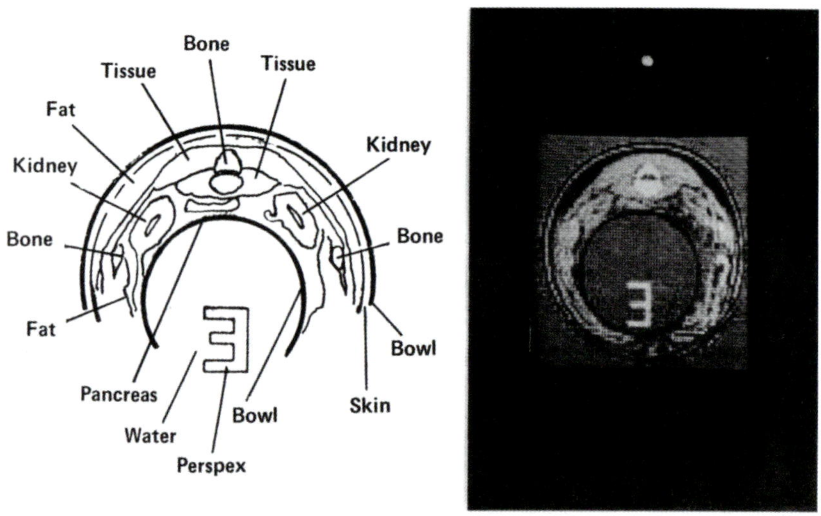

A scan through the carcase of a pig
(Copyright EMI Music)

An excellent history of the 1969–71 work on CT scanning was written in 1981 by Dr James Bull. He was known around the world as a radiologist and a teacher of neuroradiology. He trained at St George's Hospital (to which Atkinson Morley belonged) but he was not involved in James Ambrose's pioneering work. James Bull's group at Queen's Square Hospital received one of the first three production CT scanners in the summer of 1973, within a few days of the installation of a CT scanner at Manchester University Hospital where Professor Ian Isherwood worked. James Bull described the collaboration between Drs Evan Lennon, Frank Doyle, Louis Kreel, and James Ambrose: *Lennon invited Doyle, Kreel and Ambrose to submit specimens to Hounsfield: Doyle – bone, Kreel – abdominal contents, and Ambrose – brain. In retrospect it is clear that Kreel had the biggest problems – bone and brain specimens were not difficult to provide, but an abdomen was another matter.*

Ambrose was enthusiastic and indicated that preserved tissue may not give the same readings as fresh tissue. Hounsfield then visited a number of abattoirs and cut out cows' brains. The pictures of these, at first, were rather disappointing, until it was realized that hemorrhages produced by the humane killer were extending into the ventricles. This was confirmed when samples of blood were compared with ventricular fluid. Hounsfield then turned to Kosher-killed animals, sealing all arteries and veins, and making every attempt to retain ventricular fluid. Only then were good pictures of the ventricles obtained.

(Godfrey used paper clips to seal up blood vessels and to try to keep all of the fluids in the correct place in the cows' brains. Visiting the abattoirs made him move towards a more vegetarian diet. Bill Ingham recalls Godfrey's lab looking like a butcher's shop at this stage.)

Kreel was equally enthusiastic, and it so happened that his surgical colleagues at the Royal Free Hospital were engaged in liver transplants in the pig and he was assisting them. Thus he had no difficulty in obtaining material for Hounsfield, and he produced a number of fairly thin transverse sections of a pig's abdomen with most of the small and large bowel in position, held in a polythene bowl.

The first pictures showed that the polythene bowl could be clearly distinguished from the dermis, while that in its turn was distinguished from the underlying fat. There was also a distinction between muscle and bone, and the kidneys could be seen. The vertebra was well outlined, and the spinal canal was clearly visible. In spite of this encouraging result, Kreel and Hounsfield complained of the presence of gas in the tissues. This, of course, was explained by the fact that the image took 9 hours to make and considerable decomposition had taken place in the pig's tissues during that time. However, the experiment was an undoubted success and indicated that a differentiation of tissue density could be shown.

To eliminate tissue decomposition, Kreel then froze a specimen and cut a good section with a saw, having removed the bowel. On viewing the image he obtained, Hounsfield now complained that ice was spoiling his picture! In another experiment, again without the bowel, Kreel stitched the kidneys, spleen, and pancreas into their proper positions, and better quality pictures with greater differentiation of tissue were obtained. At the same time Ambrose was amassing the pictures taken of fresh bullocks' brains. These experiments, together with Doyle's work on bone, were discussed at a meeting in the Headquarters of the Department of Health on January 14th 1970. (Reproduced from Bull 1981.)

The 14 January 1970 meeting concluded that a prototype machine should be built for clinical tests. By coincidence, this came at almost the same moment as the DHSS issued its first funds to EMI. The DHSS did not deliberately delay their funding until success was certain, but it seems that EMI, and particularly Godfrey, shouldered all of the risk for the lathe-bed phase.

Peter Langstone tried to slow down the decay of tissue samples in the scanner by cooling them, but the cooling was too effective and the whole machine seized up because the water surrounding the sample froze!

On 2 August 1970, Geoff Byers (a commercial contracts manager for EMI Electronics) met Gordon Higson and obtained his agreement to provide £9,000 for further feasibility tests using the lathe bed. The work covered the period from 10 February 1970 to 10 August 1970, so the DHSS was, as usual, funding the work almost entirely after it was completed.

A letter from Byers to Higson describes this work. The main focus was on scanning fresh brains from cows in the lathe bed, and scanning various Perspex and aluminium objects to improve the accuracy of the processing techniques. Godfrey and his medical collaborators were now sure that they would see the ventricles in living brains, and they hoped (but were not certain) that they would see haemorrhages and tumours. Godfrey and Stephen were working on how to correct for the non-linear absorption of bone.

Stephen Bates and Peter Langstone confirmed that only a very small number of pictures were scanned using the lathe bed: probably about fifteen. The reasons for such a surprisingly small number may have been the very long scan time, and to save money on computer time. EMI's archive includes a printout from "Picture 6", dated 3 January 1970, which is the pig with a Perspex E inside it. However, the picture may have been taken earlier, because the pictures were sometimes reprocessed to test changes to the reconstruction. Mac Gollifer (who knew Godfrey from rambles in the 1950s) remembers meeting *a young lad with a happy face walking past me to get to the 1905 computer*; this was Stephen Bates, who was taking punched paper tapes to and fro. The archive also shows that by March 1970 the main focus moved on to designing the clinical prototype.

After the lathe-bed project, Godfrey developed a prototype scanner for clinical trials, which was then put directly into production with minimal changes. He moved in a single step from his lathe bed to a massively successful clinical scanner.

Godfrey held regular meetings with Evan Lennon, Brian Keane, James Ambrose, and Gordon Higson (later replaced by Norman Slark), and this was an important factor in the subsequent acceptance of the scanner. The meeting minutes suggest that Godfrey took the technical decisions but

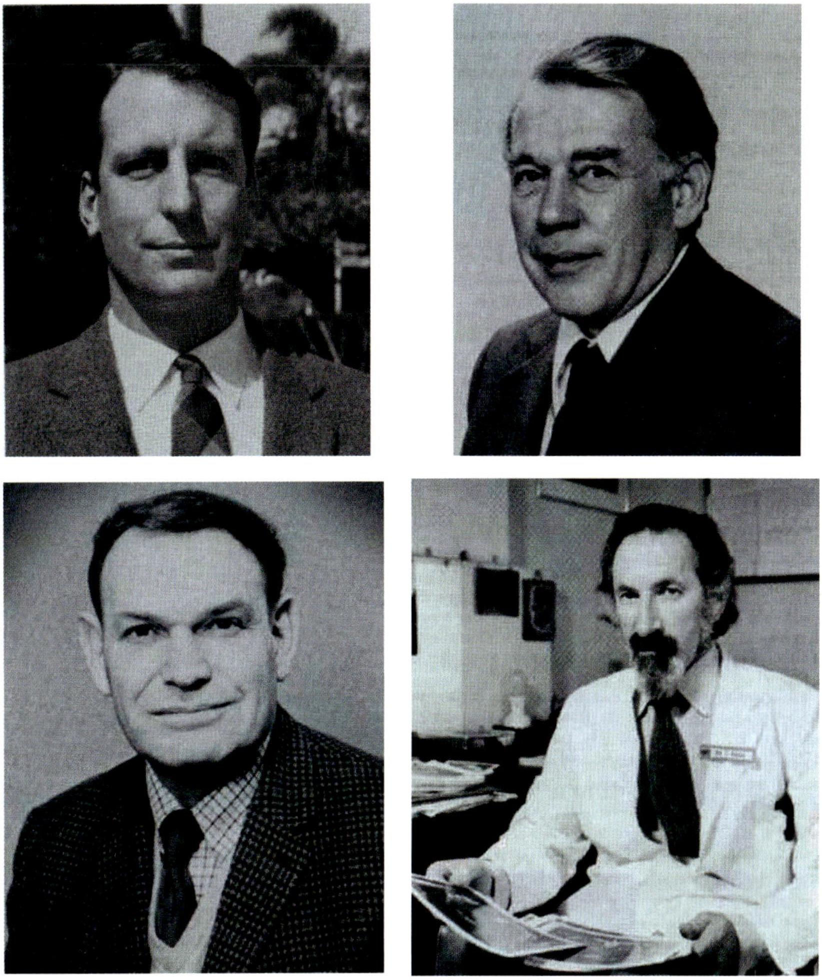

Clockwise from top left: Drs Evan Lennon, Frank Doyle, Louis Kreel, and James Ambrose
(Reproduced from Bull 1981)

deferred to the DHSS on matters of patient comfort and safety, such as the control switches, status lights, X-ray safety interlocks, the patient's table, and the water box.

The DHSS set Godfrey a target that would still be challenging today: the pictures from the scanner should cost no more than conventional radiographs and they should take no longer to reconstruct than the time taken to develop an X-ray film. We believe that Godfrey was on course to achieve this target with his design based on a relatively slow scanner and a centralised mainframe, but we doubt that any subsequent scanner has come close to this cost target. Product evolution has kept scanner prices high owing to increased scan speeds and increases in the number of detectors and in the complexity of the processing and viewing systems.

In a video interview in 1991, Godfrey recalled trying to assess the likely demand for CT scanners in about 1970. *I went round various hospitals and medical schools to see what they thought of the idea, mainly from the sales point of view, and it was very discouraging. I took our sales manager, Mr Elliot, and he was not very impressed. I talked mainly to radiologists at medical schools and unfortunately they were so steeped in their X-ray pictures that they couldn't really grasp the importance of the method. They couldn't grasp the advantages of higher sensitivity. On normal X-ray films organs are superimposed and therefore detail is obscured so that extra sensitivity would not help. I kept on saying, 'look we can get orders of magnitude more sensitivity', and they said: 'so what!' They couldn't understand that they would be seeing much more with my technique, as organs would be defined separately. It was very discouraging.*

Funding issues could have derailed the project by preventing this clinical prototype from being built. Developing a clinical prototype needed more money than could be found in the research budgets at EMI and the DHSS. The operating divisions of EMI all declined to get involved and Bill Ingham was told that he could proceed only if he got external funding, not only to pay for the new work but to recoup what EMI had already spent. Bill, Godfrey, and Gordon Higson solved this dilemma with a contract for the DHSS to buy four machines that did not yet exist. The development was funded by the margin from these sales, plus extra funding from which the DHSS would earn a royalty. Bill deserves great credit for this agreement, but instead the history has been misunderstood and his crucial role was known to only a few people. Bill and Godfrey took a big risk in doing almost all of the work before the DHSS finally signed the contract on 29 July 1971, only two months before the first clinical scan at Atkinson Morley Hospital.

Bill Ingham recalls, *It was at this stage that the funding crisis arose, as the Company decided that it was not prepared to fund the research any further. This has either not been mentioned at all in published accounts, or glossed over with a brief reference to DHSS and royalties as though all part of an ongoing plan. In fact the project was in jeopardy.*

The work had been kept going in the Research Lab, but much larger sums were now urgently required if the research was to continue. In fact things were so bad that just about the first memo that I received on the scanner research, after succeeding Broadway as Director, was from the Finance and Administration Department of the Lab, saying that the project was out of money and unless I could obtain more funds there would be no option but to terminate the research. I still have a copy somewhere I think. [That memo is in the EMI archives and is dated 13 April 1970.]

Outside CRL doubts were still being expressed within EMI about the whole thing. It was said that the device 'would be far too expensive for hospital budgets'. And we were now talking not just about a small processing business for a few machines, but a manufacturing business for high-cost products that did not yet exist and, if they did work, would not fit with existing EMI interests. To make things more difficult even the possibility of achieving on the spot processing was doubted: a mathematician at one of the leading universities in the UK was consulted (not by Central Research Labs) and said that the image reconstruction that would be required would be so complicated that it could not be achieved. There were few supporters.

The Company decision not to fund any further research may seem incredible today, after all the great successes that have followed from Godfrey's work, but to be fair it has to be viewed in the context of its own time. The financial climate was then very difficult; the Research Lab had just had a cut in overall Company financial support and a second was soon to follow. As for the X-ray work, there was of course no requirement by the operating divisions for work in the medical field: EMI was not even in the medical business except for some small products from a subsidiary company run by Rolf Schild and his Company [SE Labs, short for Schild & Epstein] *was not in any position either to provide the support that would be required or to make a scanner even if the funds were made available. It was said that if the work continued the only EMI division capable of handling such a complex product would be Systems and Weapons Division, but this was a division engaged mainly on cost-plus defence contracts and there was little interest. The reaction of the commercial divisions, engaged in other activities, was 'Here is Ingham talking about a product that doesn't exist, will be very costly if it does work, and is not in our line of business anyway. Would he please go away.'*

So I was told that the Company was not prepared to invest any more money in the project, as the limited funds would be better used on something the Company and the product divisions wanted. Furthermore, if I went ahead in spite of this I would have to get outside funding not only for all the future research but ALSO to cover all the investment that the Company had made up to that time. The situation had been made clear, the divisions were not interested (and the Company has always accepted this), there would be no more funds and if I went ahead with the research my head would be on the block. This was not an unknown situation for the Director in the history of the Central Research Laboratory from the time of the pioneering work on television.

The options were rather limited. NRDC funds could be a problem, and although NRDC had held brief discussions with me at an earlier date it would have taken time to open up this source. We did not have any time. The DHSS was already involved but the Department was not set up to provide large sums to support electronics research, which was what was now required.

However we realized that DHSS could purchase equipment. So what we did was to invent a performance specification for a product that did not exist, and then negotiated a deal with DHSS in which they would buy scanners if the idea worked and if the performance specifications were met. This was somewhat risky, but it was the only way.

Of course I had total faith in Godfrey and his brilliant team and lost no sleep on whether the research would be successful. The risk was in presenting the research as though it was production, and specifying the timescale and the costs not only of the research but also of building scanners, when these things were not yet known.

We made a careful assessment of the likely cost of completing the research and of constructing a scanner that would go to Atkinson Morley Hospital for the first exploratory tests. This was a real problem because no one could be sure of the figures, and the numbers kept changing almost as soon as they were written down as people had further ideas and second thoughts. Nevertheless Godfrey Hounsfield and Bob Froggatt (who was Assistant Director for the Systems Group at that time) did a great job in helping to assess the likely effort, and together we came up with a figure. To this we had to add the amount already invested by the Company in order to comply with the instruction that, if we went ahead, this must be recovered. It was obvious that ends would not meet with the sale of a single scanner.

Two other factors also had to be considered. One was that in covering the research cost as if it were a sale we would, in fact, be setting a precedent for the price in the commercial sales that we were sure would follow. This was an additional constraint. The other point was that it was clear to us in Central Research Labs that EMI would need a machine for itself when the trials were successful and others finally saw the light. We had to work out some arrangement that would leave the Company with a scanner.

So we proposed to DHSS a deal in which, if the specification were met, they would buy the 'prototype' machine and three further scanners. Another part of the agreement was that DHSS would also pay half the cost of the remaining research and would receive a small royalty on sales. This was an arrangement that could be built in to the overall 'purchase' agreement, and the whole thing allowed us to cover all the cost and left EMI with a scanner (which was not one of the ones sold to DHSS).

It was at ***this*** *stage that a royalty was agreed with DHSS, not in the early low cost studies as stated incorrectly in a paper on CRL and since often repeated. In later years, when the scanner was being sold in hundreds (and everyone was then an enthusiast), I received some criticism for agreeing a DHSS royalty - though without it there would have been no scanner business. How quickly things can be forgotten!*

In constructing the proposal and in negotiating the deal I had the important help of Geoff Byers of Commercial Electronics. He worked with us throughout the preparation of the estimates and took part in the negotiations as our 'commercial contract officer' (as of course we did not have one). The deal was put together and negotiated in great haste whilst the work of Godfrey and his team was continuing; fortunately the deal was concluded satisfactorily and financial cover obtained (so long as the estimates and ultimate performance turned out to be correct).

The deal was put together with much reference to defence contract procedure as DHSS had nothing suitable. It was negotiated with Gordon Higson of DHSS and it is a pleasure to record his contribution, for without his foresight and willingness to enter into such a revolutionary deal it could not have happened.

Peter Hayman gave us advice on the level of a 'sale price' (as opposed to CRL costs); it was at this stage that the ball park price was effectively set, not, as some reports have stated, in a much later meeting following the US announcement to confirm the price of the initial batch of manufactured scanners. Rolf Schild continued his interest and valuable support.

Well, Research Labs did go ahead and the first experimental system went into Atkinson Morley Hospital, with the magnificent co-operation of James Ambrose, for the exploratory medical work. [...] The performance specification was met, DHSS did agree to buy the scanners, and the world of medical imaging was changed for ever. (Quotation by kind permission of Bill Ingham and the Royal Society.)

Godfrey's team was extended to include Tony Williams on mechanical design, although initially he was only on loan, and Godfrey had to struggle to stop him being called away to work on another project. The June 1970 report shows that work on the design of the clinical scanner was well under way.

A letter from H. R. Marcuse arrived at EMI on 17 March 1971, having been posted in Amsterdam on 2 February but delayed by a postal strike in the UK. He invited Godfrey to give a fifteen-minute talk at the Second Conference of the European Association of Radiology, 14–18 June, in Amsterdam. Marcuse worked in Academisch Ziekenhuis Radiotherapeutische Afdeling – the university hospital's radiotherapy department. He wrote that his team saw Godfrey's recently published patent application *as a remarkable achievement in Röntgen technique and believe that with further development it also opens perspectives for more economic utilisation of the absorbed dose delivered to the patient in order to get the largest quantity of information.* (Wilhelm Röntgen discovered X-rays in 1895 and he won the first Nobel Prize for Physics in 1901.)

Marcuse deserves credit as he seems to be the only person who found and fully understood Godfrey's patent at this stage. Godfrey went to the conference and read a paper showing the lathe-bed scans of the pickled brain, the pig, and human vertebrae, and a picture of the clinical scanner, which was then nearing completion. He expressed confidence that tumours would be detected. He did not yet have scans of live patients, his paper missed the printing deadline, and no one took any interest. This was probably just as well, otherwise potential competitors could have started work ten months earlier!

The preliminary mechanical design for a complete clinical machine for examining the head, neck and limbs is being studied and is being drawn. Provision has been made for modifying the machine in order that it may be sold as an experimental machine for investigations over the whole of the body.

Since the proposed machine will deal mainly with pictures taken of the brain it has therefore been necessary to be more certain of its capabilities on fresh brain tissue which has in the past been difficult to obtain (fresh tissue tests have been carried out on the body of pigs only).

A picture has been taken of a bullocks brain but this was only a partial success as considerable tissue change occurred while the picture was being taken. It is hoped to take another picture of a bullocks brain on the same day of killing. If this is successful, it is proposed to take another picture of a bullock's brain in a human skull.

The Ministry of Health have been kept in touch with the revised specification and are satisfied with the progress of preliminary design drawings.

Godfrey's monthly report, June 1970
(Copyright EMI Music)

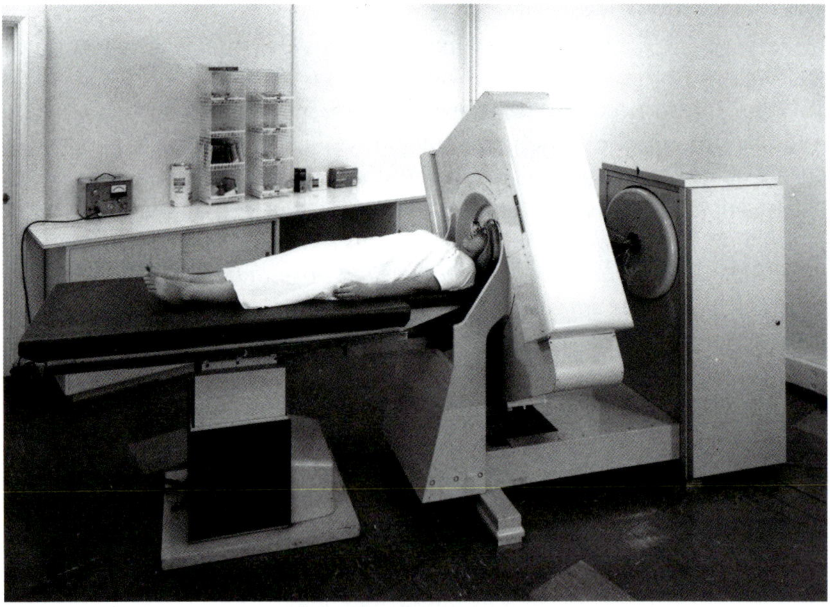

The Mk1 EMI-scanner
(Copyright EMI Music)

The Mk1 EMI-scanner took a scan in four and a half minutes. The large frame that surrounds the patient's head rotated as the scan progressed. The X-ray tube and detectors were mounted on this frame. They went backwards and forwards, making a noticeable thumping noise each time they hit the springs, which helped them to change direction.

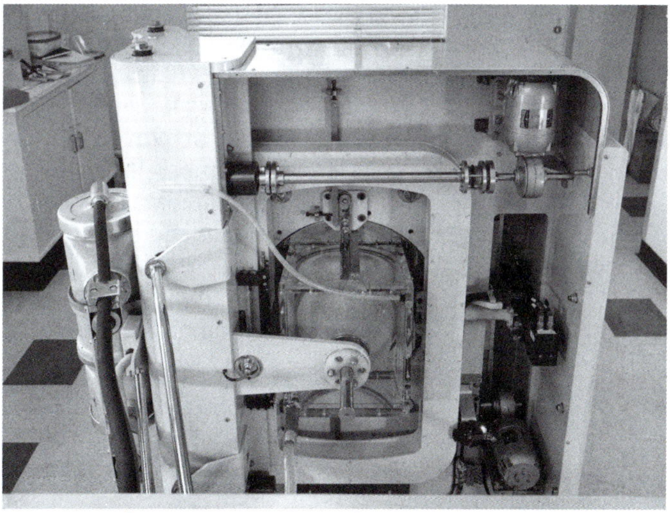

Mk1 EMI-scanner with covers removed
(Copyright EMI Music)

The X-ray tube (above image, on the left) is about to move in an up and down direction, driven by the motor at the top right. In the centre of the photo is a rectangular box made out of Perspex, holding water. A flexible rubber membrane in the far side of this box enabled the patient's brain to be surrounded by water while remaining dry. The water box in this scanner was needed to keep the level of detected X-rays reasonably constant as the beam scanned across the brain. Without it, the X-rays would vary by about a factor of a thousand. Modern CT scanners can easily cope with such a range, but they use integrated circuits which were not available in 1971.

The design and use of the water box needed care. The water was warmed to body temperature using the heating element from a kettle. The water pressed on the patient's head, needing straps to stop the patient gently sliding out of the scanner. Air could get trapped between the head and the rubber membrane and gradually escape during the scan, but in spite of these issues the water box gave good scans for tens of thousands of patients.

Perhaps the most dramatic issue with the water box was that if the membrane split then water would leak onto the patient, so it was removed as soon as the detector electronics could cope without it. Godfrey slightly regretted its passing, because as well as keeping the X-ray signals within a small range, it also controlled the hardening of the X-ray beam, which produced very accurate numerical values in the CT picture. Godfrey and James Ambrose were very interested in the numerical values. Everyone could see the diagnostic value of a picture that showed the location of a tumour, but at that stage nobody knew whether or not the numerical values held valuable diagnostic data.

Getting the scanner ready for the first scan of a live patient was delayed by the general problems inherent in developing a new machine. Events conspired to make the completion date slip. Godfrey used an X-ray tube from Pantak, which mostly supplied industrial rather than medical markets. At a late stage the lead shielding that prevents X-rays from escaping in unwanted directions failed to meet the more stringent standards for medical use, so upgraded shielding was needed urgently. One of Godfrey's sodium iodide crystals failed and his supplier had no better replacement. He had no spare part because of his tight budget, so he and Peter Langstone needed to find alternative suppliers. Eventually they dealt with the last of these snags, and scanned the first patient.

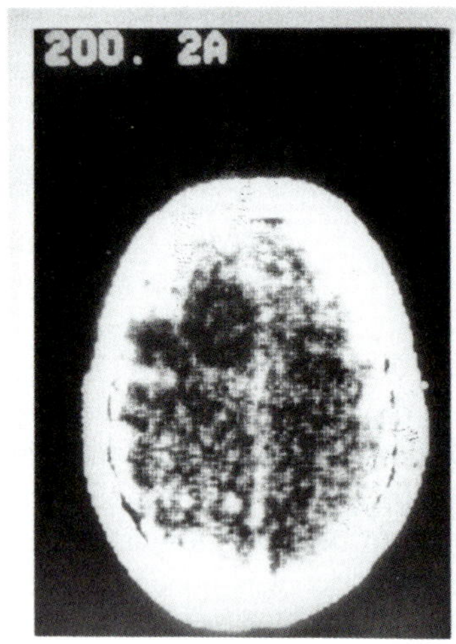

Image "200.2A"

This is Godfrey's first clinical CT scan of a live patient. It was taken on 1 October 1971. There is a circular cystic tumour in the frontal lobe. (The image is 160×160. The iterative system in use at that time could produce this, but normally an 80×80 picture was used for faster processing.)

In the "Scanner Story" film, James Ambrose says, *This is the very first CT scanner which was ever made. It was installed here in 1971 and on October 1st we scanned our first patient. This was actually a middle aged female patient with a suspected tumour in the left frontal lobe and we saw the brain in a great deal more detail than we'd expected. We were able to identify cortex, white matter, the ventricular system, and the cystic tumour which was present in this patient's frontal lobe. This was successfully operated on, and this was the result which caused Hounsfield and myself to jump up and down like footballers who had just scored a winning goal.*

Godfrey had reached this point on a budget of only £69,000. When scanners of this design were sold, the sale price (admittedly including the £12,000 computer) was about £130,000. That is incredible: the budget to design and build the first clinical CT scanner was roughly half of the sale price. Could anyone else have done it? As Bill Ingham says near the end

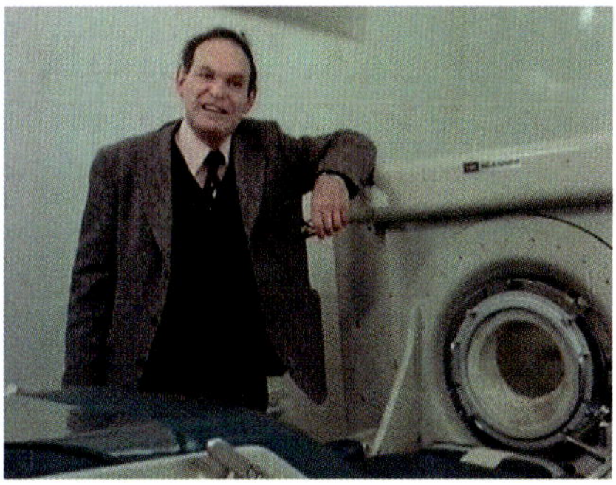

Dr James Ambrose in the "Scanner Story" film
(Copyright EMI Music)

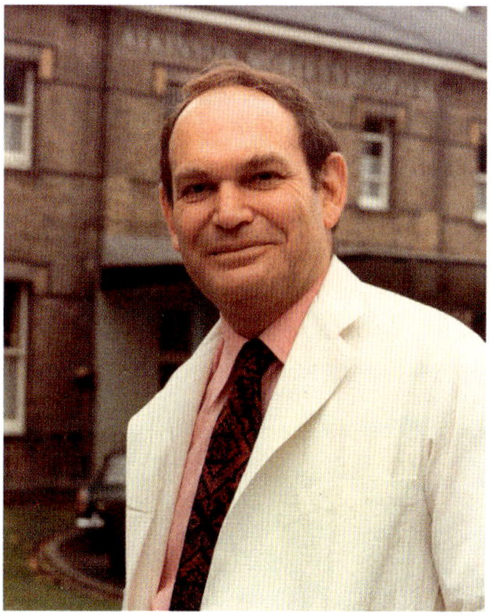

Ambrose outside AMH
(Courtesy of Sheena Ambrose)

of his document: *These notes [...] reveal the difficult climate in which Hounsfield worked. The lack of support in the early stages of the scanner research is reminiscent of Whittle and his jet engine, one of the other great inventions of the century.*

Around this time, Stephen Bates left CRL to join a small part of EMI called SE Labs, which worked at the leading edge of computers and software. So far Stephen had developed software for Godfrey on an as-needed basis: Godfrey could not afford to use him full time, but he did not need to be full time to keep up with Godfrey's needs. When Stephen moved to SE Labs, Godfrey viewed the software as finished, and it ran unchanged for several months. Around the time of Christmas 1971, Godfrey and Bob Froggatt became interested in sending data between EMI and the hospital by phone lines instead of magnetic tapes, and they asked Mac Gollifer to investigate that, and also the option of using a mini computer to process the scanner data in the hospital, rather than processing it at EMI.

In autumn 1971, Godfrey reported another problem: he bought ten rubber membranes for the water box and only one was left. The supplier would not send any more until EMI paid for the first batch. Was this Godfrey's fault? EMI would not pay the invoice until Godfrey signed it, stating that the membrane was satisfactory. With so much going on it would be understandable if he forgot to do so. Whatever the truth, it was probably a mistake, because invoices were not routinely left unpaid. But these little issues paled into insignificance when compared with the results from the scanner.

Godfrey took magnetic tapes backwards and forwards between the hospital and Hayes. EMI charged a £10 fee for processing each scan on their mainframe computer. Even this relatively low price deterred James Ambrose from taking too many pictures. Budgets mattered in the NHS then, as they do today. About 200 pictures had been scanned by the end of February 1972.

Godfrey describes the excitement as the first few scans emerged: *I remember seeing the first pictures being printed out from the computer with all sorts of diagnostic features which were showing up very interesting things. I didn't know what they were, but I was pretty certain that they were diagnostically useful. It was very exciting. I was working day and night because I would scan the patients in the hospital and then come back to Hayes with the tapes, staying overnight watching them being processed.*

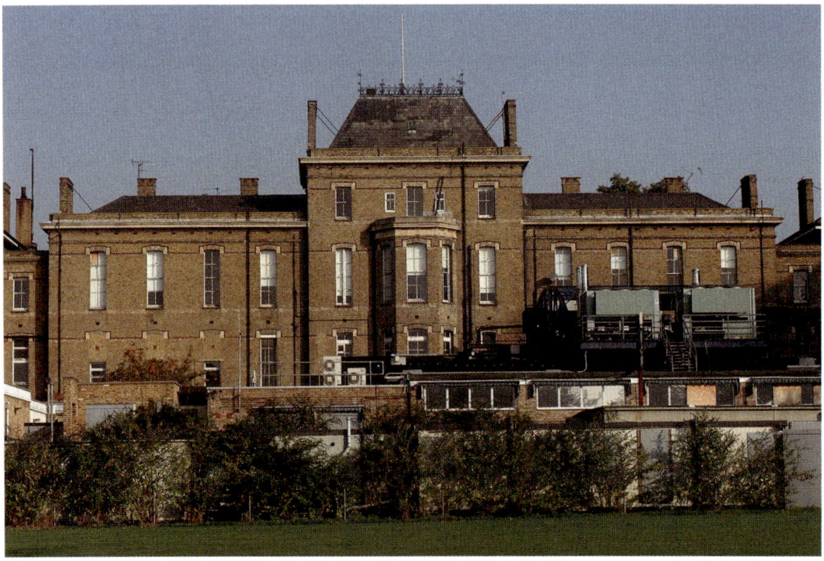

Atkinson Morley Hospital
(Courtesy of the Wimbledon Guardian)

Chapter 7
Doubters become believers

First public announcements and their consequences

The first publication of clinical CT scans converted all of the doubters into believers. On 20 April 1972, James Ambrose and Godfrey spoke at a BIR conference. This followed a press briefing at EMI's London headquarters on 19 April at which Bill Ingham and Godfrey spoke to sixty journalists.

EMI news

from EMI Electronics and Industrial Operations, Blyth Rd., Hayes, Middlesex. Telephone: 01-573 3888

43/72

EMBARGO UNTIL 18.00 HOURS
THURSDAY, 20TH APRIL

NEW EMI SYSTEM REVOLUTIONISES THE INVESTIGATION OF BRAIN DISEASES

Accurate, Detailed Pictures of Brain Tissue Possible for the First Time

A new British equipment for the investigation and diagnosis of a wide range of brain diseases, such as tumours, cysts and haemorrhages, is expected to revolutionise clinical and research work in this challenging field of medicine. This breakthrough in the investigation of cerebral diseases follows a three-year research and development programme by the Central Research Laboratories of EMI, at Hayes, Middlesex, in conjunction with specialists from the Department of Health & Social Security. These are based at Atkinson Morley Hospital which contains the neurological and neurosurgical units of St. George's Hospital, Wimbledon.

By combining the speed and accuracy of the digital computer with highly sensitive X-ray detectors, the system enables 100 times more information to be extracted from the X-ray photons than with conventional X-ray methods. It provides information on brain conditions with a sensitivity and detail hitherto unobtainable.

Part of the handout to journalists on 19 April 1972
(Copyright EMI Music)

In the conversation between Godfrey and Bill Ingham that was filmed in 1991, Bill talked about the impact of this announcement: *Well after that it really just took off. All the doubters in the medical profession and the doubters in the company were all suddenly believers. We'd struggled to keep this project alive and now we had the problem of coping with the enormous demands on the research lab.* The story appeared on BBC radio and in major UK newspapers: The Times, Financial Times, Guardian, and Daily Telegraph. Seventy-five per cent of the national newspapers attended EMI's press conference, in comparison with only thirty-two per cent of the medical journals.

Thirty-Second

ANNUAL CONGRESS

SCIENTIFIC EXHIBITION

IMPERIAL COLLEGE OF SCIENCE AND TECHNOLOGY
DEPARTMENT OF MECHANICAL ENGINEERING
EXHIBITION ROAD, LONDON SW7

20-21 APRIL 1972

THE BRITISH INSTITUTE OF RADIOLOGY

The first publication of CT scans of living human patients
(Courtesy of the BIR)
Bill Ingham and Rolf Schild were the only people from EMI who attended this meeting. It was the 32nd Annual Congress of the British Institute of Radiology.

Bill Ingham's handwritten notes on the day said, *FRS and knighthood predicted!* FRS means Fellow of the Royal Society, which is a very prestigious award. *Even allowing for the natural enthusiasm of scientific specialists I think that it is certain that we have a new device that really can be called a breakthrough & EMI and Central Research Labs can be proud to give birth to it.* Later Bill wrote, *The other papers being read at this meeting were the usual ones reporting work aimed at trying to improve conventional X-ray systems, which was all that medical science knew. When Hounsfield and Ambrose read their paper on the scanner, and on the results obtained at Atkinson Morley, the impact was stunning: one felt sorry for the people who had to follow them as no one was interested in the normal X-ray any more.*

It must have seemed to Godfrey that the company now wanted him to do everything at once. They wanted him to launch a product based on his prototype as soon as possible, to develop faster methods of reconstructing the pictures, and to develop better brain and body scanners. At the same time they wanted him to support sales efforts, visit potential customers, accept awards, and speak at every conference. He was under immense pressure.

SCIENTIFIC PROGRAMME
Thursday, 20th April 1972

LECTURE THEATRE A — **DIAGNOSTIC SESSION**

14.15 NEW TECHNIQUES FOR DIAGNOSTIC RADIOLOGY

Chairman: Dr. G. H. du Boulay

Dr. J. Ambrose, Mr. G. Hounsfield, Atkinson Morley's Hospital	*Computerised axial tomography (A new means of demonstrating some of the soft tissue structures of the brain without the use of contrast media)*
Dr. G. M. Ardran, Nuffield Institute for Medical Research	*The value of high kV techniques for chest radiography*
Dr. L. Rosen, University of California Los Alamos Scientific Laboratory	*Possible use of negative pions and negative muons in therapeutic and diagnostic medicine*

15.45 Tea

Dr. D. K. Bewley, Hammersmith Hospital	*Radiography with fast neutrons*
Dr. V. R. McCready, Dr. C. R. Hill, Royal Marsden Hospital	*Constant depth ultrasonic scanning*

LECTURE THEATRE B — **JOINT RADIOTHERAPY AND RADIOBIOLOGY SESSIONS**

Chairman: Professor J. Rotblat

14.15 DRUG-RADIATION INTERACTIONS IN CANCER THERAPY

Dr. G. E. Adams, Mount Vernon Hospital	*Background and present status of use of radio-sensitisers for clinical radiotherapy*
Prof. N. M. Bleehen, The Middlesex Hospital	*Clinical trials of combined chemotherapy and radiotherapy—a critical review*
Prof. G. Hamilton Fairley, St. Bartholomew's Hospital	*The place of combination chemotherapy in the treatment of malignant disease*

15.45 Tea

HEAD AND NECK CANCER

Dr. G. H. Fletcher, M. D. Anderson Hospital and Tumor Institute, Texas	*Clinical dose response curves of human malignant epithelial tumors*
Mr. J. S. P. Wilson, St. George's Hospital	*Some aspects of the treatment of cancer of the head and neck*

8

Extract from of the 32nd Annual Congress of the British Institute of Radiology
(Courtesy of the BIR)

EMI had a good public relations department, in which Colin Woodley was working throughout the CT years. He deserves credit for attracting journalists to the press conference and for the resulting coverage in national newspapers. Recalling the scanner years, he said, *One day I hoped I might become involved again in something which is technologically as much of a breakthrough, but also one that would have the same terrific social advantage. I'd be very lucky to find that sort of lightning striking again.*

Unsurprisingly, EMI now wanted to be seen as having backed Godfrey's invention from the start, which slightly glosses over the ups and downs described in earlier chapters. The DHSS was always given credit for its support, and received good royalties, but without mentioning the details of the crucial agreement between Geoff Byers and Bill Ingham at EMI and Cliff Gregory and Gordon Higson at the DHSS.

Godfrey was always very grateful to the DHSS. He was quoted in EMI's 19 April 1972 press release as saying, *The development of this machine owes a great deal to the co-operation and support of the Department of Health & Social Security, and particularly its specialists at Atkinson Morley Hospital. This machine, which I believe will make a real contribution to improvements in the investigation of brain diseases, is a significant example of the benefits which can result from close collaboration between specialists in the electronics and medical spheres.* It is a great example of collaboration between government and industry, as well as between medical and electronics spheres.

The impact on diagnosis of brain problems was profound. Dr Ivan Moseley said in the "Scanner Story" film: *The most common condition which can occur after head injury is a collection of blood between the brain and the skull itself, which presses on the brain and can, indeed, result in death. To show this before CT would have meant carrying out cerebral angiography, with injections of rather toxic substances into the arteries leading to the brain, but here very quickly and easily within ten minutes of the patient coming into hospital we had the answer. This was an alcoholic who fell in the street, and you see here this large collection of blood* [top left in the photo] *and it is displacing the ventricles away to this side* [the right-hand side] *and compressing the whole of the brain. This is a life-threatening blood clot.*

CT gives a diagnosis that is fast enough to save a life and to preserve quality of life, because irreversible brain damage happens quickly in such situations. Another huge benefit is that CT gives an accurate diagnosis, so that any surgical operations are performed in the right place to relieve the blood clot, and are not performed at all in cases where they are not likely to be beneficial. The need for exploratory surgery is greatly reduced by CT.

Ian Isherwood said, *News spread rapidly but not always accurately. One request was addressed to the 'Cat skinning department'!* Ian and his team worked on dual-energy scanning, subtracting scans at two different X-ray tube voltages. This technique gave greater insight into chemical composition inside the patient.

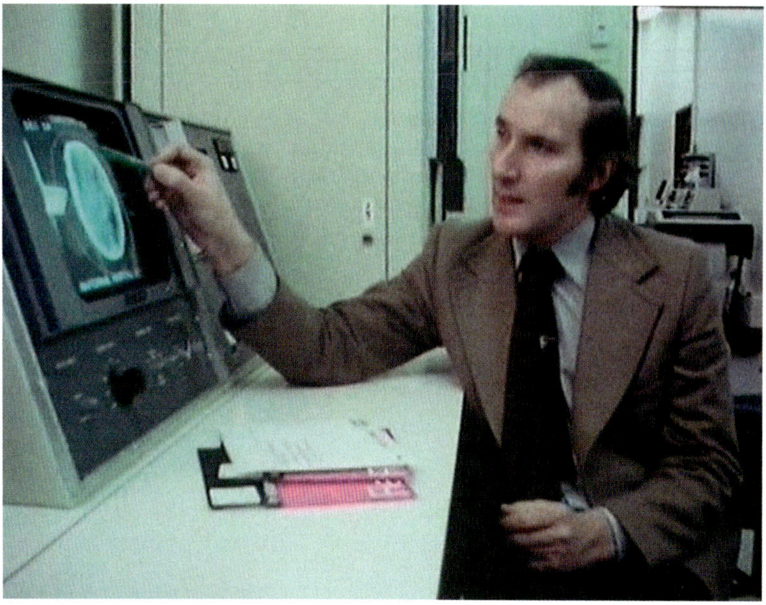

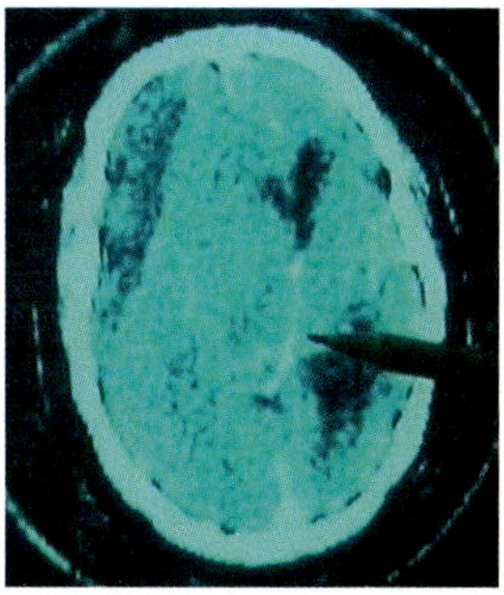

Dr Ivan Moseley
(Copyright EMI Music)
Speaking in the "Scanner Story" film. EMI, 1977.

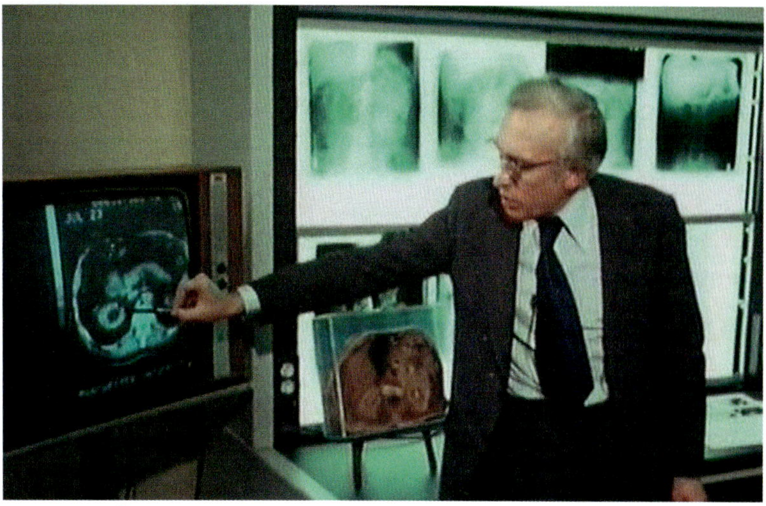

Professor Ian Isherwood in the "Scanner Story" film
(Copyright EMI Music)

An early "believer" was John Powell, who joined EMI in the autumn of 1971 as group technical director and who became involved with the EMI-scanner by March 1972. John Powell was an important man throughout the subsequent history of the EMI-scanner. He claimed responsibility for the decision to manufacture scanners rather than license the technique. His role in the company grew at the same time as the medical business. As a result, some people take the view that he was over-stretched. By 1974 he was managing director of EMI, while still remaining the only reporting link between the US and UK sections of EMI's medical business. John Powell played a major role in setting the strategy of EMI's medical business, until it hit the rocks and he left the company in 1979. He was a persuasive and coherent speaker, and the EMI archive includes video of him presenting a Faraday lecture, as detailed in Appendix 2, and a transcript of his interview with Professor Charles Süsskind.

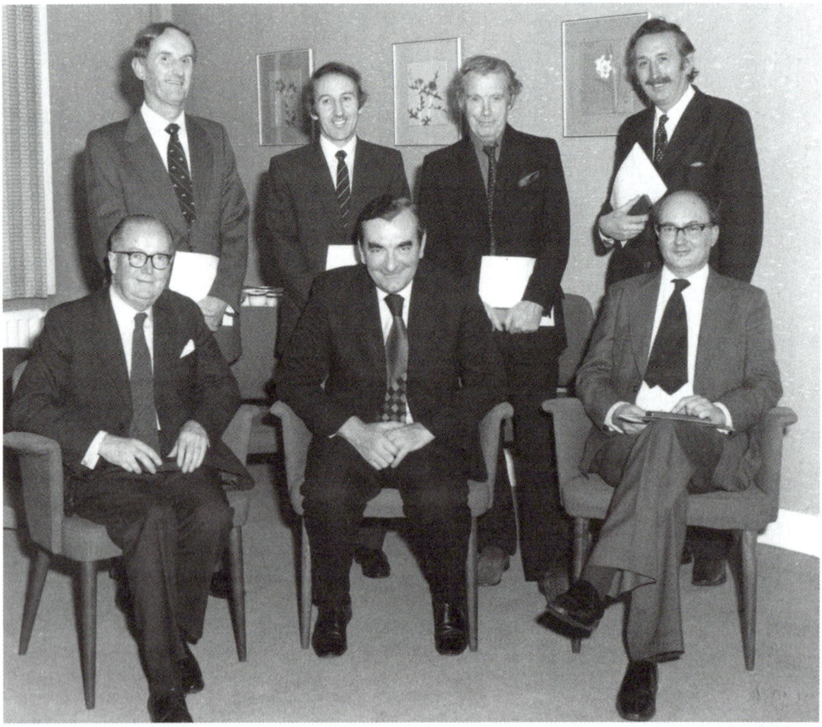

Presentation of twenty-five-year service awards by Dr John Powell to Godfrey and others
(Copyright EMI Music)

The above photo shows several people who played important roles in the story, although in different years from each other. On the left of the front row is Geoff Byers, who played a pivotal role in reaching a successful agreement with the DHSS in 1971, then John Powell and Jim Lodge, who wrote a history of CRL after working there for many years. The back row contains John Wardley (known as Jim in those days), John Griffiths, Douglas Palmer, and Godfrey. The back of the photo is stamped

7 November 1974, which is two years ahead of this point in the story, but the photo is included here because it shows John Powell and Geoff Byers and others.

In April 1972 EMI had no CT manufacturing division. Many parts of the first twenty scanners were built in the research labs, while early recruits such as Eddie Gowler, Anthony Strong, and Dave King became familiar with the product while working alongside Godfrey. Manufacturing moved into other buildings a few hundred yards away on the Hayes site in the summer of 1973, while still relying on advice from Godfrey's team and using metalwork made in CRL's workshop.

The decision to make scanners rather than issue manufacturing licenses or form partnerships with existing suppliers was debatable. A note by Geoff Byers in April 1972 says that licensing was under review, but it was hampered because the drawings were not at production standard. He said: *As we do not possess the full asset to offer to proposed licensees (i.e. the complete package of production drawings and related information) we should prepare an Outline Agreement with more sales appeal rather than a fully detailed legalistic draft at this stage. I am therefore attaching a suggested draft outline intended for a USA Licensee.* Byers recommends manufacturing for the UK and Europe markets but licensing for the USA and Japan. In practice, the decisions were taken by John Powell rather than by Byers. By October 1972 Powell had decided to manufacture.

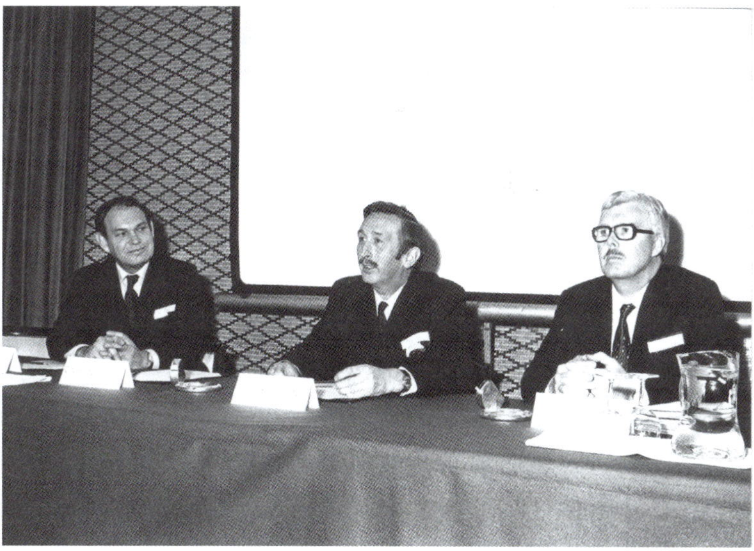

MacRobert Award press conference
(Copyright EMI Music)
Left to right: Dr James Ambrose, DMRD, FRCP, of Atkinson Morley Hospital; Godfrey Hounsfield, DFH, AMIEE; William Ingham, BSc, CEng, FIEE, Director of EMI CRL.

The MacRobert Award was presented on 22 November 1972. It is the most prestigious award for engineering in the UK. The prize was a gold

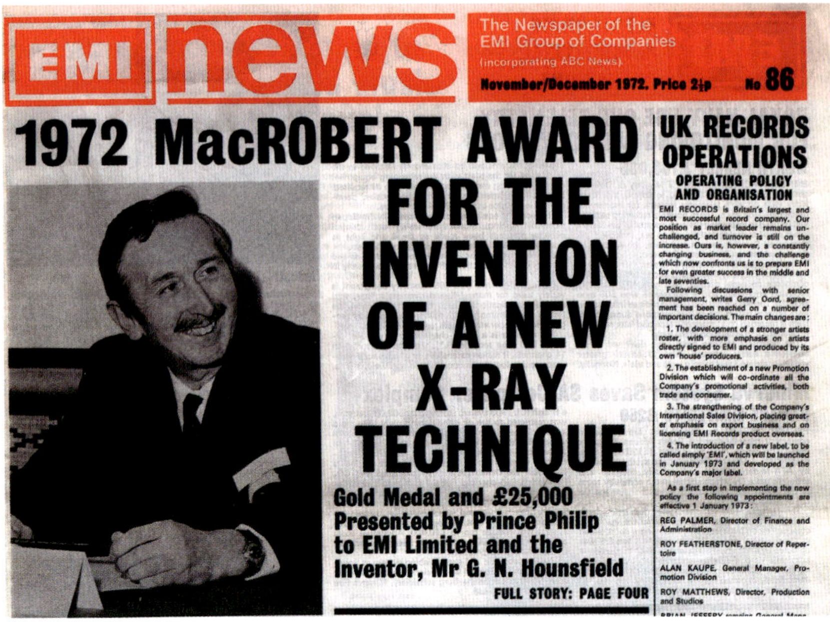

EMI news

The Newspaper of the EMI Group of Companies (incorporating ABC News)

November/December 1972. Price 2½p No 86

1972 MacROBERT AWARD FOR THE INVENTION OF A NEW X-RAY TECHNIQUE

Gold Medal and £25,000 Presented by Prince Philip to EMI Limited and the Inventor, Mr G. N. Hounsfield

FULL STORY: PAGE FOUR

UK RECORDS OPERATIONS

OPERATING POLICY AND ORGANISATION

EMI RECORDS is Britain's largest and most successful record company. Our position as market leader remains unchallenged, and turnover is still on the increase. Ours is, however, a constantly changing business, and the challenge which now confronts us is to prepare EMI for even greater success in the middle and late seventies.

Following discussions with senior management, writes Gerry Oord, agreement has been reached on a number of important decisions. The main changes are:

1. The development of a stronger artists roster, with more emphasis on artists directly signed to EMI and produced by its own 'house' producers.

2. The establishment of a new Promotion Division which will co-ordinate all the Company's promotional activities, both trade and consumer.

3. The strengthening of the Company's International Sales Division, placing greater emphasis on export business and on licensing EMI Records product overseas.

4. The introduction of a new label, to be called simply 'EMI', which will be launched in January 1973 and developed as the Company's major label.

As a first step in implementing the new policy the following appointments are effective 1 January 1973:

REG PALMER, Director of Finance and Administration

ROY FEATHERSTONE, Director of Repertoire

ALAN KAUPE, General Manager, Promotion Division

ROY MATTHEWS, Director, Production and Studios

MacRobert Award
(Copyright EMI Music)

medal and £25,000. To set that in context, the salary of the chairman of EMI was £21,000 in the financial year ending in June 1974.

Lord Hinton who chaired the award Evaluation Committee wrote, *One of the medical referees consulted during the evaluation stated that no comparable discovery has been made in this field since Röntgen discovered X-rays in 1895, and we agree with him.*

The EMI-scanner system developed by Mr. Hounsfield within the Central Research Laboratories of EMI is epoch-making, because it breaks away from the photographic techniques for recording X-ray pictures which in principle have remained unchanged since Röntgen's day. These techniques have the inherent defect that they seek to show a three-dimensional object in a two-dimensional picture, without the benefit of perspective. This confuses the information recorded on the film. Also, details of healthy and diseased brain tissue, which have low absorptive characteristics, are masked in X-ray pictures by the surrounding, denser bone of the skull.

As well as overcoming these obstacles to the diagnosis of disease in the brain, the EMI system avoids the need, associated with other diagnostic techniques, for injecting the patient with substances such as radio-opaque fluids, which are not without risk to the patient.

With this new system, the patient is not put at risk, and is no more inconvenienced than by a chest X-ray. Without the need for unpleasant injections, 100 times more information is extracted from the X-ray photons than is possible using conventional means.

The technique has, as yet, been applied only to cranial examination but the MacRobert Award Evaluation Committee believes that the principle of this invention can be widely used.

There is another aspect of EMI-scanner which is remarkable. In these modern days it is rarely that one finds great developments which are the work of one man. The EMI-scanner is different: the submission for the MacRobert Award was prepared not by the inventor, but by EMI, who stated, 'Mr. Hounsfield has been the guiding expert throughout all aspects of the work. The EMI-scanner was as much a one-man invention as anything can be these days.' (From a Press Release on 22 November 1972 by the Council of Engineering Institutions, courtesy of the Engineering Council.)

Godfrey's niece Lynda Hounsfield says, *there is a lovely story when he won the MacRobert award: he goes along to the bank with this cheque, I can't remember how much it was, about £25,000 or so, wasn't it? Well they called in Security and had him checked out, because they thought it wasn't kosher! Don't you just love that! We just laughed – it was the way he told the story you know – and he said 'don't tell anybody, I was a bit embarrassed you know' and it was just such fun.*

Anthony Strong joined Godfrey's team in 1972: *I remember Godfrey as a brilliant intuitive engineer. Where the rest of us had to grind though the mathematics to prove what we wanted, he was able to give the answer directly and was always right. He was always kind and helpful. Like all truly great people he was never pretentious. He was perhaps a little commercially naive in a positive sense as he would willingly discuss scientific matters with anyone.*

In my early days at EMI I used to lunch with Godfrey and he used to write on the back of the menu the details, diagrams and equations I needed. The documents not only had the vital data but on the front the menu and critically the date. They were a useful set of references. I remember him as someone not enthusiastic about writing things down. The lunch room was the one place where I had a captive audience!

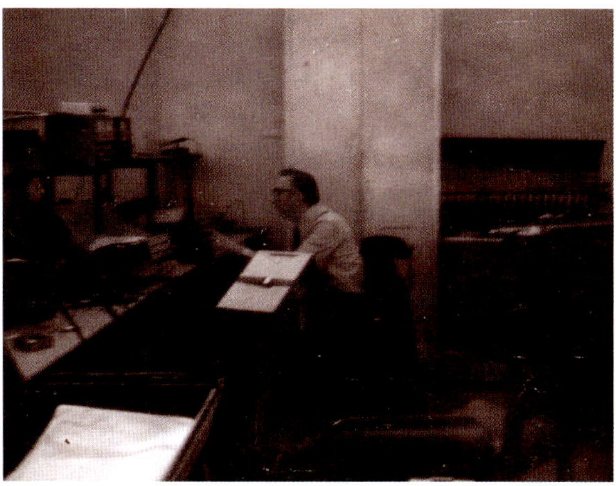

Godfrey at work
(Courtesy of Ian Fairbairn)
This is how his colleagues saw him, at a cluttered bench in the corner of a lab. The focus of the photo isn't sharp, but it reflects very strongly the focus of the man.

Godfrey liked working at the bench, trying to understand the science. Awards were not important to him: they were about the past, whereas he was searching for the next breakthrough.

Mac Gollifer moved the CT reconstruction program on to a Data General "Nova 820" minicomputer, having shown Godfrey that this would be faster than the rival PDP-11. He persuaded Godfrey to include a disk drive instead of relying only on a tape deck. This allowed the scanner to deliver a picture within five minutes, rather than waiting for it to be processed by the mainframe computer at EMI's Hayes site. This made immediate diagnosis possible, which made the scanner even more beneficial and saleable.

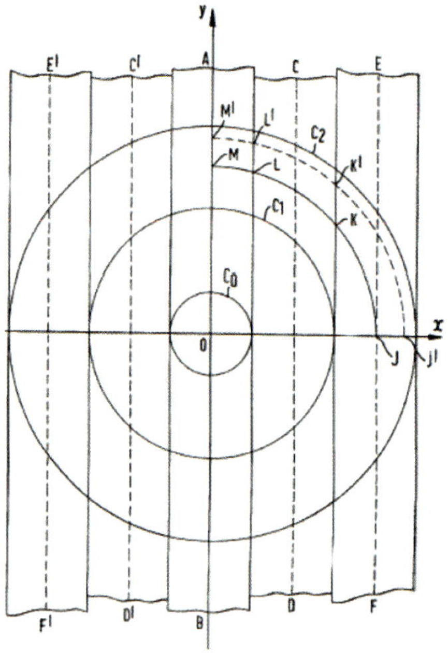

$L_0 = 1.00000$
$L_1 = -0.44447$
$L_2 = -0.01498$
$L_3 = -0.02548$
$L_4 = -0.002699$
$L_5 = -0.006653$
$L_6 = -0.004478$
$L_7 = -0.003331$
$L_8 = -0.002552$
$L_9 = -0.002022$
$L_{10} = -0.001639$
$L_{11} = -0.001356$
$L_{12} = -0.001140$
$L_{13} = -0.0009717$
$L_{14} = -0.0008381$
$L_{15} = -0.0007306$

Christopher LeMay's circle method

Christopher LeMay was brought in (on loan from another department) to find new and faster ways of reconstructing the image. In January 1973 Christopher produced a "circle method" which got the answer right first time, rather than by successive approximation. This is now called "filtered back-projection".

The effect of overlaying readings from many angles is to attenuate the fine detail in the picture, and this can be compensated by a high-frequency boost. The diagrams from US patent 3924129 give an indication of this.

Christopher LeMay wanted to calculate the absorption at the centre of the circles in this diagram. His method states that beams that pass exactly through this point must be multiplied by one. The "next door" beams that just miss the inner circle must be multiplied by –0.4447, which is shown as L_1 in the diagram. The beams that miss the centre by two beam widths must be multiplied by L_2, and so on. Christopher worked out the numbers for L_1 and L_2 by calculating how much time the central beam spent in the surrounding circles as the scanner rotated. The details can be left to the mathematicians, but the important point is that this method gets the picture right first time. This makes it faster than Godfrey's iterative method, although the resulting pictures are very similar.

The nearby beams have the largest effect. Looking at the diagram we can see that L_0 and L_1 will have more effect than the other numbers which are much smaller values. So Christopher's method applies two sharp negative peaks, one on each side of each beam.

Mac Gollifer remembers, *Godfrey asked me to look at what the iterative reconstruction system was doing, so I simulated a picture with just one pinpoint object in it, and looked at what was happening as the iterative system processed this. I got two sharp peaks which looked like a mistake in the test, until he asked me to test Christopher's proposal a few weeks later, which put very similar sharp negative peaks on each side of the main beam.*

John Ryan transferred back from SE Labs to work with Godfrey in the research labs in February 1973, and Stephen Bates followed about a month later, after direct intervention by the chairman, Sir John Read. John Ryan recalls Godfrey and Christopher LeMay returning from lunch deep in conversation, and pausing in the corridor outside John's office. A few minutes later they were drawing diagrams on the wall of the corridor!

The patent process moves very slowly, and Godfrey's patent application from 1968 was being inspected by the examiner at the USA Patents and Trademarks Office in the early months of 1973. In January 1973, Allan Logan wrote a memo to Godfrey saying that the claims had been modified in light of Cormack's work in 1963, which the patent examiner was now aware of. He mentioned a document published by Ramachandran in 1971, which was dated after Godfrey's work. Allan said that both of these people had found "one-shot" techniques (although their maths would run slowly on a 1973 computer), and that methods of getting the picture right first time were worth investigating. In fact Christopher LeMay had already done that, and had found a faster method a few weeks before Allan suggested it. In March 1973, Allan Logan wrote to John Powell, Bill Ingham, and others to say that the US patent was about to be granted, which was a significant event for EMI.

In April 1973, a dialogue began because William Oldendorf thought (incorrectly) that Godfrey's work was based on Oldendorf's patent, but the relationship moved into more positive territory with Oldendorf becoming a consultant to EMI. He and Godfrey worked in similar ways and shared similar interests. They also shared the Ziedses des Plantes Gold Medal award in 1974 and the Lasker Award for Clinical Medical Research in 1975. They both liked to solve engineering problems in simple and economical ways; Oldendorf's method is intuitive and completely eliminates any mathematics, which matched two of Godfrey's preferences.

Unfortunately, it is inefficient in its use of the X-ray dose, which means that it would expose the patient to hundreds of times more radiation than a CT scan. More detail on the work by Godfrey's predecessors can be found in Appendix 7, to show that there are many difficult steps between having ideas about a CT scanner, as his predecessors did, and making the breakthrough. It was Godfrey who put in all of the hard work to convince the world that CT scanning could detect tumours and other disorders at an acceptable X-ray dose and cost. There is **much** more to being a genius than simply having ideas.

Godfrey's next objective was to design a body scanner. He knew that a short scan time was essential, and his team looked at a "rotate-only" design. Rotate only means that there was no side-to-side movement of the detectors, and that a large number of detectors collected information across the whole width of the patient's body at the same time. The X-ray tube and detectors just rotated around the patient. This project was codenamed "Diamond", which set the pattern for naming projects after precious stones, rather than using names that described the goals of the work.

John Ryan recalls those days: *Steve and I shared an office and Brian Lill was next door with Tony Williams further down the corridor. Steve and I managed to obtain a second-hand whiteboard for our office. Every day Godfrey was sorting out problems on the brain-scanner in the morning and then he joined us sometime between 11:00 and 2:00 when we would discuss Diamond. I suspect that these discussions were mainly in our office because of our whiteboard. Brian would usually join us from next door and sometimes Tony. I wondered whether I had done the right thing by leaving a good job at SE Labs, because these seemingly endless discussions went on for most of that year with not much to show. In retrospect of course it was quite different, i.e. having discussions with a future Nobel laureate at the height of his creativity. Godfrey would write his proposals on the whiteboard in random positions with a blue pen and we would discuss/argue. When the whiteboard was full we had to agree whether part, or all, of it could be erased. For this reason I wonder whether there was much recorded on Diamond. During that period the problem of detector stability and the ring-artefact problem was identified. Godfrey was in some ways repeating what he did on the brain-scanner by building up detailed knowledge and solving all the problems before proceeding, but the management were concerned that the competition would catch up, so we were eventually asked to produce Emerald as an interim measure!* (Emerald was the prototype for EMI's largest selling body scanner.)

After one bank holiday weekend Godfrey returned to say that he had had a brilliant idea, but unfortunately he had forgotten what it was. Over the next few days we went through all of the issues we had been discussing the previous week to try to trigger his memory, but to no avail. During this time the team had several new ideas, and I believe some PQs [patent queries] *were written, but we never discovered what the brilliant idea was. I wondered if this was an innovative technique by Godfrey to stimulate us to come up with ideas.*

Godfrey always worked from first principles. Pocket calculators were just becoming affordable, but Godfrey clearly distrusted them and often after one of our sessions on the whiteboard he would return the next day having worked out his own solution via log tables. On one occasion Godfrey did not believe the results we were getting and went through the calculations several times with the same result. Eventually we pointed out to him that he was not checking the principles, but only that log tables gave the same result as the pocket calculator.

Godfrey often made the point that the correlated information on the absorption values adds up linearly, whereas the Gaussian noise adds up 'RMS-ically'. I find myself using this term today when summing interference sources.

He became worried about the effects of scatter, so he decided to run an experiment using the X-ray source on the original lathe-bed, but how was he to measure the scatter in the surrounding space? All of his team wore radiation detectors (X-ray film inside badges) which were changed monthly, and sent away to be checked. Godfrey's idea was to borrow the radiation badges from his team and place these around the test-bed and then rely on the data from monthly monitoring to reveal the amount of radiation at each location. Certainly the company doctor would have been surprised by our increased exposure to radiation. Bob Froggatt thought this was highly amusing but managed to persuade Godfrey that it was not a good idea.

Paul Beaven had joined Godfrey's team, and he recalls, *Godfrey lost the petrol cap from his car, and he was too busy to find a replacement. He was driving around with a piece of mutton cloth in the petrol filler pipe, just like a Molotov cocktail.*

John Ryan adds another story: *Godfrey had been so busy he had forgotten to tax his car. As he was getting quite well known the management decided that this might reflect badly on the company, so it was decided that he should have a company car, which he would not have been entitled to on his grade. In the meantime his old Triumph 2000 remained in the car park, rusting away. After several months he went over to the mechanics at the Jet garage and gave them the key saying that if they could get it through the MOT they could have the car.*

One of the cleaners (Bill?) was handicapped and also had severe speech impediment such that few of us could understand him at all. On one occasion I returned after lunch to find Godfrey in deep discussion with Bill, who he had cornered in an office. Godfrey liked to bounce his ideas off anyone who would listen, whether they understood it or not. For quite different reasons I doubt that either could understand what the other was saying, but this did not seem to matter to Godfrey.

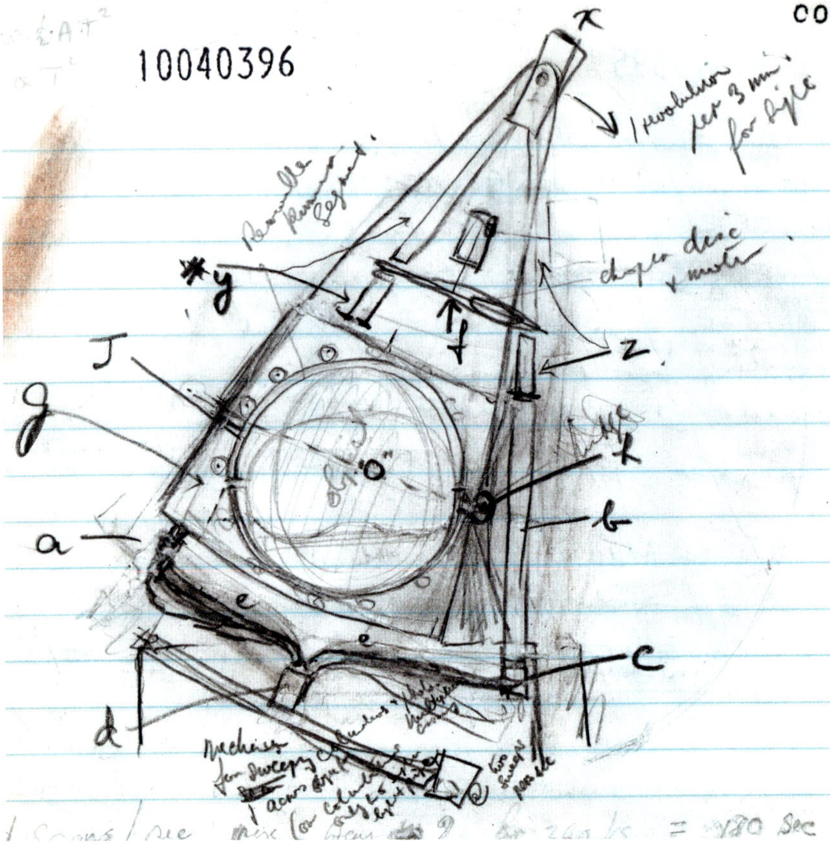

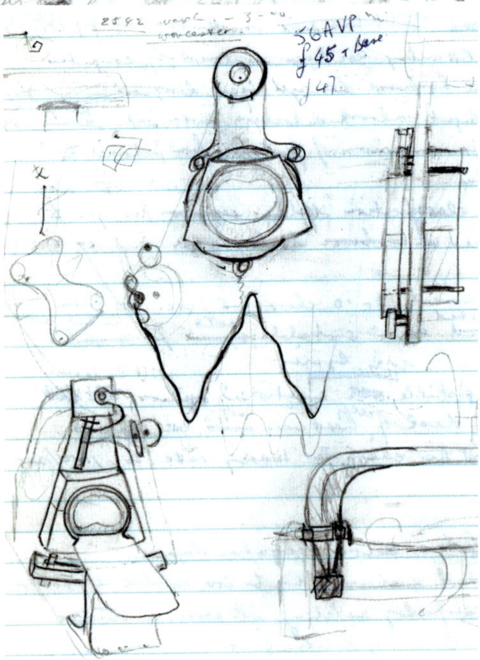

Godfrey's daybook contains sketches of early ideas for body scanner design
(Copyright EMI Music)

The first body scan at EMI was on 19 November 1973, when Dave King adapted an Mk1 brain scanner to take a picture of the slimmest available volunteer, who happened to be Tony Williams. Dave removed the water box, and used an inner tube from a car tyre instead, which he filled with water. It was not a particularly good picture, because nobody can hold their breath for four minutes. Colin Oliver says, *It was a toss up between me and Tony Williams, and I decided to let Tony have a go on that! I don't think they went around measuring waists, they just looked at me and Tony and said you look thin enough: two likely victims! I didn't fancy it, so I let Tony have the X-ray dose and the glory.*

The Diamond project quickly reached the conclusion that variations in gain between one detector and another would need to be controlled to within 1 part in 5,000 to avoid ring artefacts, in which the picture becomes corrupted by unwanted black and white rings. So the work to develop body scanners split into two paths: Emerald was a translate–rotate machine with a twenty second scan time, designed as a stop gap while a faster machine was developed. The second path was Ruby, later called Topaz, which was a faster rotate-only design using an X-ray tube with a magnetically deflected focal spot to overcome the ring artefacts.

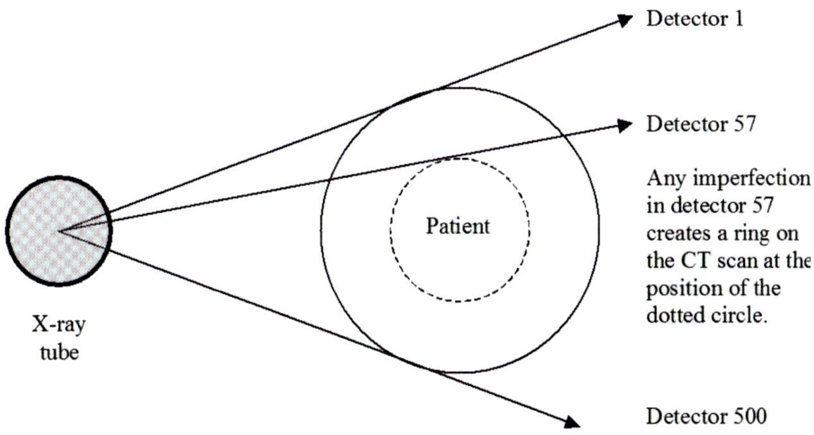

The ring artefact problem

Richard Gillard recalls working on the body scanner prototype (Emerald) in 1974: *one evening Godfrey was wanting to go through some computer printouts of detector readings with me, in the early days of the body scanner development. I was tiring as the time went by, and it was getting late. Eventually he suggested going to a Chinese restaurant. This sounded a good idea, but as soon as the meal had been ordered the printouts reappeared and off we went again!*

When Emerald was designed in 1974 computers were in their infancy. The next photo shows a "Teletype" as the user interface: it printed messages from the computer on a roll of paper in place of the screen that one would expect today.

Brian Lill worked with Paul Beaven on the problem of rapidly calculating exactly how much each edge reading intersected with each pixel in the scan. This included a different way of implementing Godfrey's "jacked-up sine wave" interpolation between the beams. Stephen Bates had used a look-up table for that task, because that was very well matched to the ICL 1905 computer. Brian and Paul found a method that was more suitable for the Nova minicomputer, or for use in bespoke hardware. Paul and Brian say, *we developed a way of performing this task, but when we described it to Godfrey, he didn't believe it could work. It took several hours and lots of drawings to convince him that it was a viable technique. The next day Godfrey came into our office and said that he had been thinking about our technique and he didn't believe it would bring the performance gains we intended, so we had another lengthy debate convincing him it worked correctly. Yet another day passed and again Godfrey re-appeared, saying that he'd thought it over at home and still didn't think it could work. So another lengthy session ensued and we again managed to convince him that the idea worked with the performance we needed. We wrote up the technique and sent it off to the patent department. How Godfrey's name came to be on the patent we don't know, but when he was subsequently awarded the Nobel Prize, it gave us the claim to fame that we shared a patent with a Nobel Prize winner.* The puzzle is that some heads of department routinely added their own names to all patents invented by their staff, but Godfrey did not.

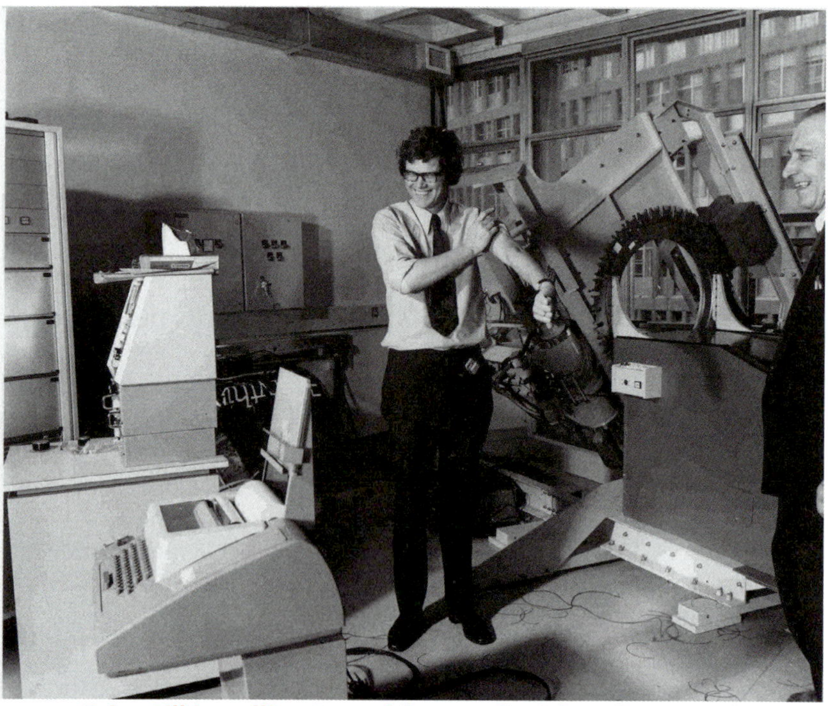

Brian Lill installing Emerald at Northwick Park Hospital
(Copyright EMI Music)

It is difficult to be sure why Paul and Brian found it so hard to convince Godfrey that this new idea worked. Certainly, he cared deeply that the new method should not degrade the performance of his jacked-up sine wave: the importance of that had been burnt into his memory during the lathe-bed phase. It seems likely that he was not thinking along the same lines as Paul and Brian. He did not share their university maths background, and he often gravitated towards his own analogies and mental pictures rather than following the way in which someone else described an idea. In simple terms, he was not listening well, but in his defence we should remember the enormous pressure that he was under.

A challenge when working with Godfrey was that his memory was selective: some things stuck and others did not. He could easily remember that he had reached a conclusion but he was notoriously bad at remembering **why**. He might confidently reinvent a reason, but sometimes he made a complete hash of it. It made the youngsters smile at the time, saying, *Godfrey is right for the wrong reason*, but as we get older some of us can see it happening in ourselves.

Godfrey could be generous in acknowledging contributions from others, as Don McLean recalls, *The question was how do you see the detail in the liver? It looks like a flat area unless you turn the contrast right up, but then you can't see the structure anywhere else. So he came up with the idea of using colour to enhance the low frequency information in the scan, and display it as a colour wash over the normal greyscale picture. But he was really generous, he named me on the patent, but frankly he didn't have to because the idea was all his. The other topic which we worked on was a 3D display: he wanted to see the structures inside the body which you can't get a good picture of from a single slice. He came up with an idea for making the 3D structure more visible. He arranged for large transparencies of consecutive CT slices. I put these in a big cardboard box and rigged it up so that they could be lit in different ways. So the lighting gave you a way of dialling in the layer which you wanted to see. It was very simple and effective.*

Brian Lill was working out how to drive the scanner backwards and forwards. *I decided on a permanent magnet motor, ordered one and later showed it to Godfrey. He immediately said that it was not big enough and I should order a larger one. I was quite happy with my choice as I had applied a large safety margin to the design, and Godfrey was remembering motor sizes from earlier magnet technology.*

I fitted the motor and a gear box to a wooden bench for testing. Before I had done any testing Godfrey had a look and said that he did not think it would give the required performance. The next morning Godfrey said that he had done some calculations and that it would be OK. I went to the lab to start testing and found his calculations written on the wooden bench!

Development of single-purpose brain scanners continued parallel to the new body scanner. It was still unclear whether or not a body machine would be clinically worthwhile, and in any case there might still be a market niche for a specialist brain machine. Initially, the focus was on improvements that could fit (and preferably retrofit) onto the existing Mk1 scanner, including the "Pearl" upgrade, which used Chris LeMay's methods and the Lill/Beaven technique to increase processing speed and to give a 160×160 matrix. This was in operation by October 1974.

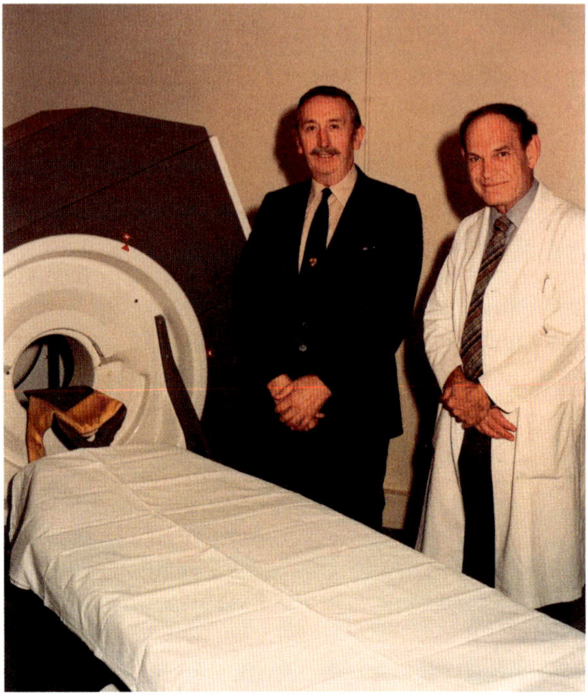

Godfrey and James Ambrose in about 1976
(Photo ownership is unknown)
They are standing next to a CT1010 brain scanner, which was developed in the Super Opal project.

James Ambrose made a most important contribution in 1970–71 by helping Godfrey to make the design of the prototype match the practical needs of the hospital. The above photo shows the CT1010 brain scanner, which was better for patients than the Mk1 EMI-scanner. The patient typically spent only four minutes on the table rather than twelve. There was no water box, so the doctor could scan areas such as the brain stem, and the patient felt more comfortable.

The Super Opal project developed this CT1010 brain scanner, which gave the best pictures of any EMI-scanner. It used the same X-ray detectors as the Emerald body scanner: sodium iodide crystals coupled to photomultipliers. The output from these would today be converted into numbers by a single silicon chip, but in those days it needed about twenty electronic components. The prototype went to Atkinson Morley in April 1975 and the production version, the CT1010, followed in 1976.

Godfrey was not a born manager, although, at crucial times for both the EMIDEC 1100 and the EMI-scanner, he was put in charge of large teams because his enthusiasm and determination was exactly what was needed to drive through a large inventive project. He had no desire to run a department for an extended time: what he wanted was to run an interesting project, with whatever team it needed – fifty people for one project but then perhaps only two for the next. At times, his unusual approach puzzled his staff.

Colin Oliver and Ian Fairbairn joined Godfrey to work on Super Opal. Colin says, *Godfrey was much more like a playing captain in a football team than a manager. Godfrey often said 'let's have a meeting about that' but it never came to pass. He seemed to find ways of deciding without any meetings.* This was probably a good thing because meetings waste a lot of time. Ian recalls how much Godfrey liked to get involved in the detail: *I applied to work in the Research Labs again. Godfrey interviewed me and offered me a job. As I was pushing a trolley full of my paraphernalia out of the engineering building, one of the secretaries asked me where I was heading and I told her I was going to work for Godfrey Hounsfield. She looked shocked: 'Do you have to? He'll drive you mad!' A year or so later I'd modified a circuit and after updating a copy of the diagram I sought Godfrey's approval. He agreed with the design changes and in the top right-hand corner of my modified copy of the drawing simply wrote: 'Latest'.* (It is better to write the date, to avoid confusion if two are marked "latest".)

On a later occasion when I was working on Topaz, after a long session discussing a design detail with Godfrey he finally left the office saying: 'You decide, Ian'. I escaped to the library to continue my work there knowing he'd be soon back to have another go at persuading me to change to his preferred approach. And sure enough – Colin Oliver told me he'd come back shortly after I left! But I never found Godfrey to be dictatorial.

Alan Harwood says, *I joined his section and didn't see him for the first few days. The following Monday he rolled in and he told me about Super Opal, and what we were going to do. He sat with me for about half a day, and then on the way out he said 'we're delivering it in October', and it was September already! So I'm thinking that we must have some facilities here! But it was late of course. He wanted a large gear wheel, about half a meter across, with specially cut teeth. The rest of us were sure that standard teeth would be fine, and far cheaper. So we made both, and they both worked, but he was very happy to change to our suggestion.*

Doug Jackson recalls, *As a very junior member of the operational team I presented myself and the suppliers of the fluorescing crystals, Rank Laboratories, to the door of Geoffrey's office. After some technical discussion we retired to the Blue Anchor pub for lunch as was the practice in those days. After steak, chips and a pint we looked to our host, Godfrey, to pay the bill. Godfrey didn't carry or bother about money. Being the only other EMI person there I dug deep (no credit cards then) and coughed up, Godfrey saying he would settle with me later. After further meetings with Godfrey when nothing was mentioned about the money I gathered up courage and asked him directly: the reply was 'Follow me. We will go and get some.' We walked to Hayes High Street and into the Post Office where Godfrey produced his passbook and withdrew the exact amount. As a young engineer this was a strange experience as I knew that Godfrey had won the £25,000 MacRobert Award and my salary was very small compared to that. None of this was important to him of course, other things were.*

A lot of CT-related work was carried out by other departments in CRL. Nigel Johnson first met Godfrey when he demonstrated his "frame buffer" viewer for CT pictures – it was a great improvement on the previous viewer. *This was something I'd spent quite a long while working on and it was the first time it had been exposed to people outside of the video group where it was designed and built. Everybody was in the lab and 'oohing and aahing' over the brilliant quality of the pictures which they were seeing for the first time on live television. Godfrey came into the room at that point, took one look at the picture and pointed to the greyscale down the left hand side of the image. He pointed at the bottom step of the greyscale and said 'That's too bright!' and then he walked out without making any comments on the actual image itself. Luckily I'd been forewarned as to Godfrey's nature and, along with the others in the lab at the time, was amused at this observation which demonstrated Godfrey's ability to focus on to the details. Godfrey was always very careful in setting the brightness and contrast of the display screen. That was my first personal encounter with him and something I'd never forget.*

Stephen Bates put this into context: *Godfrey was central to CT during (and beyond) the whole of EMI's involvement. Throughout it all he was tireless in his attention to detail and determination to see his vision materialise. Nothing he did was for personal gain but only to see the job done. He was a mild-mannered man who was a joy to work with. He could also be difficult to work with, and would sometimes drive people to near despair with his single-mindedness. He would sometimes come to ask me if I knew what was upsetting some member of the team or other, and could genuinely not see that his desire to be involved in every*

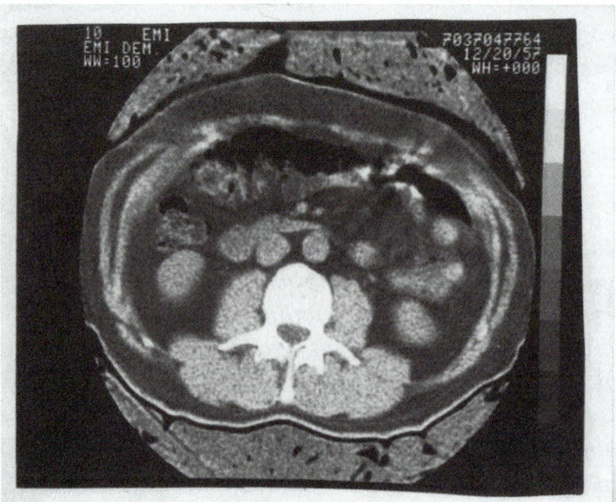

Godfrey's abdomen, December 1974
(Copyright EMI Music)

aspect of the work might be the problem. But he was a caring person and everybody in his team respected him and above all it was a privilege to work with him.

The image of Godfrey's abdomen shows the first CT scan taken using the Emerald body scanner. Godfrey claimed to recognise his lunch in this picture, although this seems doubtful. His lunch was crisps and beer in the Blue Anchor pub. His kidneys are visible either side of the spine. Above the spine are the pancreas, blood vessels, and part of the digestive system. The packing material around Godfrey's abdomen was used to keep the detector readings within range.

In March 1975, Bob Froggatt wrote to tell the research staff how well the first Emerald pictures were received by the medical community: *Godfrey Hounsfield and I attended the Computed Cranial Tomography International Symposium and Course in Bermuda. [...] The Management of EMI have been concerned with the rise of possible competition in this field in recent months and it was decided that something about our progress in research on Emerald should be revealed to potential future customers. It was therefore arranged that a special talk should be given by Hounsfield at 8.00am on Friday 14th March. Speculation was rife and we were worried that expectations would outstrip the achievement. Never was anybody more wrong, Godfrey outlined the progress on body scanning, showing pictures, from the pig, through the 80×80 and 160×160 Tony Williams picture to the 320×320 slice of himself.*

The audience actually gasped at this and broke into applause and for the rest of the conference we lived under a welter of congratulations from some of the world's leading radiologists. Dr. Powell expressed his regret that some of you whose work has contributed to this landmark of radiology (and I quote one eminent gentleman) could not have been present to witness the occasion and to realise what our work will mean to the medical profession.

We still have a lot of work to do but I think you ought to be aware of the very great regard with which our work is held by the world's radiologists, how appreciative they are of our efforts and what a lot they expect from us in the future.

Bob Froggatt spoke at the same conference, and his talk included a little sidelight: *In the early days of EMI-scanner the then Director of EMI's Central Research Laboratories, Dr. Broadway, sent a mathematician to see Hounsfield for two reasons. First, to satisfy himself that Hounsfield knew what he was doing and secondly, if this was so to give him any help he could. The mathematician, who was of the old school and prepared to invert matrices quickly and efficiently, came back slightly stunned at the novelty of the idea and had not been able to prove whether it would work or not by the time experimental vindication arrived. I think we were all then like the mathematician, slightly shattered by the invention, hoping it would work but not being sure.* We believe that this mathematician was

William S. Percival, a brilliant member of Alan Blumlein's team that developed television in the 1930s.

Emerald body scanners were working in Northwick Park Hospital, the Mallinckrodt Institute of Radiology, and the Mayo Clinic by October 1975. The 1976 production version was called the CT5000 (later CT5005).

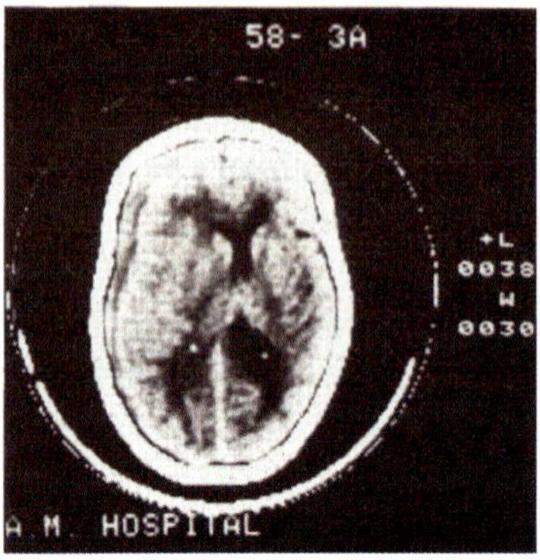

Brain scan from the Super Opal scanner

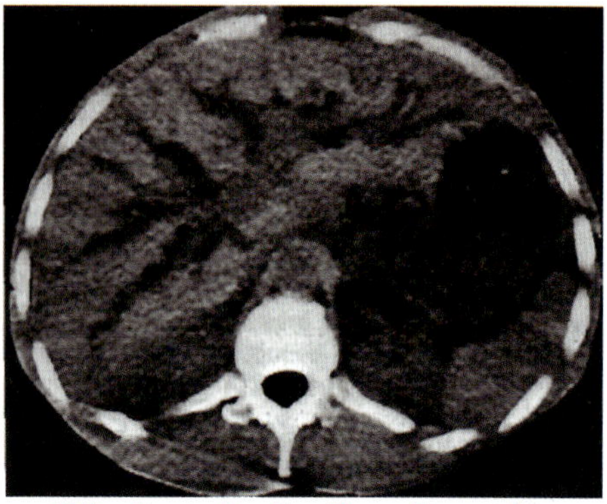

Bile ducts in the liver from the Emerald body scanner

CT quickly replaced some unpleasant diagnostic techniques. The ventricles in the brain are cavities filled with spinal fluid, and are easily seen as dark regions in a CT scan. A tumour or concussion or other abnormality may make the ventricles asymmetrical. Before CT, the ventricles could be seen using X-rays only by filling them with air. It was uncomfortable and it could be very painful: the patient usually vomited, and this was the examination that a patient described to Godfrey as feeling like being kicked in the head by a horse. CT was a very attractive alternative. Before CT, diagnosis of a liver problem was often possible only by surgical examination, whereas if a CT scan is performed first then surgery is directed only to the place where it can actually help in the cure, and patients who will not get any benefit are spared the pain of surgery.

Adrian Thomas says, *CT fundamentally changed how we practice medicine and how we use medical images. Prior to CT we used invasive diagnostic techniques and invasive therapies. CT caused a major shift towards* ***non-invasive*** *methods. Prior to CT a lot of radiology was indirect imaging: in which doctors had to* ***infer*** *the presence of something which was displacing blood vessels, or to use a barium meal to infer that a growth is displacing the stomach. With CT we do not need to infer, we can see such things directly. In Godfrey's famous first scan, instead of inferring that there may be a cyst by seeing how it is displacing the ventricles, CT lets you see the lesion directly.*

Both of the new scanners used a small fan of detectors to produce a faster scan than the four and a half minutes of the Mk1 machine. The body scanner, Emerald, had thirty detectors in a ten-degree arc, and could scan one slice in about twenty seconds. The brain scanner, Super Opal, had a three-degree fan with a total of sixteen detectors (eight per slice), and it could scan two slices in one minute.

These scanners were the last to be built mainly from off-the-shelf components. Future designs would need many newly designed components such as detectors, electronics, processors, X-ray tubes, and high voltage supply. As a result, the cost, risk, and timescale of product development increased dramatically.

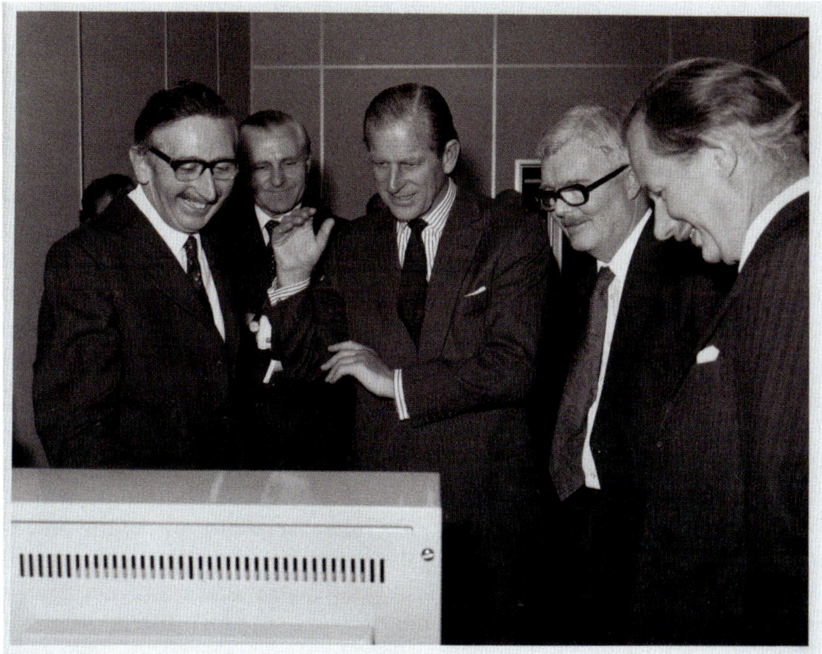

Godfrey, Sir John Read, Prince Philip, Bill Ingham, and Christopher LeMay
(Copyright EMI Music)

Godfrey was delighted that Prince Philip took a detailed interest in CT. In the above photo they are looking at a CT scan in about 1974, when Godfrey was awarded the Prince Philip Medal.

The Prince Philip Medal
(Photo courtesy of City & Guilds)
This medal was the personal gift of City & Guilds President HRH The Prince Philip, Duke of Edinburgh, for outstanding individual achievement in science, technology, and industrial development, or for exceptional proficiency in workplace skills.

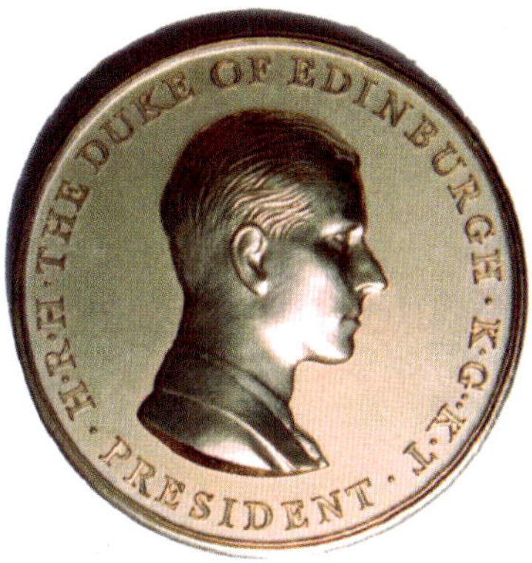

The Medal was for those who, in Prince Philip's words, had *travelled the City & Guilds path*, beginning or furthering their career with City & Guilds qualifications. The aim was to honour those who made the most of their individual talents and abilities, often overcoming initial educational disadvantages.

Godfrey still found time for IVC meetings, as John Davis recalls, *From the late 60s there was a Travel sub-club whereby once or twice a month members assembled to hear a talk, usually with slides, about an interesting trip a member had made. Around 60 people usually attended and we served coffee afterwards. For much of that period I was the Organiser but I had a committee to help, not only on the evening but to help find likely presenters and at the December meeting to help make the mulled wine to accompany the special pre-Xmas entertainment – typically a skiing film. Godfrey was on the committee and during that time struggling to get the embryo CT device to work at Atkinson Morley. Despite all his brainpower he regularly VOLUNTEERED to wash up all those coffee cups at the cramped little sink at the far end of the Victoria Room – and when I protested, he replied that it was 'nice to relax over a routine task at the end of a long battle with the equipment!' He also operated the rather decrepit film projector at the Xmas meeting – and got a lot of fun by running the film in reverse afterwards (backwards skiing!).*

One task that Godfrey did not volunteer for was speaking in public, but it was often difficult to refuse. For example, on 23 June 1976 he was in San Diego, USA, to speak at the American Academy of Achievement and accept the Golden Plate Award. On 8 July he was in Loughborough, UK, to accept an Honorary Doctorate and make a speech. On 11–14 September he travelled to the USA again to give the fifth annual Wendell G. Scott Lecture in St. Louis. On 14 October he gave the Mitchell Memorial Lecture in Stoke on Trent for the Association of Engineers. He was in constant demand.

John Ryan recalls, *As the installed base of scanners grew Godfrey began to receive more and more correspondence, but he had no time to answer it, so it built up on his desk until it became unusable. Godfrey's solution was to abandon it for the office next door and start again. Eventually it was decided that he should have a secretary, which his grade would not normally be entitled to, so Audrey Lester was recruited. Once it became known that his correspondence was being answered, the volume increased even more. Audrey was very much moved by the content of the correspondence, as we all were. A large part of it was from relatives whose loved-ones lives had been saved by his invention.*

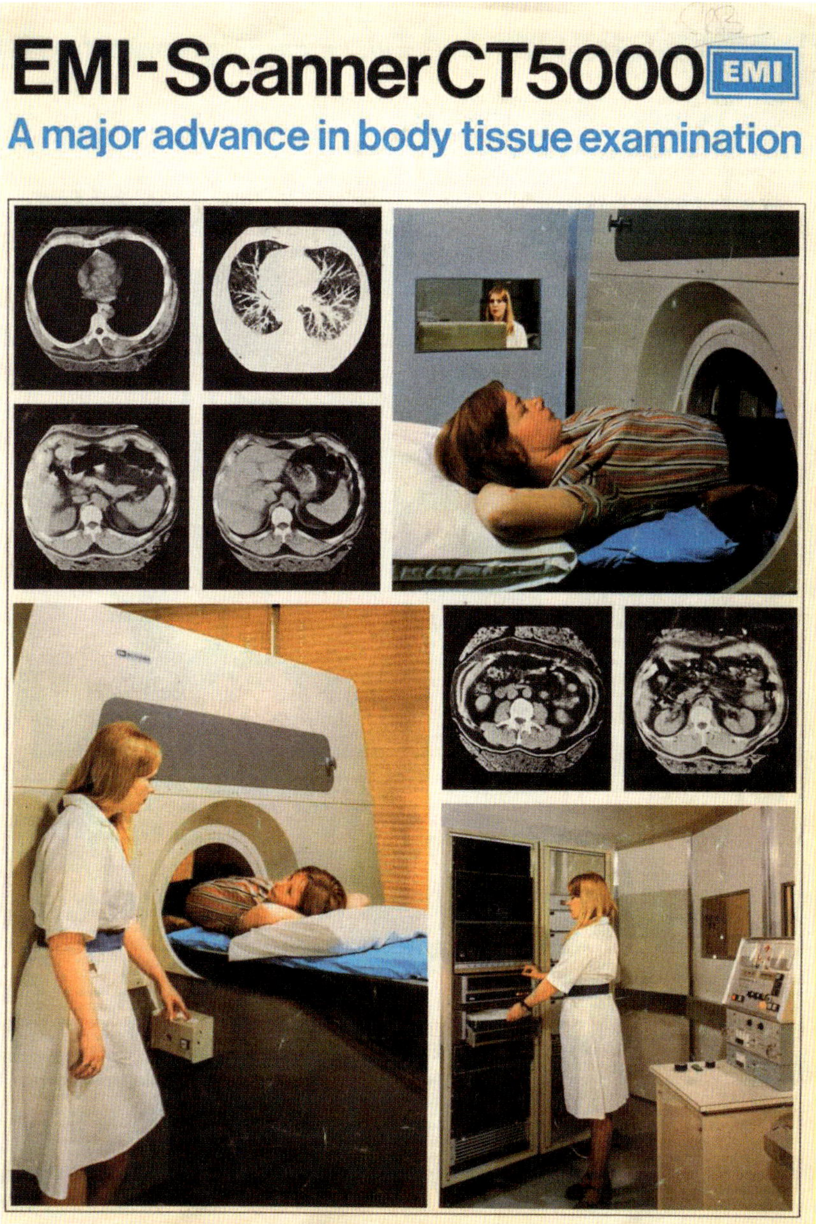

The Emerald body scanner
(Copyright EMI Music)

This photo shows Godfrey's team in mid 1975.

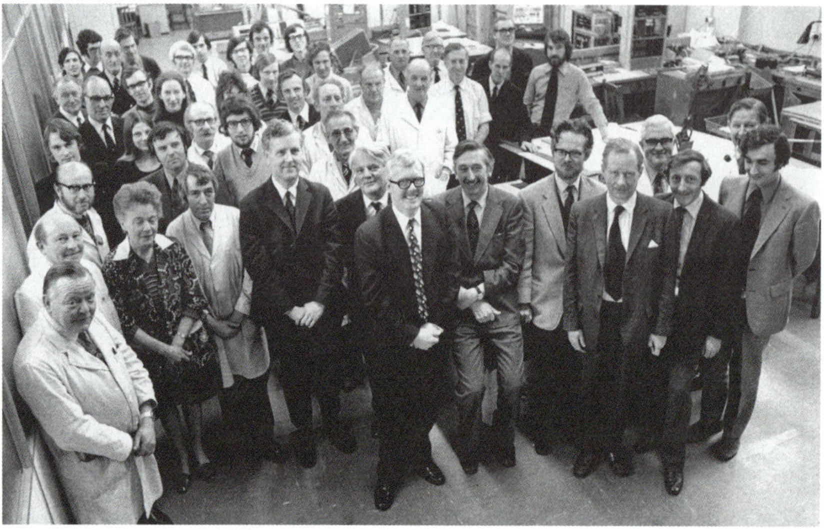

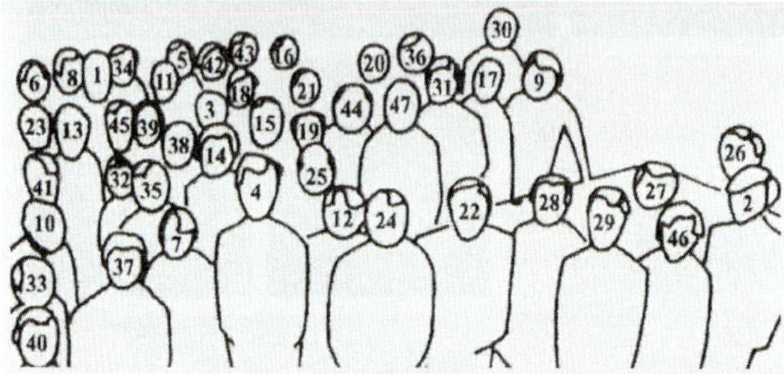

Summer 1975
(Copyright EMI Music)

Names are: 1, Peter Bade; 2, Stephen Bates; 3, Martin Bishop; 4, Alan Blay; 5, Phil Bone; 6, Dave Bradley; 7, George Brock; 8, Tony Buzzing; 9, Ken Charles; 10, George Eades; 11, Ian Fairbairn; 12, Bob Froggatt; 13, Syd Gilbert; 14, Richard Gillard; 15, Mac Gollifer; 16, Trevor Hancock; 17, Jim Harding; 18, Alan Harwood; 19, Arthur Heath; 20, Ron Henbest; 21, Barry Holloway; 22, Godfrey Hounsfield; 23, Albert Hutchinson; 24, Bill Ingham; 25, Ernie Johnson; 26, Frank Keel; 27, Ernie Kitchenham; 28, Peter Langstone; 29, Christopher LeMay; 30, Roy Luckett; 31, Peter Nevell; 32, Pat O'Brien; 33, Alec Peddle; 34, Dave Pycock; 35, John Ryan; 36, Len Smith; 37, Pam Smith; 38, Harold Snelgrove; 39, Jean Steven; 40, Peter Symonds; 41, Geoff Thiel; 42, Jeremy Thomson; 43, Richard Waltham; 44, Stan Wardlaw; 45, Roger Waterworth; 46, Tony Williams; 47, Les Witty.

Ken Charles worked with Godfrey from 1975 and recalls, *his incredible innate intelligence and depth of knowledge in so many fields, and his willingness to spend time helping even the most junior members of his team.*

The body scans were exciting, but in a sense they were pushing on an open door. The early brain scans had already converted all of the doubters into believers.

The Nobel Prize citation described how this machine *was epoch-making in medical radiology [...] with an unusual combination of vision, intuition and imagination, and with an extraordinary eye for the optimal choice of*

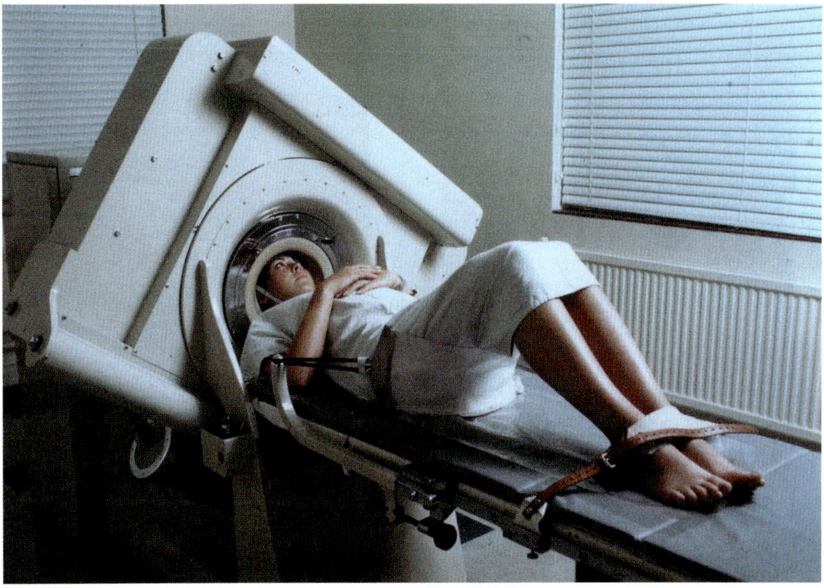

Mk1 EMI-scanner
(Copyright EMI Music)

physical factors in a system that must have offered very great problems to construct, he obtained results which in one blow surprised the medical world. It can be no exaggeration to maintain that no other method within X-ray diagnostics has during such a short period, led to such remarkable advances.

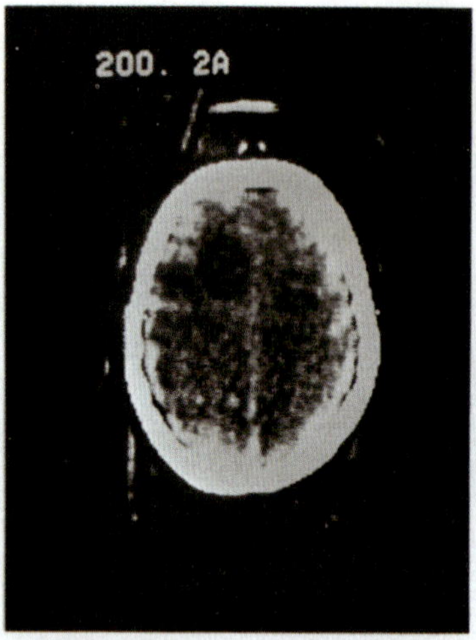

Astrocytoma III cystic left front lobe (160 x 160 matrix high-definition picture - note detection of grey and white matter patterns)

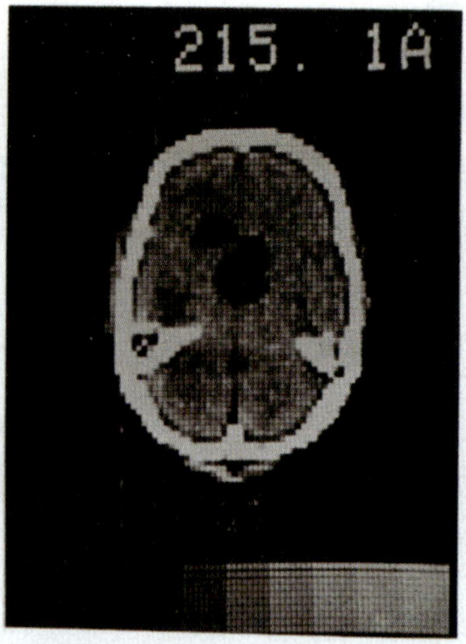

Cranio pharyngioma

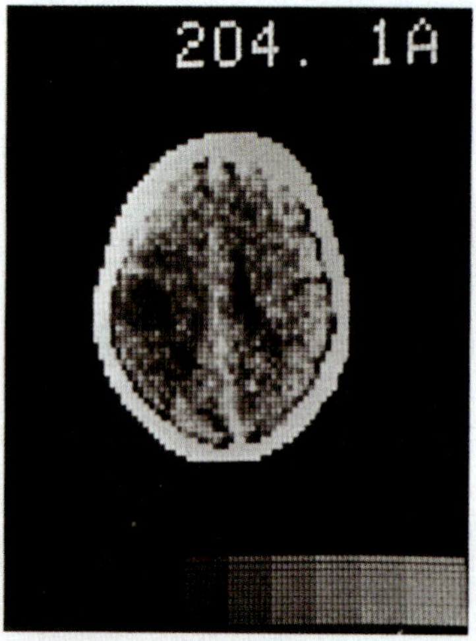

L. parietal astrocytoma grade III.

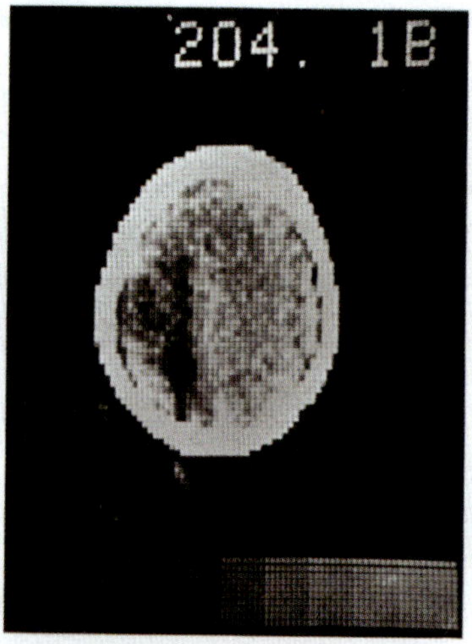

(As left) Taken 1 cm. higher on same patient.

Brain scans from Atkinson Morley Hospital

Chapter 8
America!

From a backpacker's hostel to the heart of the USA

In May 1972 Godfrey travelled to New York with Dr James Bull, who had seen the CT scanner in action at Atkinson Morley Hospital. Many eminent neuroradiologists were speaking at a postgraduate course at the Albert Einstein College of Medicine. This was a good opportunity for Godfrey and James Bull to speak, but the programme for the course had already been fixed. James Bull was already booked to speak on a different topic, otherwise James Ambrose would have presented this important talk.

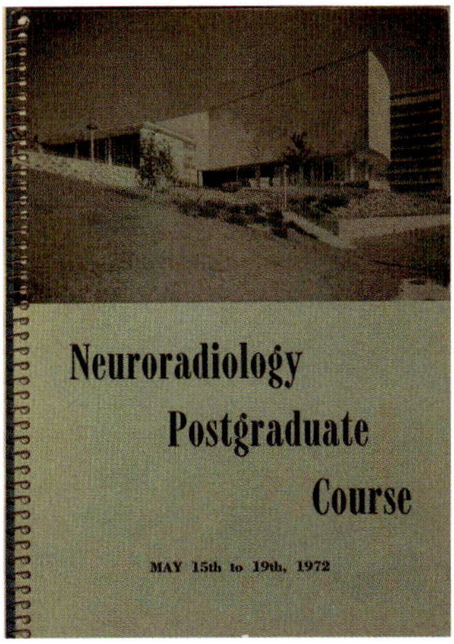

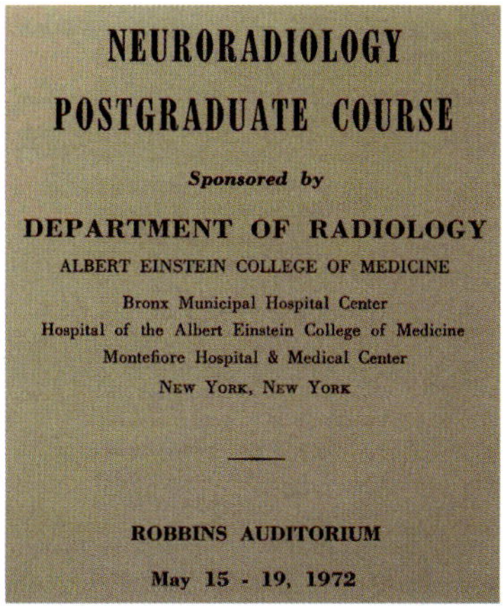

NEURORADIOLOGY

POSTGRADUATE COURSE

Sponsored by

DEPARTMENT OF RADIOLOGY

ALBERT EINSTEIN COLLEGE OF MEDICINE

Bronx Municipal Hospital Center
Hospital of the Albert Einstein College of Medicine
Montefiore Hospital & Medical Center
NEW YORK, NEW YORK

ROBBINS AUDITORIUM

May 15 - 19, 1972

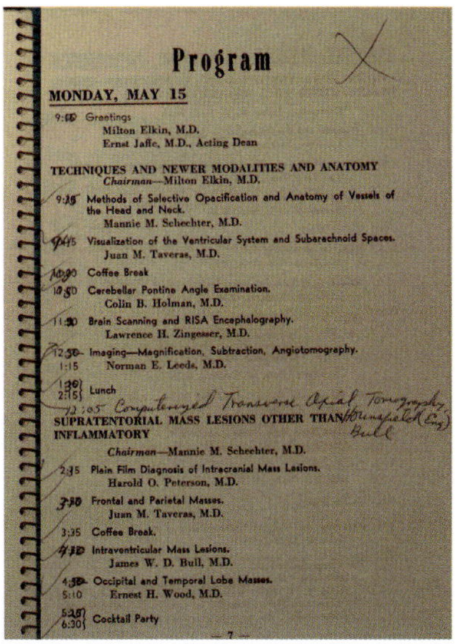

Program

MONDAY, MAY 15

9:00 Greetings
Milton Elkin, M.D.
Ernst Jaffe, M.D., Acting Dean

TECHNIQUES AND NEWER MODALITIES AND ANATOMY
Chairman—Milton Elkin, M.D.

9:15 Methods of Selective Opacification and Anatomy of Vessels of the Head and Neck.
Mannie M. Schechter, M.D.

9:45 Visualization of the Ventricular System and Subarachnoid Spaces.
Juan M. Taveras, M.D.

10:30 Coffee Break

10:50 Cerebellar Pontine Angle Examination.
Colin B. Holman, M.D.

11:30 Brain Scanning and RISA Encephalography.
Lawrence H. Zingesser, M.D.

12:30 Imaging—Magnification, Subtraction, Angiotomography.
1:15 Norman E. Leeds, M.D.

1:30
2:15 Lunch

12:05 Computerized Transverse Axial Tomography, Hounsfield (Eng) Bull

SUPRATENTORIAL MASS LESIONS OTHER THAN INFLAMMATORY
Chairman—Mannie M. Schechter, M.D.

2:15 Plain Film Diagnosis of Intracranial Mass Lesions.
Harold O. Peterson, M.D.

2:50 Frontal and Parietal Masses.
Juan M. Taveras, M.D.

3:35 Coffee Break.

4:00 Intraventricular Mass Lesions.
James W. D. Bull, M.D.

4:30 Occipital and Temporal Lobe Masses.
5:10 Ernest H. Wood, M.D.

5:25
6:30 Cocktail Party

— 7 —

New York announcement, 15 May 1972
(Courtesy of Albert Einstein College of Medicine and Dr Forrest Clore)
An enlarged version is shown on the next page.

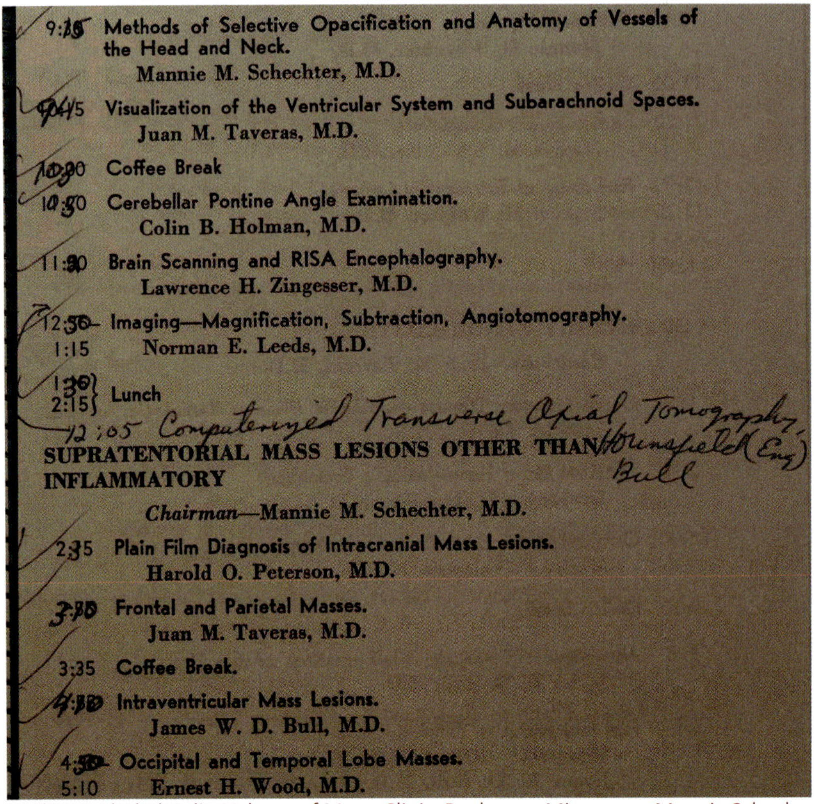
9:15 Methods of Selective Opacification and Anatomy of Vessels of the Head and Neck.
Mannie M. Schechter, M.D.

9:45 Visualization of the Ventricular System and Subarachnoid Spaces.
Juan M. Taveras, M.D.

10:20 Coffee Break

10:50 Cerebellar Pontine Angle Examination.
Colin B. Holman, M.D.

11:30 Brain Scanning and RISA Encephalography.
Lawrence H. Zingesser, M.D.

12:30–1:15 Imaging—Magnification, Subtraction, Angiotomography.
Norman E. Leeds, M.D.

1:30–2:15 Lunch

12:05 Computerized Transverse Axial Tomography, Hounsfield (Eng) Bull

SUPRATENTORIAL MASS LESIONS OTHER THAN INFLAMMATORY

Chairman—Mannie M. Schechter, M.D.

2:35 Plain Film Diagnosis of Intracranial Mass Lesions.
Harold O. Peterson, M.D.

3:20 Frontal and Parietal Masses.
Juan M. Taveras, M.D.

3:35 Coffee Break.

4:20 Intraventricular Mass Lesions.
James W. D. Bull, M.D.

4:50–5:10 Occipital and Temporal Lobe Masses.
Ernest H. Wood, M.D.

Speakers included Colin Holman of Mayo Clinic, Rochester, Minnesota; Mannie Schechter of Albert Einstein College, New York; Juan Taveras of Massachusetts General Hospital, Boston; and Ernest Wood of Columbia Neurological Institute, New York. James Bull was due to speak at 3:55 p.m. on conventional radiology.

Dr Forrest Clore attended this course as part of preparing for his radiology "board" exams. On a video made by his colleague Dr Scott Klioze he says, *This course was an annual thing and it was partly a social gathering for big-name neuro-radiologists to get together and give these lectures. It was well-attended, with more than 400 attendees. They announced about 11am that an unscheduled guest from London was going to talk during lunch-hour, so that anyone who wants to stay can listen to Godfrey Hounsfield on the topic of Computerised Transverse Axial Tomography. I stayed with a few others, probably ten or twelve, but practically every one of them were the lecturers, including Ernest Wood and Juan Taveras who were the authors of the bible of neuro-radiology at that time.*

Godfrey Hounsfield started speaking and it was interesting, until he showed some of the images that were being produced, and then it became not only interesting but ***exciting****. Up to that time we had to learn to diagnose strokes by learning all of the small arteries throughout the brain, and look for these little tiny arteries which were occluded, or diagnose a haemorrhage by seeing the same type of blood vessels* *splayed or displaced in angiograms. Tumours were also quite a challenge to diagnose. But Hounsfield was showing pictures where you could see blood as a different density to brain directly – you didn't even have to be very smart! You could just look at the image and say 'there is a haemorrhage', and you could see how big it was, and its location, and what it was pushing on. Strokes were also visible, and tumours were just astonishingly visible. It was amazing. He offered some literature so I went up to the front and I was bumping with these famous neuro-radiologists who were taking the literature and asking him questions because they could see that this was going to revolutionise neuro-radiology.*

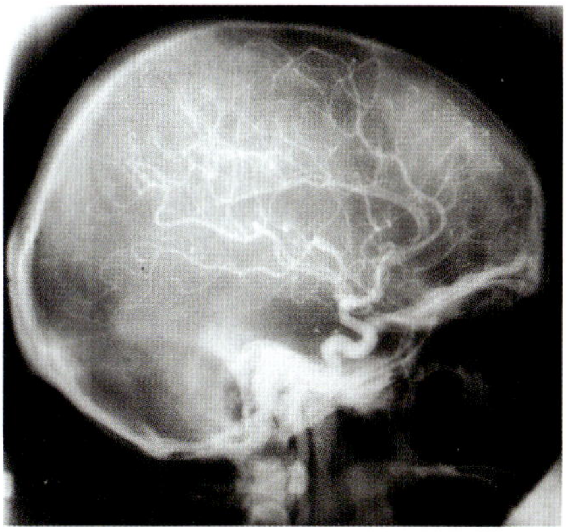

A conventional cerebral angiogram

Godfrey wrote a visit report on his return, and it starts as follows:

114 Copies to: Mr. W. Ingham. ✓
Mr. E. Gowler.
Mr. R. Froggatt.

VISIT TO NEW YORK AND BOSTON

I get the impression that many important English Doctors have moved to America and most have some connections with Dr. Bull and DHSS and the Atkinson Morley Hospital. This is greatly in our favour. Dr. Bull is known very well over there, many doctors being ex-pupils of his.

Dr. Wood of Columbia Institute suggested that there would be an evaluation period of at least a year, as in this country, and said that in the first year we would sell a minimum of three and a maximum of six in New York and about the same over the whole country. But in the five years he predicted 500 machines could be sold, i.e. every town with a population over half a million would have one (this may be an 'on the spot' exaggeration - considering the number of towns of this size, 100-200 machines is a more likely figure.)

The Chicago Exhibition is very important and he suggests we book space immediately, as it gets taken up very quickly. He says that a machine should be sent over for the exhibition, as people in America like to see what they are buying. He suggested that he bought it after the exhibition for evaluation and to help us with sales.

Visit to New York and Boston, G. N. Hounsfield, 24 May 1972
(Copyright EMI Music)

In a 1992 BBC2 television programme "Great British Inventions", Godfrey described what happened after he gave his talk: *I showed these pictures and they were very pleased with them. Afterwards a number of doctors persuaded me to go round hospitals showing the slides to the various hospitals. The result was that I hadn't brought enough money and I had to kip down at a $5 a night place where a lot of students lived and people with haversacks and so on. But it did the trick, because when I came back we had about 12 orders, which made us, really.*

His report shows that he visited seven hospitals in New York and that he visited Massachusetts General Hospital in Boston with Dr Juan Taveras, and it lists over twenty people who requested further literature. Eddie Gowler, who was copied on this report, was appointed three weeks earlier to coordinate the production and commercial exploitation of the scanner.

Godfrey was visiting New York at a time when the UK restricted the amount of money that could be taken abroad. These rules were introduced in 1939, at the start of World War 2, and (like food rationing) they persisted for a surprisingly long time afterwards. In a time of austerity the government did not want people to take a substantial portion of the national wealth overseas. Godfrey did not need exchange control permission if he took £50 or less. If he was staying only one or two nights, then it would not make sense to seek permission to take more money.

The 1991 film interview with Bill Ingham includes the following dialogue:

> Godfrey: *We had some pictures and they were very good. Everyone was very keen but we were uncertain how valuable they were. It was only when we went to the States and I gave a lecture at the Albert Einstein Hall, Dr Bull came along, an expert on detecting brain tumours and well known in the States, and he explained the pictures. It went down extremely well: when I left the lecture hall I had a queue of doctors asking me to come to their hospitals to lecture and show my slides. I agreed to visit them, but unfortunately I hadn't brought enough money so to economise I slept in a doss house for hikers in New York and I got back to England with only a few pounds left in my pocket. In retrospect I could have contacted various EMI people in New York, but I don't think that the set-up was well enough organised for that.*
>
> Bill: *You also wrote a paper in the UK with Ambrose.*
>
> Godfrey: *That's right but there was little time for writing. As soon as I arrived back we were inundated with orders. We had orders for at least a dozen machines on the table.*
>
> Bill: *People were turning up at the research laboratory, one chap came from Australia, literally just turned up and knocked on the door.*
>
> Godfrey: *That's right. Dr Juan Taveras was one of the people who came to EMI at Hayes and knocked on the door and said 'I want to place an order for a scanning machine' and was told in effect 'What machine? We don't make medical equipment here.'*

Godfrey did not **have** to stay in a doss house. Most people would have stayed for the pre-arranged time in the proper hotel, returned to the UK, and then recommended that a follow-up visit should be funded. We have already seen Godfrey improvise to get great results from a shoestring budget in designing and building the scanner, and here we see him doing exactly the same in getting the message across to potential customers.

The reception given to Juan Taveras in Hayes is regrettable, given that the company knew from an early stage that the USA would be a major territory for the CT scanner. For example, a memo in April 1970 predicted that the USA would be the best market, and one of the first five clinical prototype scanners was always intended to go there. However, EMI was a big company and news of CT had not yet spread far within it.

Rolf Schild visited the USA and Canada in September 1972, and his visit report shows that he followed up many of the people whom Godfrey had met in May, and confirms Godfrey's optimism about the prospective sales of the scanner. His report said that, *There is no doubt that the name EMI-scanner is becoming as familiar to the neurologists as the name Hoover is to the housewife, and with this, the name of EMI. Nearly all the Doctors visited have recently purchased EMI stock, as they expect EMI results to change. ... The EMI-scanner to E&I0 is as great a discovery as the Beatles were to the Record Division, with the same profit potential. ... Hospitals like the Mayo Clinic expect to examine up to 30 patients daily. This means that the Mayo Clinic will examine as many patients in one week as so far have been examined by the Atkinson Morley Hospital in Wimbledon during the whole year. ... The potential sales are high and the effort now available is hopelessly inadequate to the size of the project.*

It is interesting that doctors were buying shares in EMI, a foreign company which they had not previously heard of. This shows how strong the enthusiasm for CT was in North America, even before a single scanner had been installed in the continent. The initials E&IO stand for the Electronic and Industrial Operations within EMI. The mention of The Beatles and the music division of EMI is the only time that there is **any**

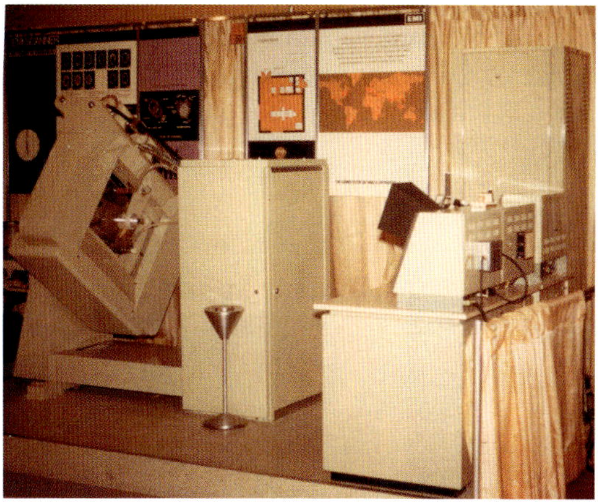

RSNA 1972 set-up
(Courtesy of Mac Gollifer)

reference to that topic in the archives: the businesses were run totally separately, and the development of CT was not funded by The Beatles or from the revenue from pop music. Rolf Schild is simply making an analogy to alert everyone to the size of the opportunity.

Godfrey's New York visit report in May 1972 mentioned an important exhibition in Chicago, organised each November by the Radiological Society of North America (RSNA). EMI booked a small stand – it was the largest that was still available.

In the previous photo, the scanner gantry on the left could move as if it was making a scan, but of course with the X-ray tube switched off. On the right are the (backs of) the viewer and the minicomputer.

Many people wanted to look at the pictures on the screen of the viewer. When the exhibition opened there was a crush of people trying to see the screen. The photo below was taken from where those people stood.

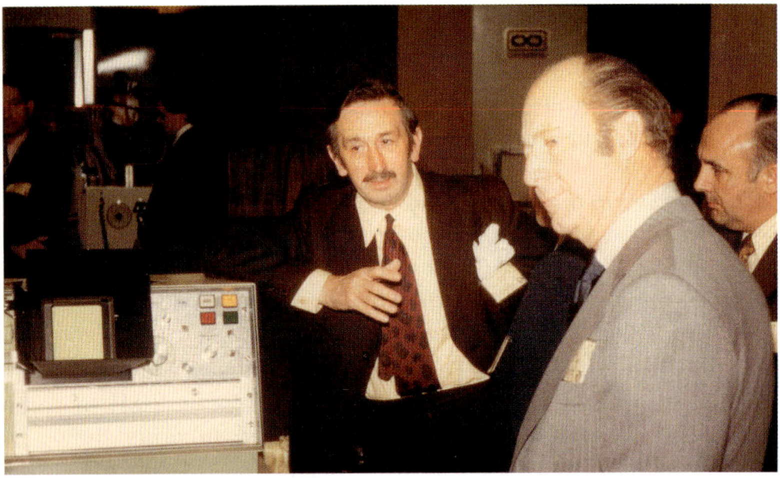

Godfrey at RSNA 1972
(Courtesy of Mac Gollifer)

The small screen on the left of the photo could show scans from Atkinson Morley Hospital. Godfrey is describing the scanner gantry, which is out of shot behind the left shoulder of the cameraman. Mac Gollifer set the computer to bring up a sequence of CT scans, and Anthony Strong, who had recently joined the team at CRL, ran the scanning gantry.

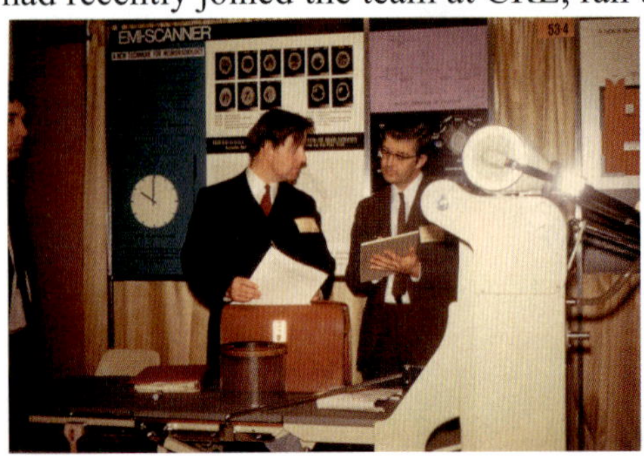

Anthony Strong operating the scanner
(Courtesy of Mac Gollifer)

EMI showed a film about the scanner in a room in the Hilton hotel every hour. The clock behind Anthony Strong in the photo shows that the next screening was at 10 a.m. Scans from Atkinson Morley Hospital were on the wall.

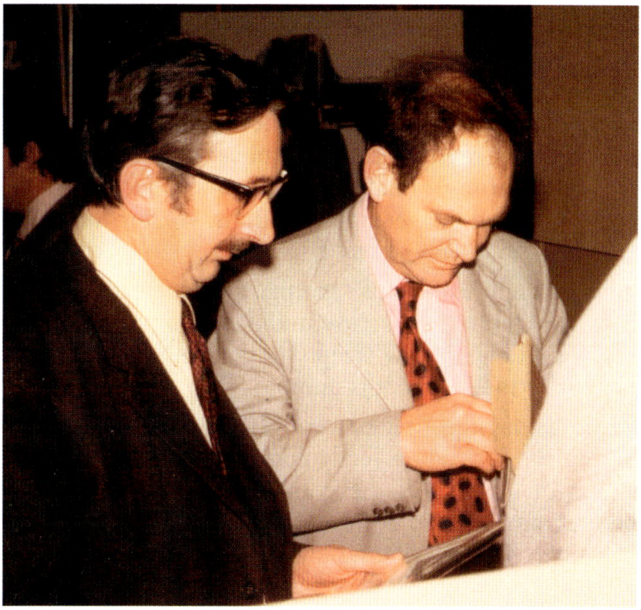

Godfrey and James Ambrose at RSNA
(Courtesy of Mac Gollifer)

The take-up of CT scanners was very fast in the USA, much faster than in the UK. There were many reasons for this, including:

- The population of the USA was then (and still is) more than four times that of the UK.
- In the UK the large majority of healthcare was funded by the state and delivered via the National Health Service and was "free at the point of use" on the basis of need, but the purchase of CT scanners was constrained by government budgets. In the USA, healthcare was funded predominantly by private insurance with state support restricted to groups such as the elderly or those with low incomes via Medicare and Medicaid.
- There was (and still is) a competitive market in medicine in the USA. If one hospital had a scanner then other hospitals in the vicinity might lose customers unless they also offered CT.
- The USA spent, on average, considerably more per person on healthcare than the UK.
- The USA was (in retrospect) at least thirty-five years ahead of the UK in the spread of medical malpractice litigation, and the USA had more lawyers per citizen than any other country. So doctors were inclined to give their better-funded patients the best possible diagnosis, rather

than risk being taken to court and asked to account for any failure in diagnosis.

- The USA was founded by pioneers, and Americans still generally admire pioneers and are receptive to new inventions.

The USA has a strong tradition of philanthropy, and this played a significant role in the early sales of scanners there. For example, in the USA, Mr Fritz Huntsinger single-handedly bought a brain scanner for his local hospital. In the UK there was less of a tradition of such huge individual donations, partly because people expected the NHS to decide what to buy. The charitable fundraising campaigns for CT scanners in the UK typically collected many small donations, so they took a substantial time to raise enough money to buy a scanner.

The mixture of high healthcare funding, medical malpractice lawyers, philanthropy, and the huge increase in diagnostic power from CT made the demand for scanners grow steeply in the USA. The waiting lists for CT scanners grew to nine months or more.

John Powell (managing director of EMI) had previously worked for Texas Instruments, a leading technology company. So he had a good understanding of how quickly events could move in the USA. From almost the first moment that he saw Godfrey's scanner, he was trying to get EMI to move faster in getting into production, and in expanding in the USA. He was a senior and very persuasive man, and he normally got what he wanted, although often not quite as fast as he hoped.

All of these forces aligned. Godfrey's talk in New York, the follow-up visit by Rolf Schild, the enthusiasm of doctors in the USA, the enthusiasm of John Powell, and the well-funded healthcare market all

The atmosphere now is one of excitement and enthusiasm! The sceptics are becoming fans and the disbelievers becoming convinced that we have something. I will not attempt to repeat all the expletives uttered around the viewing unit! Comments ranged from "If you could only show us the ventricular system, that would be a fantastic advance", to "no hospital should be without one". It is very early days yet, but I can assure you that the word will soon be spread around America. The "grape vine" appears to work quite fast here and through it I have heard many hospitals are asking about "that machine" in Rochester!

Dr. Baker is now on holiday and I have been sitting alongside Dr. Holman, one of the senior radiologists. What help I have been able to give in assisting him with diagnosis seems to have been appreciated and already he is "getting into the swing" of it. When Dave King arrives back home he will show you a set of photographs for a patient who had an operation some time ago. The diagnosis was a cystic area surrounded by a tumour, from the EMI-SCANNER. In the operating theatre this proved absolutely correct. Dr. Holman watched the operation and was very excited when he came back to the "EMI Room", as it has been named, and told me. Later I saw the surgeon and his comment was that the tumour extended a bit further back than we had said, but nonetheless excellent - it helped him a lot. On Monday I hope to have a report back on another patient with a meningioma and a large oedema area alongside.

Status report from the Mayo Clinic, 23 June 1973

pointed to the same result: Godfrey's invention was now unstoppable. The first EMI-scanner in the USA was installed at the Mayo Clinic in Rochester, Minnesota, the following summer by a team including Dave King and Peter Clarke. The first CT scan of a patient at the Mayo Clinic was on 19 June 1973. Peter Clarke's status report (which is shown on the previous page) starts by reporting comments from the medical staff who crowded around the viewing unit to look at the first scans.

The Mayo Clinic installation meant that a CT scanner was now running in one of the most prestigious hospitals in the world, located right at the centre of the North American continent. The process that Godfrey began in New York in May 1972 was now giving improved medical diagnosis to the citizens of the USA, and they loved it. His CT scanner had gone from a backpackers' hostel in New York to the heart of the American people.

Godfrey received many letters from grateful patients, but nearly all of these have been lost. A Readers Digest article about CT scanning, "Medicine's Miraculous New Eye", in June 1976 described how Pennsylvania housewife Jeanne Hancock had undergone successful surgery for removal of a massive brain tumour that had evaded diagnosis for 12 years. But for the EMI-scanner, her surgeon had explained, Mrs Hancock would soon have suffered irreversible and fatal paralysis. She wrote a letter to Godfrey saying: *My three young daughters and I thank you for preventing a most horrible future. May life treat you as well as your invention will allow many like myself to live.*

Tim O'Sullivan was part of EMI's sales team in the USA. He recalls a practical joke at one of the early RSNA meetings: *We were with Eddie Gowler at breakfast, and Eddie ordered pancakes, waffles and strawberries with cream, which I thought was a bit odd. I looked at Eddie and he just winked. The waitress asked Godfrey if he had made up his mind about his breakfast choice. Godfrey was clearly confused and seemingly did not want to make a decision but then blurted out 'I will have the same as him', pointing to Eddie, so the trap was set. When the food arrived Godfrey declared that he would not have ordered that type of breakfast and was appalled that they would have made that mistake. Of course Eddie spoke up and stated that he certainly had ordered that concoction, at which point the laughter began and Godfrey saw the funny side. He was a wonderful man and we were all privileged to work with him.*

Godfrey and EMI formed close relationships with the Mayo Clinic and with the Mallinckrodt Institute in St Louis, Missouri. The photos below are taken from a film shot at the Mallinckrodt Institute, where the medical team included Drs Stuart Sagel, Robert Stanley, and Ron Evens.

The following sequence of three photos shows an "air study" in which a patient had part of her spinal fluid removed and replaced by air. The air that was injected into the spinal cord bubbled up into the ventricles in the middle of the patient's brain. The patient was strapped into a chair and

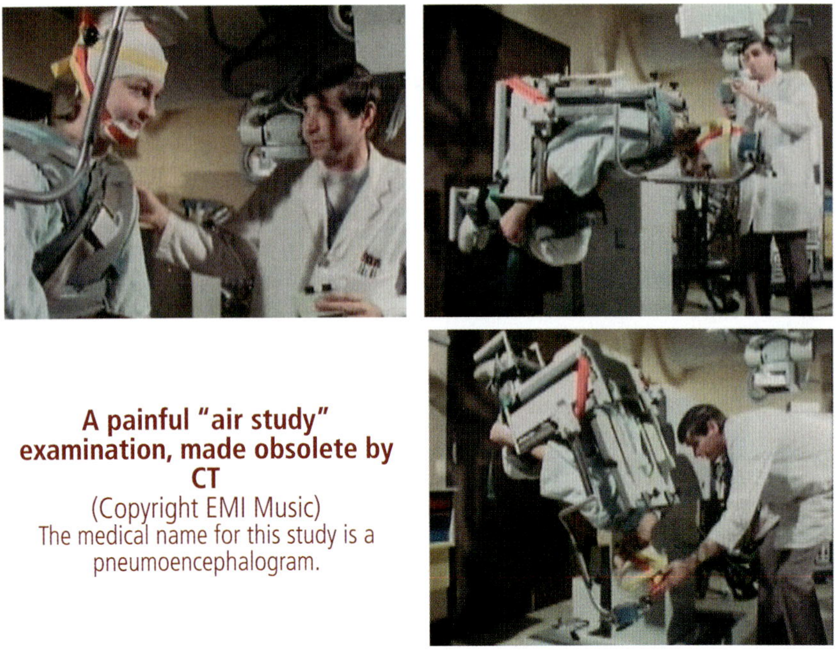

A painful "air study" examination, made obsolete by CT

(Copyright EMI Music)

The medical name for this study is a pneumoencephalogram.

was then turned upside down, so that the spinal fluid flowed back into the brain. It was a very painful procedure, the patient often vomited, and it took three months to recover from the examination, even if nothing was wrong with you. Ron Evens described this as *at the top of my list of studies which I wouldn't want done to myself.*

Two years later, in December 1975, Godfrey was at the Mayo Clinic with Dave King, Ken Charles, and Richard Waltham, investigating the performance of the newly installed Emerald body scanner. This had been installed by Ken, Peter Langstone, and Dave Bradley, and it was taking good scans of the chest and abdomen areas. Ken Charles says, *Everything was working fine except for the mode in which the scanner was slowed down from the usual 20 seconds to take a more detailed 80-second scan of the brain. This did not show quite such good performance as we hoped. We were staying in the Blondell Motel, very close to the hospital, working long days running experiments and studying the printouts. Late in the evening we'd get something to eat, and afterwards Godfrey went to bed while the rest of us would go to a nearby bar, to relax and discuss the news of the day. At breakfast Godfrey would arrive with calculations, drawings, and ideas for new experiments which he had produced overnight. Dave would arrive with new printouts, after getting up at 4am and going to the hospital to run more tests. After two weeks we had made progress in eliminating possible causes, but the next stage needed more radical tests, and Christmas was fast approaching. We dispersed, each going home to carry on working there. Dave went back to Chicago and returned to Mayo a few weeks later with two modified tanks, which contained the circuits to ensure that the high-voltage supply to the X-ray tube was a smooth waveform with a low level of 'ripple'. Somehow Dave had purloined these two tanks, which were in very short supply. He delved where most of us feared to tread, into their oil-filled interiors to modify the 140,000 volt circuitry, thus making a high voltage supply which was three times better than normal. This finally proved that the X-ray power supply was not to blame, giving a renewed spur to our search elsewhere. In the end, the culprit was a small metal bracket, which gave an unwanted earth connection, but the real lesson to me was the level of determination Dave and Godfrey showed, working at the problem in all waking hours.*

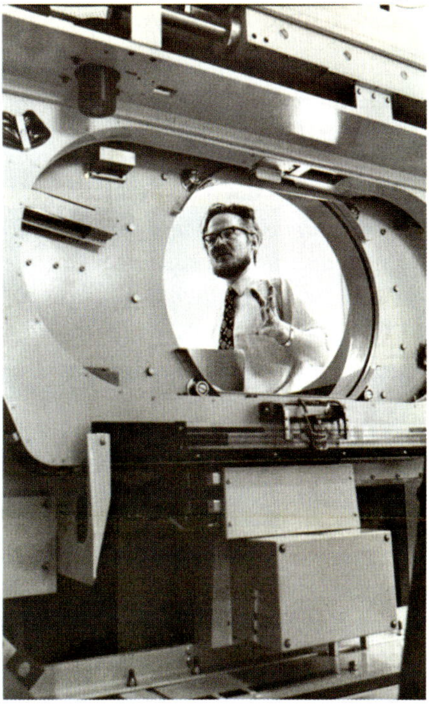

Peter Langstone installing the Emerald scanner in the Mayo Clinic, September 1975

(Copyright EMI Music)

Below Peter's hand is a glass "graticule", which acted as a ruler to measure exactly the position of the X-ray beam when each reading was taken. Below that is the box that contained the thirty detectors.

They continued working even when the rest of us were asleep. It was an inspiring example of leadership by example.

An e-mail from June 2011 says, *Tom Blondell here. We are still here and I remember the entire troupe! I was 23 at the time and am 61 plus now. Did Godfrey have an assistant who made sure he put on his socks? No disrespect intended but Godfrey travelled on a higher plane where the mundane was readily dismissed. I recall an occasion when I tagged along with Dave King while he made adjustments to the machine and he showed me an image of a brain slice captured on a black & white, instant camera, film packet. The pixels were around 3/16 of an inch with varied levels of gray.*

Stephen Bates remembers going on a tour: *Godfrey and I visited all three of the hospitals where Emerald scanners were running, two in the USA at the Mayo Clinic and at the Mallinckrodt Institute in St Louis, Missouri, and one in the UK at Northwick Park hospital in Harrow near London.*

He just never stopped, we were on the go all day every day. It was an exhausting but productive trip.

Godfrey avoided travel if he could, preferring to stay at home and focus on his work. Sometimes, as Anthony Strong recalls, he could not avoid it, and frequently something minor would go awry. *He went on a lecture tour in America. He left his Macintosh* (rain coat) *at the first hotel. It was sent on but arrived too late at the second hotel. The garment pursued him around America only catching up when he got home.*

Greg Hoeft met Godfrey in Chicago. *My earliest meeting with him was as a customer. I worked at Presbyterian-St. Luke's Hospital in Chicago and one of my roles was technical support. Just after the installation of the MK1 EMI-scanner, Godfrey came the US to visit all three of the CT scanner installations. When he visited in Chicago we met as a large group in the Scanner Control Room. The doctors involved with the CT scanner were peppering Godfrey with questions about what the CT scan images showed. Remember that the first systems had only an 80 by 80 picture matrix, an almost useless viewer and it was expected that the doctors would use numeric print-outs to make a diagnosis. This was the first CT scanner in the Chicago area. In response to the Doctor's questions, Godfrey would over and over carefully explain 'I'm not a medical man but...' and went on to teach the radiologists how to interpret the CT scan data.*

In due course I was enticed to become an early US employee of EMI, and was told that Haitch was coming for a visit and that I should stay close to him because I would learn a great deal. A few days later Godfrey arrived and we had a dinner as a group. I asked Godfrey who Mr Haitch was. You can probably guess the odd looks I got and the roar of laughter when all realized that, unknown to me, the original UK team referred to Godfrey as simply 'H'.

In April 1975 I attended a conference in Puerto Rico. I was there to support a small UK contingent and make sure that only customers gained direct access to Godfrey. We had some aggressive up and coming competitors in those days. Christopher LeMay and Godfrey both gave talks. The early full body scans were shown at this meeting.

During an afternoon break I was walking along the veranda of the hotel overlooking a beach. A typical hot and sunny day in Puerto Rico. Across the sand comes Godfrey and Chris with their suit jackets over one arm, shoes in the other, their ties snug to their necks and pants legs rolled up to their knees. They had been cooling their toes in the ocean and were heading back to the meeting room. An incredibly out-of-character image.

John Ryan says, *It was well-known that Godfrey preferred to remain on UK time when he was in the US which meant that he had to retire to bed early. He would then rise in the early hours and go jogging, usually in his suit. If possible he would then have breakfast in a transport cafe. On one occasion we were going up in the hotel lift with Godfrey at 6 pm and he looked at his watch and said, 'Oh it's late, I had better go to bed'. The Americans who happened to be in the lift looked puzzled and immediately checked their watches. On another occasion, after a late meal out, a group of us were returning to the hotel after midnight and as we entered the hotel through the main entrance we met Godfrey leaving to go for his early morning jog.*

For many years Godfrey lived in shared rented accommodation so he still regarded his brother's farm near Newark as his home, in fact this address appears on many of his patents. The US visa-waiver form contained a question on whether the applicant had been on a farm in the last 30 days to which Godfrey always answered 'no' and then filled in the farm as his home address. Inevitably this led to further questioning by US immigration. I had already been told this by others, but was able to verify this on one occasion when I was the next in the queue. Godfrey then had to turn on his not inconsiderable charm.

Godfrey owned a rather unique war-time razor. It was shaped like a modern electric razor, but was completely mechanical. In order to operate it, the body of the razor had to be rocked back and forth with respect to the head, thus causing the cutter to oscillate behind the foil. In so doing it made a loud 'click-clack' sound. When Bob Froggatt was accompanying Godfrey on one of his trips around the US he discovered Godfrey shaving with this razor in an airport men's-room with a group of fascinated Americans standing round watching him. On another occasion in Northbrook I was driving the car with Steve in the passenger seat and Godfrey in the back. I began to notice Godfrey in the rear-view mirror

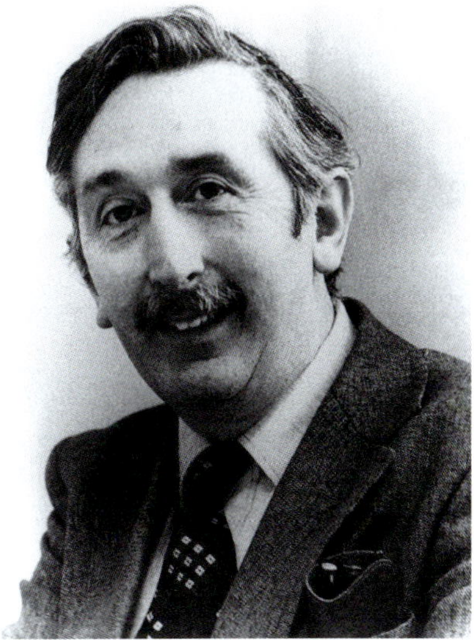

Godfrey Hounsfield
"For discoveries which have revolutionized diagnostic imaging."

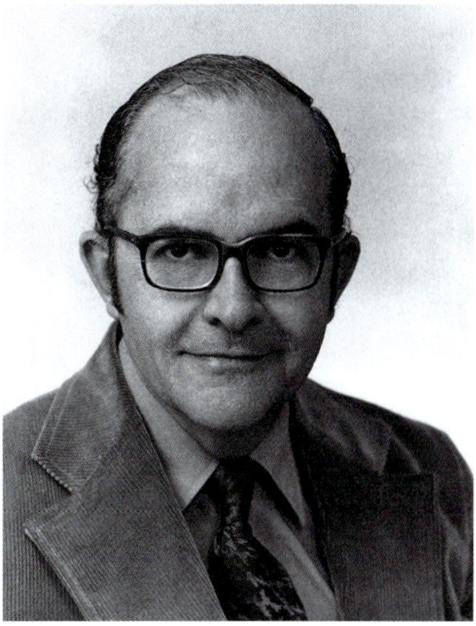

William Oldendorf
"For discoveries which have envisaged a revolution in diagnostic radiology."

(Photos and citations courtesy of the Lasker Foundation)

staring at his face and then a rasping sound as he felt his bristles. Steve said, 'you have forgotten to shave, haven't you', and Godfrey said 'yes, I think you are right'. Then I heard the click-clack sound from the back.

The 1975 Lasker Clinical Medical Research Award was shared by Godfrey Hounsfield and William Oldendorf. The Lasker Awards are among the most respected science prizes in the world.

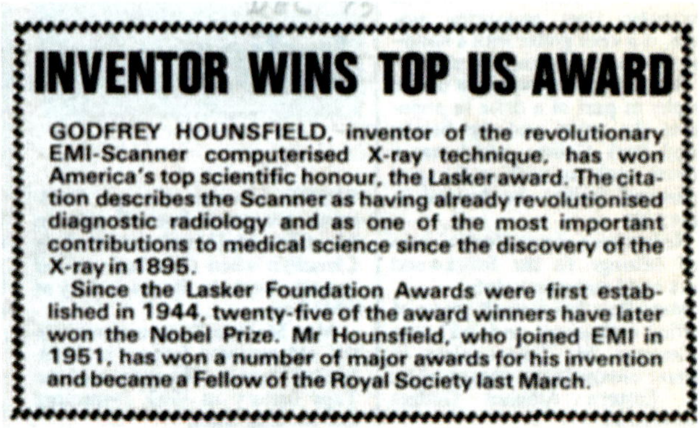

INVENTOR WINS TOP US AWARD

GODFREY HOUNSFIELD, inventor of the revolutionary EMI-Scanner computerised X-ray technique, has won America's top scientific honour, the Lasker award. The citation describes the Scanner as having already revolutionised diagnostic radiology and as one of the most important contributions to medical science since the discovery of the X-ray in 1895.

Since the Lasker Foundation Awards were first established in 1944, twenty-five of the award winners have later won the Nobel Prize. Mr Hounsfield, who joined EMI in 1951, has won a number of major awards for his invention and became a Fellow of the Royal Society last March.

The Lasker Award, as reported in EMI News
(Copyright EMI Music)

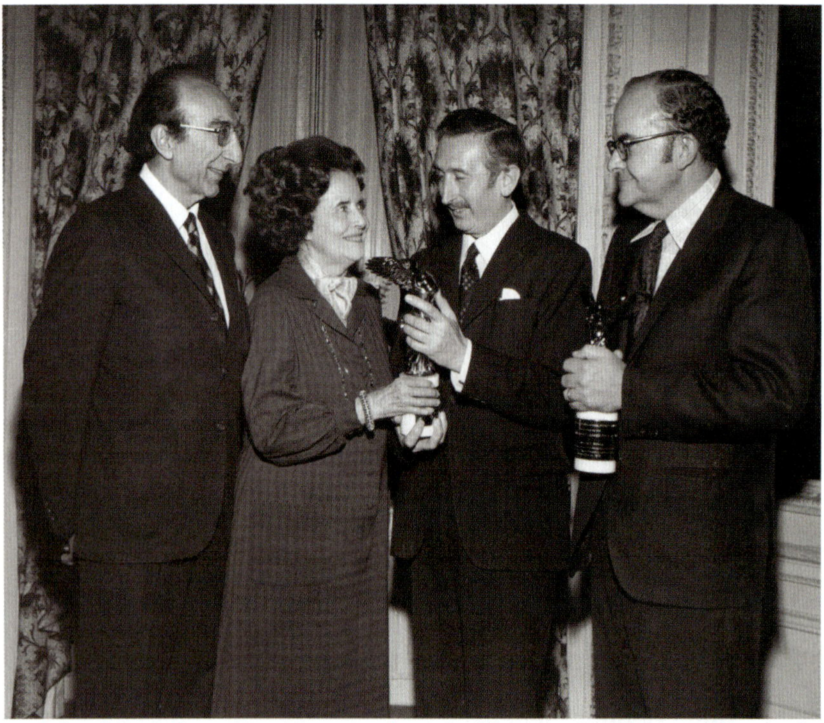

Michael DeBakey, Mrs Mary Lasker, Godfrey, and William Oldendorf
(Courtesy of the Lasker Foundation)
Michael DeBakey was the chairman of the award jury, and the winner of the 1963 award.

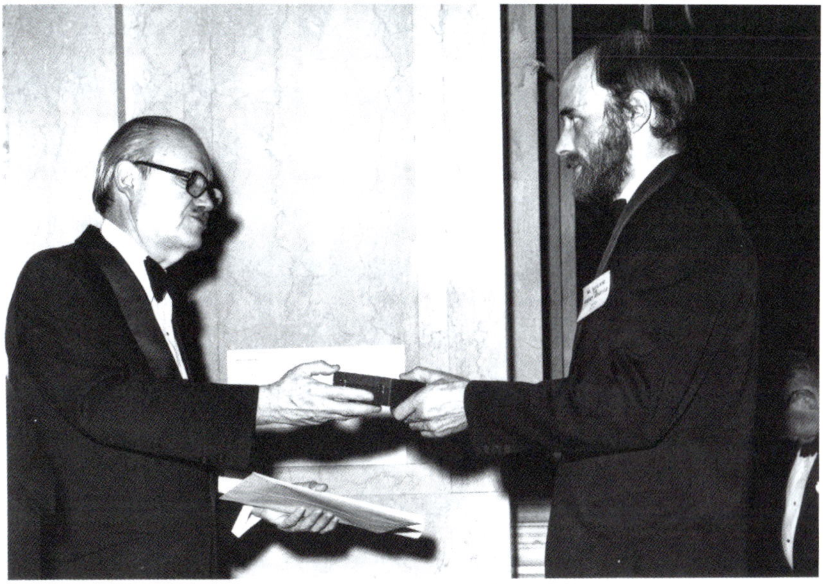

Dr Bowen C. Dees presents a medal to Dave King (right)
(Photo ownership is unclear, possibly Dr David G Kilpatrick)

This photo shows the president of the Franklin Institute in Philadelphia, Pennsylvania, presenting the Howard N. Potts medal to Dave King, who accepted it on behalf of Godfrey on 2 November 1977. It is just one of Godfrey's many awards, which are listed in Appendix 3. It is one of the few photos of Dave King in these years. He was an extraordinary man in his own right, and in addition to his great work on coronary imaging he was a concert pianist and all-England badminton champion, as well as a good friend of Godfrey. There were few people whom Godfrey would rather see accepting a medal on his behalf.

Dave King wrote in his report of this event that each award was thoroughly researched after being nominated by a sponsor from among the seventy leading scientists on the award committee: *Hounsfield's award was sponsored by Dr David G Kilpatrick, a biomedical consultant, and both he and his wife were the perfect hosts. Great interest was shown by other medallists and attendees in the CT exhibit and award.*

Godfrey and Dave had both played important roles in pioneering CT scanning in the USA, and it was now spreading across the world.

Chapter 9
The Nobel Prize
The greatest honour in science

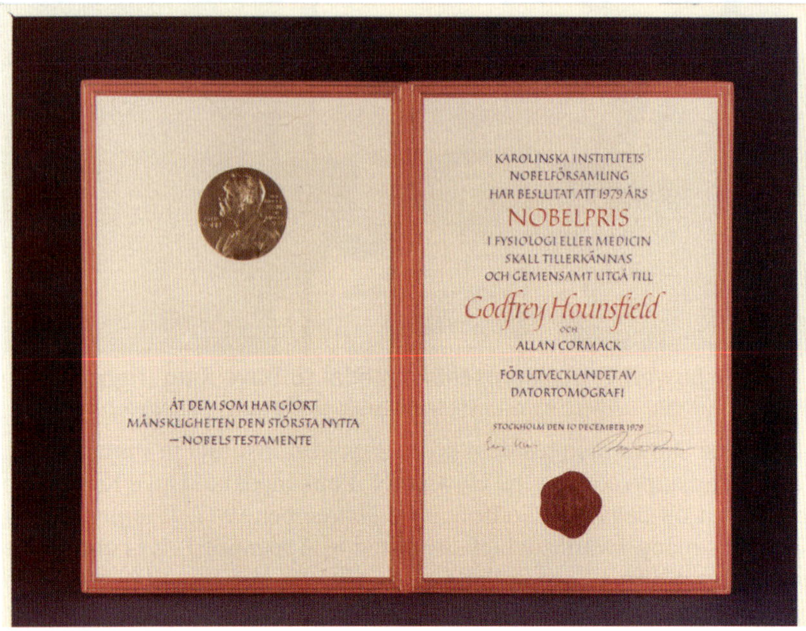
ÅT DEM SOM HAR GJORT
MÄNSKLIGHETEN DEN STÖRSTA NYTTA
– NOBELS TESTAMENTE
KAROLINSKA INSTITUTETS
NOBELFÖRSAMLING
HAR BESLUTAT ATT 1979 ÅRS
NOBELPRIS
I FYSIOLOGI ELLER MEDICIN
SKALL TILLERKÄNNAS
OCH GEMENSAMT UTGÅ TILL
Godfrey Hounsfield
OCH
ALLAN CORMACK
FÖR UTVECKLANDET AV
DATORTOMOGRAFI
STOCKHOLM DEN 10 DECEMBER 1979

Photo copyright EMI Music, medal design ® the Nobel Foundation.

On 12 November 1979 the Daily Telegraph reported that after news of his Nobel Prize reached Godfrey on 11 November, he said, *I was absolutely amazed and am still recoiling. I never expected I would be chosen for such a high honour as the Nobel Prize.*

Godfrey's reaction to the news was so typical of the man: on the one hand highly honoured to be chosen, but on the other embarrassed to receive all the attendant attention. He was genuinely pleased to have won such an endorsement of his invention but did not allow it to affect his life in any significant way. He continued to work in his normal way, and the only concession he made was to buy some modest scientific equipment in order to equip a small laboratory for his own experiments in his recently purchased semi-detached house.

The prize was awarded jointly to him and Allan Cormack for the *development of computed axial tomography a new method X-ray diagnosis particularly within brain surgery.*

Allan Cormack and Godfrey had never worked on CT together but had pursued their own research independently – Allan Cormack's work was highly theoretical and had postulated something similar, but he had not pursued his ideas as far as Godfrey did. Godfrey's engineering judgement and his remarkably fast, accurate, and dose-efficient method of picture reconstruction had started a revolution in patient care. His highly practical solution became the foundation of many forms of modern medical imaging. Godfrey was not influenced or helped in any way by Cormack's earlier work, and the two approaches were completely dissimilar. None the less, the committee responsible for awarding the prize chose to award it jointly to the two recipients. There is a long history of the Prize for Physiology or Medicine being awarded to joint recipients. In fact the majority of prizes are awarded jointly, often to people who have worked independently.

The news of the award was welcomed enthusiastically by those who worked with Godfrey at EMI and was seen rightly as the culmination of the many awards that had been given to him over the years.

Typical of the reaction is this quote from Stephen Bates (followed by several other quotes from the same source): *CRL was, despite the inclusion of Cormack, delighted for Godfrey. He had received many awards for CT, but the award of the Nobel Prize for Medicine to an engineer showed how significant the scanner had become to the world of medicine.*

Godfrey was visibly pleased to have received the Nobel Prize but never used it as a factor for establishing himself as any different to others. He still had his somewhat diffident approach in explaining his various thoughts and ideas to colleagues and never used the Nobel Prize as an ally in winning his arguments.

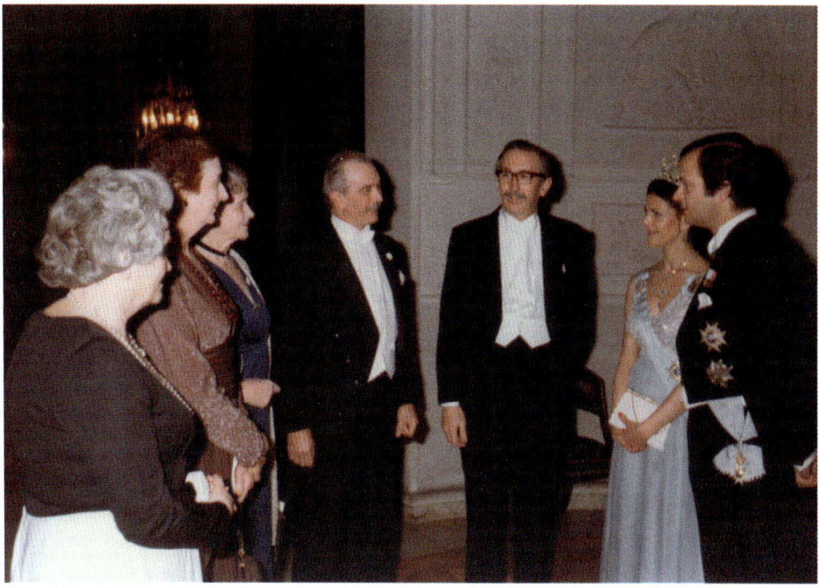

Godfrey's family (Mary, Joan, Molly, and Michael) meet the King and Queen

The awarding of the Nobel Prize occurred in the beginning of December in Stockholm. It was a significant event. The "celebrations" lasted a full week and included various functions, culminating in a Royal Banquet hosted by the King of Sweden.

Godfrey had invited as his guests his sisters Molly and Joan, his brother Michael with his wife Mary (all pictured on the previous page with Godfrey meeting the King and Queen of Sweden), his brother Paul (who was sadly unable to attend), and Stephen Bates.

I was honoured to be the only person, outside of Godfrey's immediate family, to be invited as his guest at the Nobel ceremonies. It was an experience not to be forgotten, VIP treatment as Nobel guests, cars placed at our disposal, a Royal banquet, and a diplomat from the Swedish ministry to look after us.

The man from the Swedish ministry was nicknamed 'Mr No Problem' by Godfrey's family. Everything that they asked of him received the same reply – 'No problem', and he was there waiting for us every morning. Such was Godfrey's dislike for the limelight and attention that one morning at breakfast he said that maybe we could do something without the man from the ministry. I said that I had always wanted to see the Vasa (the 300 year old wooden warship that had been raised and was being preserved in Stockholm), so we evaded the ministry man, walked across Stockholm, and spent the morning visiting the warship. We returned to find the ministry man in some panic having lost his key charge.

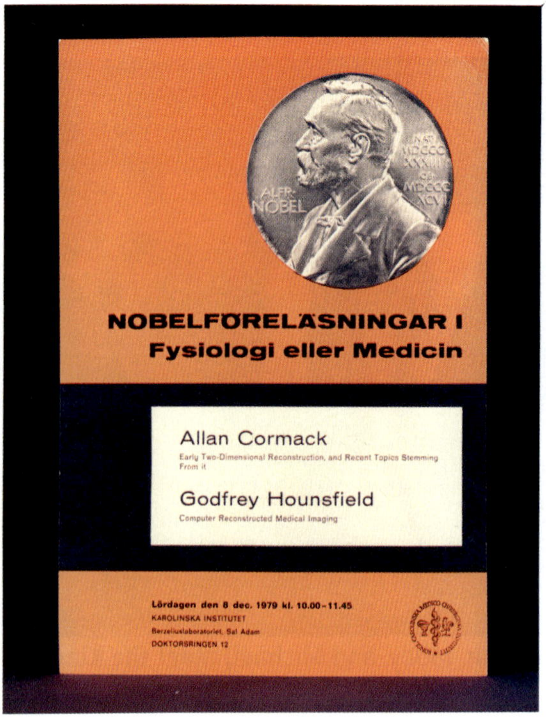
ALFR. NOBEL
NOBELFÖRELÄSNINGAR I
Fysiologi eller Medicin
Allan Cormack
Early Two-Dimensional Reconstruction, and Recent Topics Stemming From it
Godfrey Hounsfield
Computer Reconstructed Medical Imaging
Lördagen den 8 dec. 1979 kl. 10.00–11.45
KAROLINSKA INSTITUTET
Berzeliuslaboratoriet, Sal Adam
DOKTORSRINGEN 12

The Nobel Prize for Physiology or Medicine
(Photo copyright EMI Music, medal design ® the Nobel Foundation)

On 8 December, Godfrey (and Allan Cormack) gave presentations at the Karolinska Institute in Stockholm.

Godfrey's Nobel Lecture was initially wooden and uninspiring. He had no love of speaking in public but had prepared his lecture with great care and copious notes. He started out reading from these notes and his delivery was terrible. In the audience I was feeling increasingly uncomfortable as he proceeded, but then Godfrey dropped his notes. Retrieving his notes from the floor it was obvious that they had become out of sequence and that he had lost his place. He placed his notes on the lectern and proceeded to talk naturally, aided only by his sequence of slides, about the subject that he so obviously knew and loved. From that moment on his lecture was excellent.

10 December saw the award of most of the Nobel Prizes (the award to Mother Teresa of the Peace Prize took place in Norway). It was a very grand occasion with a large audience including all the Nobel laureates' guests. The King of Sweden presented the Prizes to each winner individually, as shown in this photo.

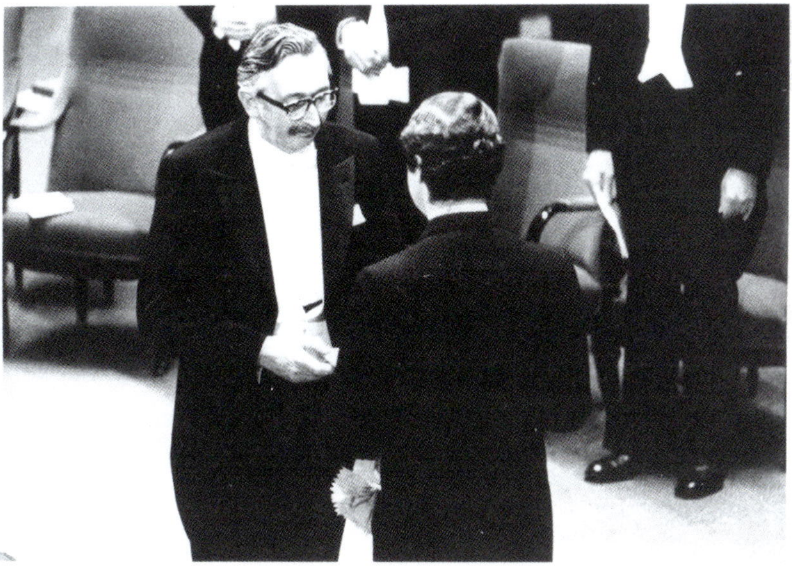

Presentation of the Nobel Prize
(Copyright is uncertain, although we have searched diligently)

There was a Royal Banquet later that same day attended by some 1,200 people. It was again a spectacular event and did even more to reinforce the dignity of the week of celebrations. Godfrey could not fail to be impressed by the whole proceedings.

Perhaps the most impressive part of the banquet was when the lights were dimmed and a long line of serving staff appeared carrying trays with the Parfait Glace Nobel which included a spun sugar swan lit by a candle. All tables were served simultaneously! An impressive sight!

SOLEMN FESTIVAL
OF THE NOBEL FOUNDATION

Monday December 10th, 1979, at 4.30 p. m.
in the Grand Auditorium of the Concert Hall

PROGRAMME

"Trumpet Voluntary" . . . . *Jeremiah Clarke*

The Laureates take their seats on the platform

Speech by *Professor Sune Bergström,* Chairman of the Board of the Nobel Foundation

Ouverture to "Candide" . . . . *Leonard Bernstein*

Presentation of the Nobel Prize for Physics 1979 to Sheldon L. Glashow, Abdus Salam and Steven Weinberg, after a speech by *Professor Bengt Nagel*

Presentation of the Nobel Prize for Chemistry 1979 to Herbert C. Brown and Georg Wittig, after a speech by *Professor Bengt Lindberg*

Allegretto scherzando from Symphony No. 8 . . *L. van Beethoven*

Presentation of the Nobel Prize for Physiology or Medicine 1979 to Allan M. Cormack and Godfrey N. Hounsfield, after a speech by *Professor Torgny Greitz*

Pomp and Circumstance No. 4 . . . . *Edward Elgar*

Presentation of the Nobel Prize for Literature 1979 to Odysseus Elytis, after a speech by *D. Ph. Karl Ragnar Gierow,* Member of the Swedish Academy

Greek dance No. 5 "Kleftikos" . . . . . *Nikos Skalkottas*

Presentation of the Bank of Sweden Prize in Economic Sciences in Memory of Alfred Nobel 1979 to Sir Arthur Lewis and Theodore W. Schultz, after a speech by *Professor Erik Lundberg*

The Swedish National Anthem: "Du gamla, du fria"

While the guests are leaving the auditorium, "Festival Music" by *Hugo Alfvén* is played.

Music performed by
the Stockholm Philharmonic Orchestra
Conductor: *Sixten Ehrling*

The decoration flowers are graciously offered by
the Azienda di Soggiorno e Turismo di Sanremo

The above programme of the ceremony gives some insight into the day.

The Nobel Week was a fitting tribute to all that Godfrey had done to further medical imaging, and he was rightly pleased with the whole episode while still feeling slightly embarrassed, to the extent that maybe he might have wished that it had not happened. None the less, he clearly saw it as a momentous occasion, as evidenced by his desire to have his family attend the proceedings. But despite that, he still continued to be the shy and diffident inventor he had always been.

The December 1979 IVC Bulletin gave the facts about Godfrey's Nobel award, and the Editor added the following personal note: *The Editor has been inundated with requests (letters, press cuttings, telephone*

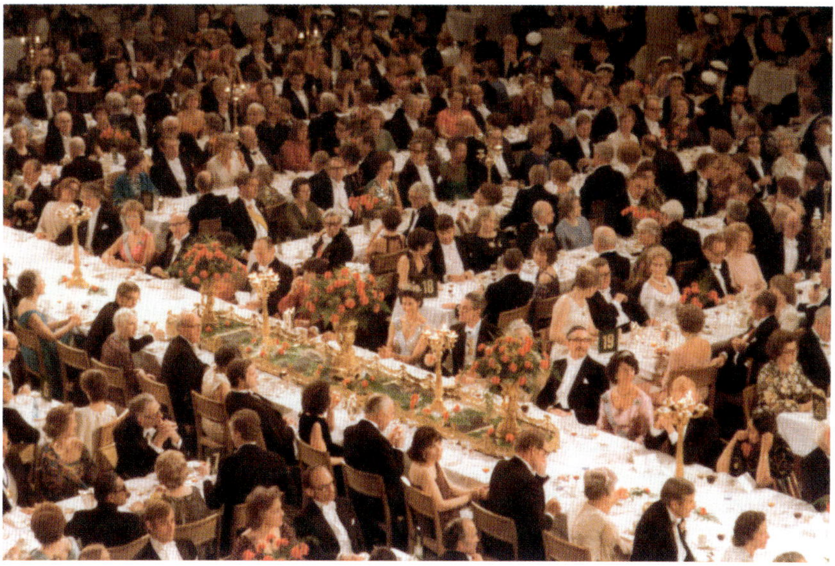

Part of the Banquet Hall

(Copyright is uncertain, although we have searched diligently)

Godfrey is sitting at the centre table alongside Princesses Lily and Desiree, and opposite the King of Sweden.

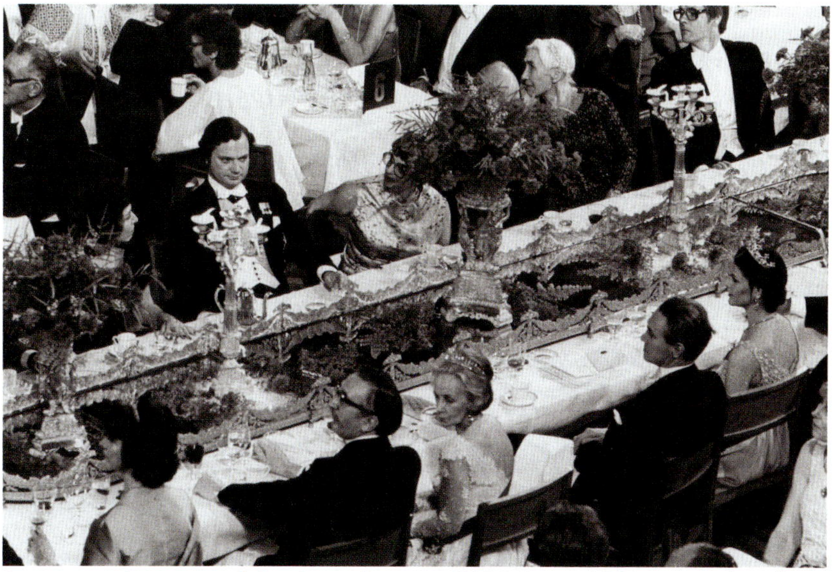

A stamp on the reverse of the above photo says "A&A Kamerabild Ronny Karlsson". We apologise for not obtaining his permission: we tried to find him without success.

calls, and personal visitations) to 'put something in the Bulletin about Godfrey'. This is a reflection of the respect and affection with which he is regarded and the pride which his friends and fellow members take in his achievement.

Godfrey received many letters as a result of the Nobel Prize, and about three hundred of these survive. Some asked Godfrey to help regarding medical problems, including a heartbreaking letter from someone whose seventeen-year-old son had been diagnosed with a fatal brain disease. Godfrey personally drafted very sympathetic replies to all such letters, although as an engineer rather than a medical expert there was not much he could say beyond offering his sympathy.

There was a letter from an eleven-year-old boy in North America who collected autographs of famous people and who could not imagine anyone more famous than the winner of a Nobel Prize. Many similar letters requested photographs or autographs, all of which received a reply. Letters of congratulation came from medical institutions, universities, and ambassadors or embassies. Godfrey must have been glad that he had Audrey Lester to help him with all of these letters.

A letter from Isaac Shoenberg's son, Professor David Shoenberg, offered warmest congratulations. David wrote, *My father was always very proud of the achievements of the research lab at EMI, and he would have been particularly proud of this conspicuous recognition of your outstanding work. He was in his later years somewhat sceptical of the benefits that television had brought to the world, but I am sure that he would have approved of the contribution your own work is making to human welfare.* David's sister, Elizabeth Shoenberg, wrote a separate letter: *As a doctor, I have been thrilled with the benefits of your work, and have seen it used to save life, and to avoid painful and dangerous radiological and surgical investigations. I am very happy that for once great merit has been appropriately acknowledged.*

A letter arrived from Joseph Gerald Stanford (known as Bill) who was joint managing director of EMI until 1972. He had seen Godfrey's lathe-bed prototype and was on EMI's committee that authorised Dr Broadway to continue the work. He wrote, *although I am of course completely non-technical, I have seldom been more impressed with the correctness of voting more funds for development work than I was on that occasion. A feeling that was strengthened that night when I related what you had shown, and told me, to my wife (who happens to be a doctor).*

I have followed the career of your wonderful invention as best I can from the non-technical Press over the years since I retired. I have noted that its real fulfilment has seemed at times to be clouded by the interferences of the basic 'commercial' influences here and overseas, but have never doubted that your brain and your efforts have made an incalculable contribution to medical success throughout the world.

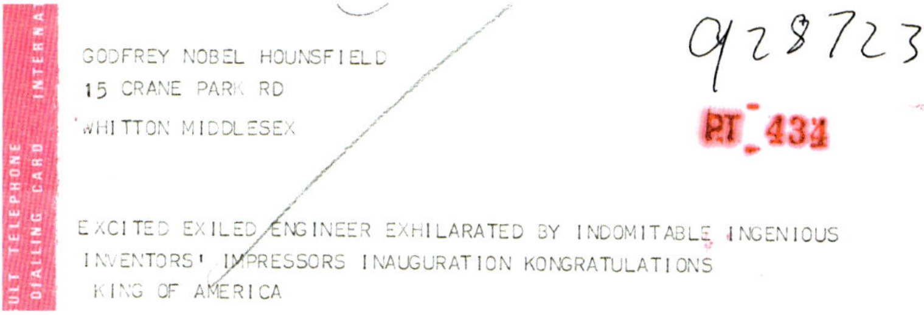
UIT TELEPHONE DIALLING CARD INTERNA

GODFREY NOBEL HOUNSFIELD
15 CRANE PARK RD
WHITTON MIDDLESEX

EXCITED EXILED ENGINEER EXHILARATED BY INDOMITABLE INGENIOUS INVENTORS' IMPRESSORS INAUGURATION KONGRATULATIONS
KING OF AMERICA

928723

PT 434

Dave King sent a telegram: *Excited exiled engineer exhilarated by indomitable ingenious inventor's impressors inauguration kongratulations. King of America.*

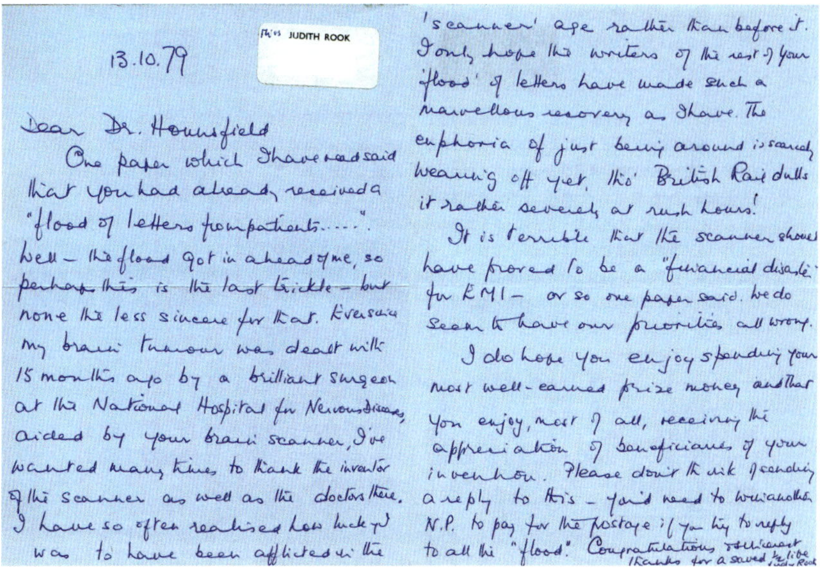
Miss JUDITH ROOK

13.10.79

Dear Dr. Hounsfield

One paper which I have read said that you had already received a "flood of letters from patients....". Well – the flood got in ahead of me, so perhaps this is the last trickle – but none the less sincere for that. Ever since my brain tumour was dealt with 15 months ago by a brilliant surgeon at the National Hospital for Nervous Diseases, aided by your brain scanner, I've wanted many times to thank the inventor of the scanner as well as the doctors there. I have so often realised how lucky I was to have been afflicted in the 'scanner' age rather than before it. I only hope the writers of the rest of your 'flood' of letters have made such a marvellous recovery as I have. The euphoria of just being around is scarcely wearing off yet, tho' British Rail dulls it rather severely at rush hours!

It is terrible that the scanner should have proved to be a "financial disaster" for EMI – or so one paper said. We do seem to have our priorities all wrong.

I do hope you enjoy spending your most well-earned prize money and that you enjoy, most of all, receiving the appreciation of beneficiaries of your invention. Please don't think of sending a reply to this – you'd need to win another N.P. to pay for the postage if you try to reply to all the "flood". Congratulations & sufficient thanks for a saved life
Judith Rook

Letter from Judith Rook
(Copyright Judith Rook)

A grateful patient, Judith Rook, wrote that her newspaper reported a flood of letters from patients. *Well – the flood got in ahead of me, so perhaps this is the last trickle – but none the less sincere for that. Ever since my brain tumour was dealt with 15 months ago by a brilliant surgeon [...] aided by your brain scanner I've wanted many times to thank the inventor.*

Albert Hutchinson had made parts for Godfrey's lathe-bed prototype in 1968, and he had been promoted to be in charge of the workshop of CRL when the scanner work reached a peak from 1972 onwards. Albert's letter recalls Godfrey giving him a rough sketch, asking him to copy the shape but saying that the dimensions did not matter. When he heard about the Nobel Prize, Albert had retired, and he wrote to Godfrey from his new home a hundred miles away. The notes at the bottom right in the picture below are by Godfrey's assistant Audrey Lester. The diagonal line across the letter was her way of marking that they had sent a reply.

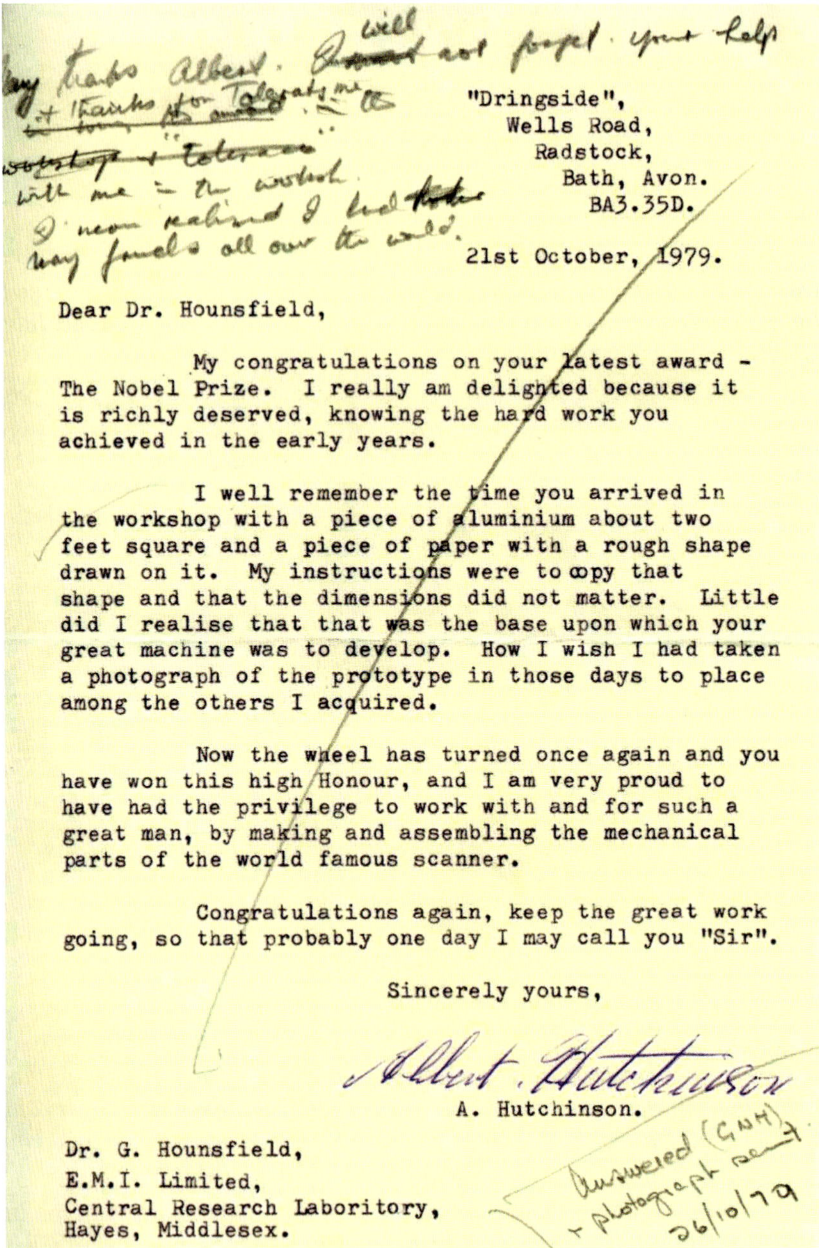

"Dringside",
Wells Road,
Radstock,
Bath, Avon.
BA3.35D.

21st October, 1979.

Dear Dr. Hounsfield,

My congratulations on your latest award - The Nobel Prize. I really am delighted because it is richly deserved, knowing the hard work you achieved in the early years.

I well remember the time you arrived in the workshop with a piece of aluminium about two feet square and a piece of paper with a rough shape drawn on it. My instructions were to copy that shape and that the dimensions did not matter. Little did I realise that that was the base upon which your great machine was to develop. How I wish I had taken a photograph of the prototype in those days to place among the others I acquired.

Now the wheel has turned once again and you have won this high Honour, and I am very proud to have had the privilege to work with and for such a great man, by making and assembling the mechanical parts of the world famous scanner.

Congratulations again, keep the great work going, so that probably one day I may call you "Sir".

Sincerely yours,

Albert Hutchinson

A. Hutchinson.

Dr. G. Hounsfield,
E.M.I. Limited,
Central Research Laboritory,
Hayes, Middlesex.

Answered (GNH) + photograph sent. 26/10/79

Letter from Albert Hutchinson
(Copyright Albert Hutchinson)

Albert's letter correctly forecasts another honour: *Congratulations again, keep the great work going, so that probably one day I may call you 'Sir'.* Godfrey's handwritten notes at the top of the letter show that he replied, *Many thanks Albert. I will not forget your help, and thanks for tolerating me in the workshop. I never realised that I had so many friends all over the world.*

Chapter 10
The commercial trajectory
Godfrey's role in the turbulent years 1976–81

Godfrey received much thanks from patients for inventing the scanner, and thus helping their diagnosis and recovery. The following letter came from Rachel Nelson, who worked for Colin Woodley in EMI's Head Office in central London. It is rather impressive that someone made a special visit to say thank you in person.

To: Godfrey Hounsfield

From: Rachel Nelson 22 September 1976

A gentleman came into EMI House the other day whose wife had been to the Brook Hospital, Greenwich last Friday, had an EMI-scan and was operated on at the beginning of the week.

He was obviously very worried about his wife, but relieved that the cause of her illness had been diagnosed.

The purpose of his visit was to ask if we would convey his thanks to you personally for inventing the EMI-Scanner.

Rachel.

Visit of thanks
(Copyright EMI Music)

In June 1976, Godfrey became a CBE, Commander of the British Empire, but the empire had dispersed in the years 1947–70. His team pulled his leg about his new title, but were pleased he had it.

IR.100

EMI **Central Research Laboratories**
A Division of EMI Limited
Shoenberg House, Trevor Road,
Hayes, Middlesex, UB31HH, England.
Telephone: 01-573 3888 Ext:
Telex: 22417 Cables: Emisearch, London.
Telegrams: Emisearch, Telex, London.
Our ref.
Your ref.

15th JUNE, 1976

DEAR GODFREY, DFH, FRS, M.D., D.Sc., FRCP, AND THE REST.

THE MEMBERS OF THE MEDICAL X-RAY DEPARTMENT OF CENTRAL RESEARCH LABORATORIES WISH TO CONGRATULATE YOU ON YOUR APPOINTMENT AS COMMANDER OF THE BRITISH EMPIRE. IF IT HAD ONLY BEEN SOONER WE MIGHT STILL HAVE ONE TO COMMAND.

Registered in England: 255852
Registered Office: Blyth Road, Hayes, Middlesex

The international music, electronics and leisure Group.

Congratulating Godfrey on his CBE
(Copyright EMI Music)
Signatures are: Trevor Hancock, Colin Oliver, Peter Langstone, Geoff Thiel, Doug Hodgkiss, Peter Nevell, Ian Fairbairn, Brian Lill, John Ryan, Mac Gollifer, Jean Steven, Dave Pycock, Richard Waltham, Steve Bates, Peter Reid, Jeremy Thomson, Phil Bone, David Bradley, Richard Gillard, Jim Barnes, Derek Smith, Barry Holloway, Alan Harwood, Don Paine, Tony Williams, Len Smith, Roger Waterworth, Dave Watson, Audrey Lester, Graham Ward, Bob Froggatt, and Chris Loughlin.

In 1976, EMI's medical business was growing fast, it was profitable and heading towards employing four thousand people worldwide at its peak. But the following years were turbulent times, and by the end of the decade it was all in tatters. That story is interesting in its own right, but most of it is not directly relevant to Godfrey, and it has been documented elsewhere, albeit with errors and omissions. Bill Ingham gives his inside view of those aspects in Appendix 4. Godfrey did not run the commercial side of the medical business. His role was to develop new ideas for future products, not to manage the production and marketing of products that had already been designed.

After 1976 Godfrey was involved in the design of faster CT scanners and in improving the performance of existing scanners. He investigated other medical imaging methods. He was a witness in litigation regarding his CT patents. He was pressed into giving lectures, visiting potential customers, and receiving awards, although he far preferred to be working, and somehow he found time for a few social outings.

Denise De Rome Asen went on an outing organised by the IVC in the summer of 1978. *Dear Godfrey. He was courteous and shy in an oddly worldly way, and yes, he drove at a snail's pace all the way from Morden tube to near Taunton, but he was an absolute whiz at skittles, which we played in a Somerset pub: fast, focused and enthusiastic! Maybe the scrumpy helped! He loved the gardens at Montacute, and I remember going round with him and talking to him about the glorious planting and design.*

Skittles are a traditional rustic version of ten-pin bowling, usually played with nine pins on a wooden floor in a room that is part of the pub. There is no machinery, and the wooden floor is uneven, being deliberately curved down at the sides to penalise poor aim, and also having random dents from being hit by bouncing balls. You need to bowl fast to overcome the uneven surface. Scrumpy is an unsanitised version of cider; a rustic drink fermented from apples without any pasteurisation. The unexpectedly slow driving may have been linked to the pressure that Godfrey was under at work. He complained of being unable to work as well as he wished owing to tablets prescribed for stress-related symptoms. In any case, it seems better to be fast on the skittle alley than on the motorway, and it sounds like an excellent night in the pub.

The words "fast" and "focused" would not be appropriate to describe the patent litigation that involved Godfrey and many others. EMI had offered licenses to the patents, but competitors were making scanners without paying the license fees. Much of the burden of patent litigation fell on patent experts such as Allan Logan and Ivan Kavrukov, while Anthony Strong fielded many of the technical questions that might otherwise have landed with Godfrey. However, there were questions about the early years of his work in 1967–71 that only Godfrey or Stephen Bates could answer, and both were interviewed as witnesses. Every available document was brought into the litigation process, no matter how distantly it might relate to the core issues. At one stage there were over 100,000 documents in the "evidence room". It is difficult to see how more than 100 of them could be important, but the legal process requires full disclosure, and it dragged on for years. Part of the litigation involved a company that was based in Ohio, USA. Godfrey was interviewed by its counsel in December 1976 and again in August 1977. It seems to have been a painful event for all concerned. Godfrey struggled to remember exactly what steps he had followed nearly ten years before, and to explain them to someone who was only just becoming familiar with CT. The counsel became steadily more impatient, thinking that Godfrey was being deliberately obstructive, and he interrupted so often that Godfrey became even worse at answering the questions. Ivan Kavrukov helpfully suggested that it might be worth letting Godfrey think and talk in his own way, without interruptions, and this produced a better outcome for them all. The opposing counsel received the best possible answer, and Godfrey suffered a slightly less uncomfortable grilling, but he had to repeat all of this anew for each new legal action.

Ivan Kavrukov makes one of the best attempts at describing Godfrey's unusual thought processes: *One impression I have of Godfrey, reinforced by many examples, is that when it came to technology and particularly CT, when faced with a problem he seemed to just know what the solution would be, and most of the time he was right, but for the life of him he could not explain in logic that others could understand why it would work and what were the logical steps on the way from the problem to the solution. When he felt obligated to give an explanation, as in deposition testimony, and even to me when preparing with him for deposition testimony, he did so very humbly and in a way that perhaps was endearing, but certainly not in the conventional logic of a rigorously trained mathematician or physicist. Still, his solutions of problems that had long bedevilled those professionals worked and did so elegantly and, in the end, this is what really mattered to people who needed what his inventions brought about and benefited from them.*

Magnetic resonance imaging (MRI) was just emerging from university work by Sir Peter Mansfield and others. Sir Peter recalls his first meeting with Godfrey when he was giving a lecture at EMI, but Godfrey was not in the audience because he was not told that the lecture was happening: *I kept asking ... where was Godfrey Hounsfield? ... (Alan) Blay said 'Well, you don't know Godfrey but when he gets a bee in his bonnet about something, and I think he is going to get a bee in his bonnet about NMR imaging, he is likely to be distracted from CT. We don't really want him to be diverted in this way.'* (NMR imaging is now known as MRI.)

As I was being ushered out of the Shoenberg building that evening ... In the foyer they had the actual device which Sir Godfrey had built with his own hands. ... I thought this is about as close as I'm going to get to him. Just as I was about to leave, Godfrey came along ... somehow they felt that their visitor was going now, and he couldn't possibly keep Godfrey long. So they introduced us. When I met him it was about five o'clock ... and he said 'Look, have you got a while, can you come to my office?' So off I went to his office and I was there until 7:30 – a two-and-a-half hour lecture he had from me. It was a replay, with additions, of my talk. (Extracted from "Wellcome witness to 20 century medicine" Volume 2. London: Wellcome Trust; 1998.) It was typical of him to work late, and to assume, unless they said otherwise, that others would happily do so. It was also typical that he would be interested in new ideas, regardless of how daunting the technology or the maths was.

The patent battle and the social outings took less of Godfrey's time than the work to develop the next generation of CT scanner, which was a long, complicated, and ultimately not very fruitful process. One problem was that all of the easy improvements had already been made. In addition, the company was probably unwise to set up a development group in Chicago without giving them the benefit of experience from previous scanner research.

The focus of research and development on the CT scanner from 1976 was to produce a faster and better body scanner. Almost every item needed to be built from scratch, as a new design. The earlier scanners were built mostly from off-the-shelf parts, such as the X-ray tube and the minicomputer; only the software, the metalwork, and a small number of printed circuit cards were designed and built from scratch. Designing the next generation of scanners was a much larger challenge.

In a normal X-ray tube the X-rays radiate from a fixed location inside the tube. The Topaz design used a "scanning" X-ray tube, in which the X-ray source was steered electronically.

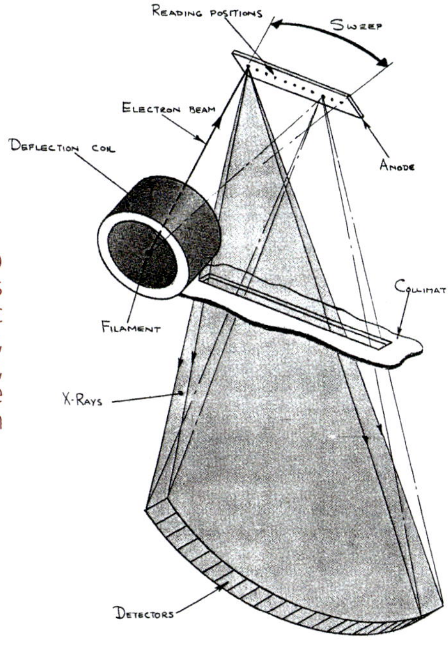

Topaz diagram
(Copyright EMI Music)
The scanning X-ray tube is similar to the type of television screen that was used before flat screens. A magnetic field deflects a beam of electrons, and when these hit the metal target, labelled "anode", they generate X-rays. You can steer the X-ray beam by adjusting the magnetic field.

The scanning X-ray tube spread the intense heat from generating X-rays over a larger area; therefore it could emit a brighter beam of X-rays without overheating, and (unlike the rotating-anode tubes that were available in those days) it did not need to cool down between scans. This was essential for rapid multislice scanning.

The main benefit of this scanning X-ray tube was its ability to calibrate the detectors continuously and avoid the ring artefacts that were described in Chapter 7. Two different detectors read exactly the same path through the patient a small fraction of a second apart. Richard Waltham recalls, *Colin Oliver asked me to help with choosing the best way to line up the beam paths for the detector calibration, which turned out to have implications across much of the scanner system. Godfrey got involved with this, and I spent many evenings working on it with him. At the end of a sequence of calculations covering maybe 45 minutes we reached a point where the answer was 15 divided by 3. I looked at it and said 'the answer is five, Godfrey'. He fell silent, looking very doubtful. For an instant I wondered if he had lost all powers of arithmetic, but he hadn't. It gradually dawned on me that he had some strong reason to believe that the answer was not five. He had an intuitive way of knowing that, but it was unrelated to the method which we had used for the calculations, exactly as Ivan Kavrukov told me in better words thirty years later. I noticed him doing this on other occasions, but I rarely found out how he was doing it, and I can't remember if he was right or wrong in this case. He often was right.*

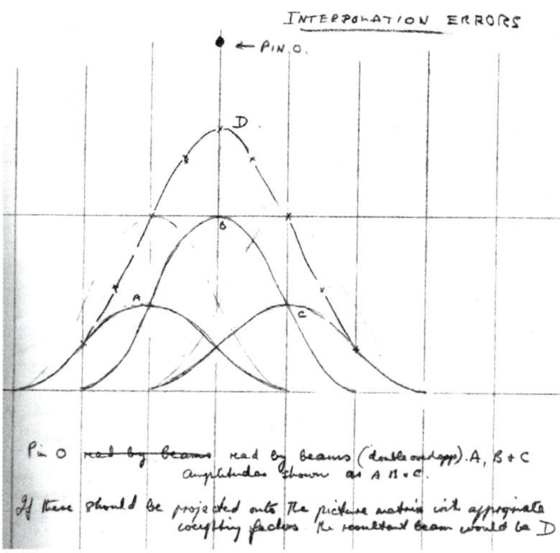

Beam addition

(Copyright EMI Music)

Godfrey often used pictures and diagrams, as in this example of adding three beams. No arithmetic was needed: he built up the sum using a second piece of paper to copy the heights from one part of the diagram to another.

Godfrey used diagrams such as the one above to work out the required sampling intervals, both the required number of angles and how often the X-ray beam needed to be measured as it traversed across the patient. He got the answer exactly right.

What Godfrey did with pictures and diagrams can be done by maths or by computer simulation. But Godfrey's shortcuts saved time and often gave a better insight than techniques that others might regard as more accurate.

Godfrey was interested in the long-winded techniques, but if they conflicted with his simple models then he would not easily change his view. If someone found a flaw in his model he would improve the model and continue using it. He also took shortcuts on machining prototype parts: Tony Williams drew the cartoon below after being irritated and very amused by the shortcut. It was fun but challenging to work with Godfrey.

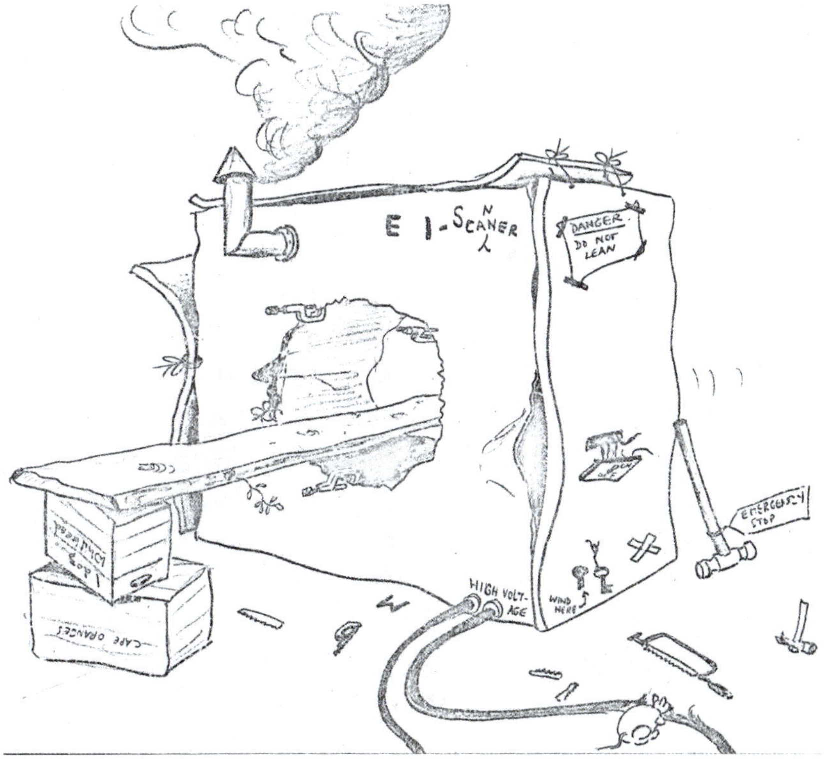

It is amazing what can be done with a hacksaw and micrometer
(Copyright Tony Williams, based on a saying by Godfrey in 1977)

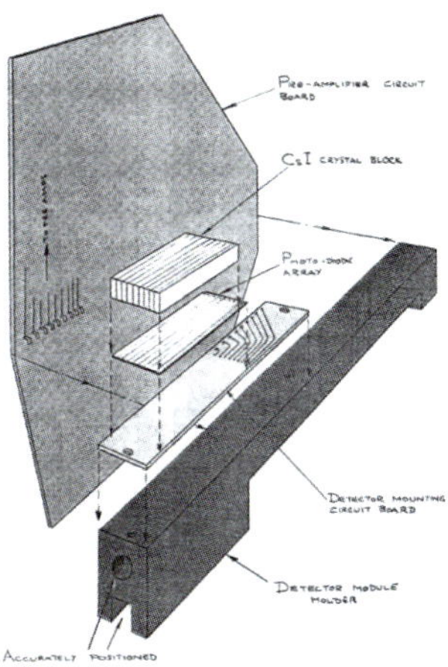

Detector card for Topaz
(Copyright EMI Music)

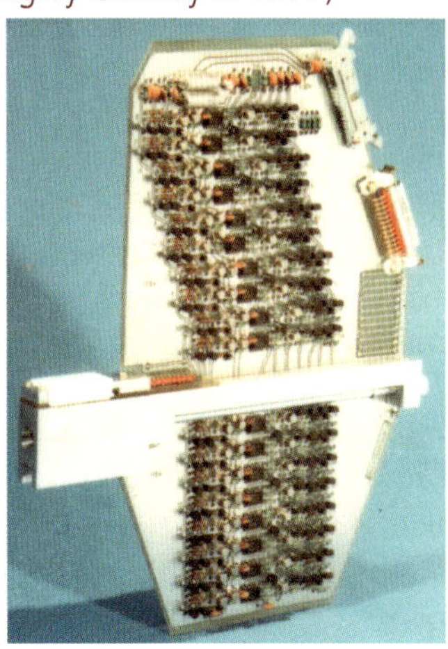

The detectors for Topaz used caesium iodide crystals to convert X-rays to light. The light was converted to electric current by specially designed photodiodes, followed by low-noise amplifiers.

The scanner generated a large amount of data in a short time, so it needed a specially designed fast processor and a multisurface disk drive.

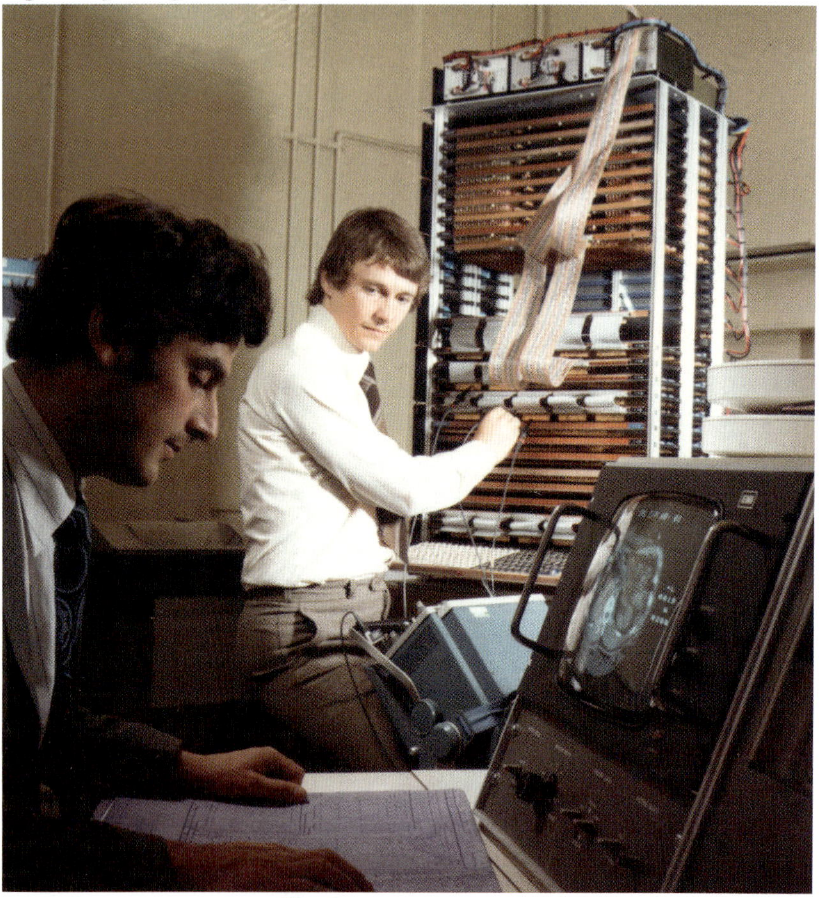

The image processor
(Copyright EMI Music)

Dave Watson is on the left and Geoff Thiel is on the right in the above photo. John Ryan led the Image Processor team, which also included Doug Hodgkiss, Graham Ward, and Derek Smith. Dave Watson says, *Geoff Thiel and I were very proud of the image processor and in particular the amount of heat it dissipated from its arrays of RAMs. Godfrey was looking around it one day and we said to him 'How much power do you think they take then Godfrey?' Godfrey holds his hand over the top of them and replies '200 watts' (at least I think that's what it was) – right to within a watt – a really intuitive engineer.*

Geoff Thiel recalls, *Godfrey needed a photo of a scanner, but the only available camera was a Polaroid set to focus on the viewer screen at about 160mm. He chose the best spectacles from the people nearby, put them over the camera lens and took a sharp photo at his first attempt!*

One other thing I remember about Godfrey was the interview at which I got the job at CRL. It was very brief – just about the only thing he asked me was 'have you ever invented anything or had any good ideas'. The only thing I could think of at the time was an idea I had about digital recording – which was that there would be no need to use fancy CRC error correction if people just used delta modulation instead PCM (because if there was a digital error it would not be a very big one and hence not noticeable). He tore this idea to shreds and terminated the interview shortly thereafter. I thought I had failed the interview and was very surprised when a job offer turned up a few weeks later. I think this illustrates Godfrey's character – I don't believe he was particularly highly qualified but he valued people like himself who could generate ideas.

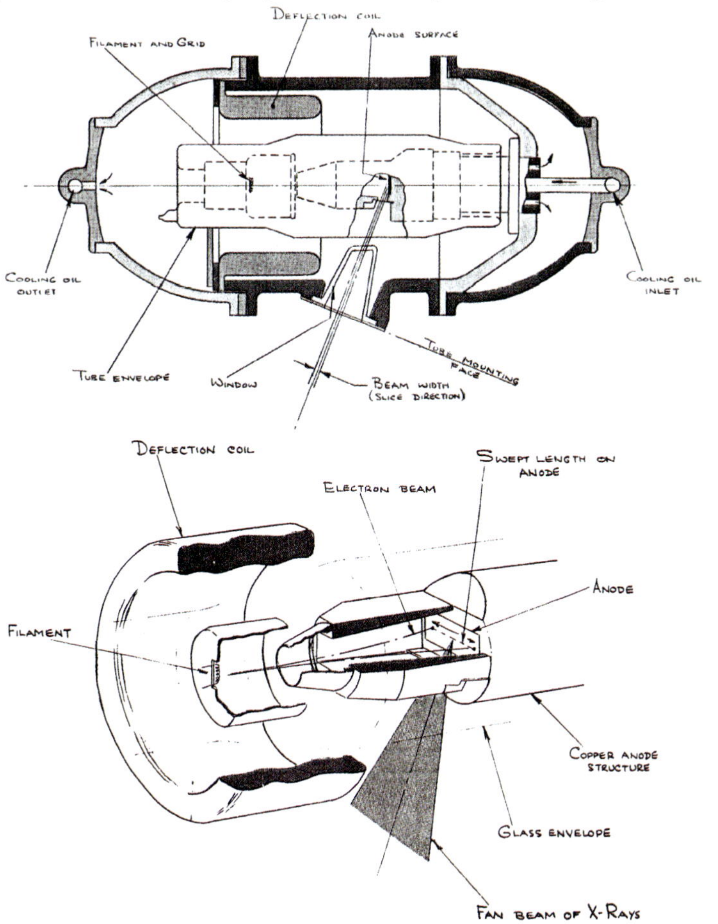

Inside the X-ray tube

(Copyright EMI Music)

Every part of the X-ray tube was designed and built from scratch, including the metalwork, glassware, and the deflection coil that steered the X-ray focal spot.

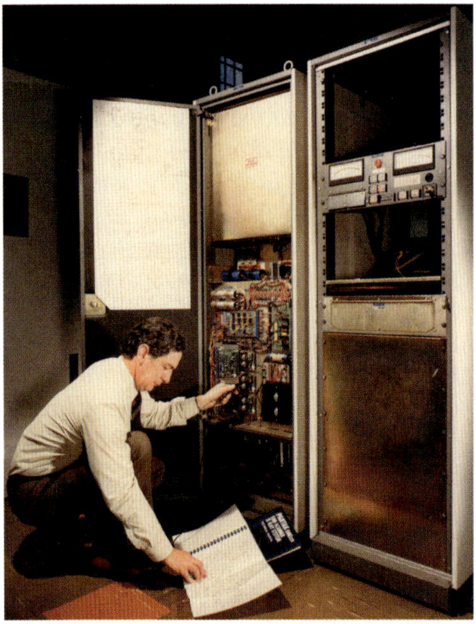

Bespoke Topaz sub-systems
(Copyright EMI Music)

The X-ray tube was switched off for a few milliseconds each time the electron beam was "flying back" to the start position, and this required major modifications to the 140,000 volt power supply.

Left: Arthur Harvey and the heavily modified 140,000 volt power supply. Below: Ian Fairbairn with the Data Acquisition System.

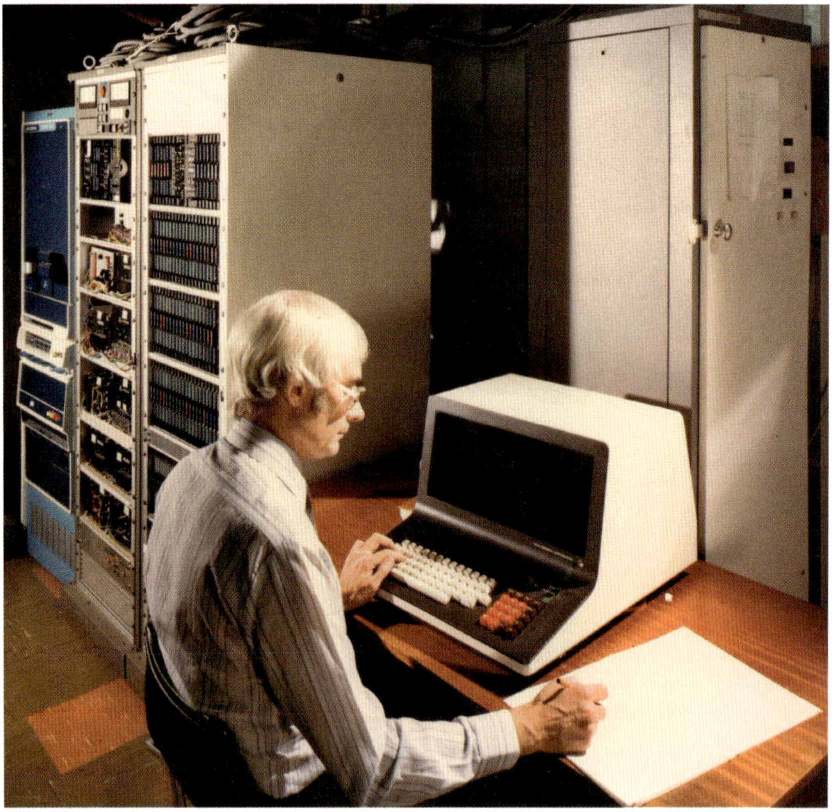

It also shows that he was not a great PR man – if he got what he wanted in a 5 minute interview, it wouldn't occur to him to spend any more time 'selling' the job at CRL to a candidate. This was just one of the many things I learned from Godfrey and I have used the same question myself ever since when employing engineers. It is a great interview question for finding 'ideas' people, but remembering how I felt after the interview with Godfrey, I do spend more than 5 minutes with the candidates.

The electronics cabinets shown on the previous page converted the X-ray signals from 630 detectors into numbers. Ideally a CT scanner needs eighteen-bit digital numbers. The best available integrated circuits offered twelve bits, so they were preceded by an analogue floating-point circuit.

The Topaz scanner
(Copyright EMI Music)
The detectors are at the top and the X-ray tube is at the bottom. They rotated around the patient and the X-rays were moved magnetically thirty-six millimetres from side to side.

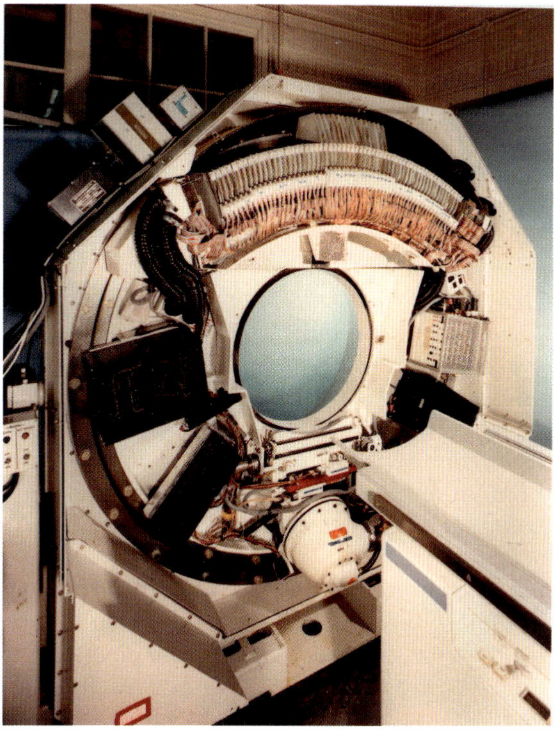

Anthony Strong says that Godfrey liked to take big leaps, not small steps: *I remember Godfrey telling the story that his ultimate ambition was automatic diagnosis by his CT machine. He would build a continuously rotating machine with a trackway through it. Patients would be loaded onto trolleys and pass through the system as it rotated. After diagnosis a set of points in the track-way would divert the patient to the appropriate department, such as Operating Theatre, Radiation Treatment Planning or Mortuary. This story is possibly the earliest description of what later became known as Spiral Scanning. The date would have been around 1978. Another idea of Godfrey's at a similar date was to put a neutrino detector in a satellite and take cross-sectional images of the Earth. He wanted to detect oil and other mineral deposits.*

Meanwhile the production division was making, selling, and refining Godfrey's previous three scanner designs. EMI Medical rapidly expanded its manufacturing capacity in Hayes. It was in profit by 1974, and those profits grew until 1977 when they were about $27 million which was about twenty per cent of EMI's total profit. During the same period, EMI's music business was also growing strongly. Both of these trends reversed sharply in 1978 and 1979, when EMI Medical made losses that wiped out about two-thirds of the profits which it had made previously. A range of factors caused this: some were external, while others were self-inflicted. Part of the problem may have been the management structure. John Powell, the managing director of EMI, was an early supporter of the scanner business and remained so throughout. Perhaps unwisely, he tried to coordinate the various parts of the EMI Medical business himself, as well as being managing director of EMI, which contained music, cinema, TV, leisure, and defence businesses as well. With hindsight, he was attempting two full-time roles.

Stephen Bates says, *One particular problem that emerged as EMI Medical grew was one of co-ordination. Separate organisations were formed to deal with the head scanner, one to deal with the body scanner, and one in the USA called EMI Medical, Inc. This caused some concern to those of us in CRL, as many of the parts of the head and body scanner were the same (computers, detectors, X-ray tube etc.). There appeared to be no one in overall control of these disparate organisations. I remember one meeting in early 1977 held at the Selfridges Hotel (part of EMI surprisingly) where some of us, including Godfrey, had been asked to express our concerns to John Powell who was now managing director of EMI as a whole. John Powell was very late getting to the meeting and apologised for his late arrival saying that he had to deal with terminating the contract with the 'Sex Pistols' (a punk rock band) after they had used four letter words on BBC television. During the meeting Alan Blay (an assistant director of CRL) had expressed his concern that there was no one in overall charge of the different parts of EMI Medical, John Powell replied saying that he was that person. We discussed after the meeting our alarm as to how somebody with such a broad role in EMI could possibly have the time to deal with co-ordinating the complex and fast moving EMI Medical.*

Around 1977, the US government greatly bolstered the "certificate of need" controls on healthcare spending. The impact of this fell mainly on scanner purchases. At the time there were suspicions within EMI that it was deliberately aimed at impeding imports of EMI-scanners until local companies had developed their own products. It certainly had that effect, even if the intentions were pure. Sales by EMI Medical Inc. (the subsidiary which was based in Northbrook near Chicago, USA) fell from £64.5 million in 1977 to only £22.3 million in 1978.

Competition grew quickly. Bill Ingham's view that EMI originally had about an eighteen-month lead is a realistic figure. By September 1976 there were seventeen manufacturers engaged in CT, which was not sustainable because of the escalating cost of research and development. Today, only a few major companies make and sell medical CT scanners worldwide.

Bill Ingham says that asking for a thirty per cent deposit at the time of order was a mistake, and began to hurt as competitors arrived. Gordon Higson took the same view. This was aggravated because EMI's delivery time was over six months and schedules sometimes slipped well beyond that. The company acquired a reputation for arrogance in some quarters, but it also exceeded expectations in looking after customers with low-cost or cost-free upgrades, and in the expert support offered by key staff such as Dave King.

The USA took about seventy per cent of EMI-scanners sold by 1977. Two special factors applied in that market: the first was that Americans often distrust anything that comes from outside the continental USA. To address this, EMI rightly set up local sales, installation, service, and support from 1973, and by 1976 was setting up local manufacture. The second factor was that many hospitals had single-supplier agreements with one of the major suppliers of conventional X-ray equipment. The arrival of EMI upset these agreements, and the suppliers wished to restore the previous exclusive arrangements quickly, so these entrenched competitors poured money into scanner research and development. EMI was in an exposed position because it made only scanners, and did not offer conventional X-ray equipment.

Possibly this would have been a good time to consider licensing and an orderly scaling back, perhaps focusing on specialist scanners, as discussed by Godfrey and Bill Ingham in the film that was made in 1991. This path was not followed.

In 1976, EMI started to invest heavily in manufacturing facilities in the USA, at EMI Medical Inc. in Northbrook near Chicago. At an early stage the management at Northbrook started to establish their own design team, and this was a much more questionable strategy, particularly as they intended it to operate without any input from the UK except for cash. Bill and Godfrey said that this approach of starting from scratch threw away the only advantage that EMI had, which was the eighteen-month lead in research and development. The decision to set up a design team in the USA was influenced by Normand Provost, who John Powell recruited, having previously worked for him at Texas Instruments. Provost worked for EMI Medical Inc. for nine months before dying of a heart attack in April 1976, and John Powell said that his death was a significant factor in the subsequent problems and delays. The key date was 3 December 1976, when it was decided that Northbrook should develop what became the 7070 scanner, and that work on Topaz should cease. This decision was based on a plan showing a working prototype within seven months and several scanners working before the November 1977 RSNA exhibition. These timescales proved to be over-optimistic by a factor of four. As a result, EMI Medical Inc. had an expensive and underused manufacturing site. The market had been promised a new machine but no production 7070s were installed until autumn 1979, by which time the business was in dire straights and it was too late for any new product to turn it around. The proposal approved on 3 December 1976 had turned out to be unreliable in every important respect.

The delays in the 7070 scanner became alarming, and so Topaz was resumed, albeit on a small budget. By July 1977 the 7070 scanner had several serious problems, and it looked unlikely that it would be working before the November exhibition. Godfrey and a team from the UK were called in: finally, the US and UK design teams were allowed to work together. However, the scanner design was already fixed and the commercial pressure was intense. The only changes that were acceptable were those that could be made within ninety days. The UK-designed image processor was available and it was used in the 7070 scanner as well as in Topaz.

Over the next three years Godfrey made about twenty visits to the USA to improve the 7070, usually accompanied by one or more of Stephen Bates, Mac Gollifer, John Ryan, Jean Steven, Geoff Thiel, Richard Waltham, and Peter Guyton from the production division. The photo below was taken during a weekend on one of these trips.

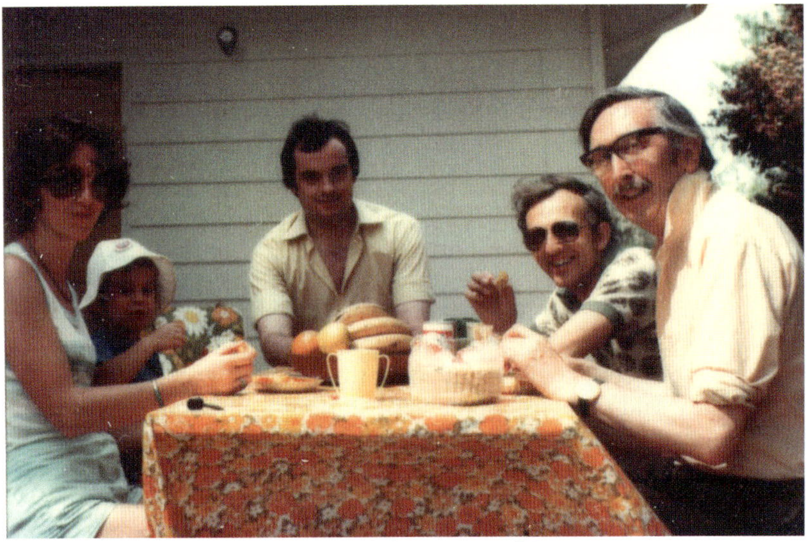

At Dave King's house in Chicago
(Photo courtesy of Matt King)
Jackie and Matt King, Richard Waltham, Mac Gollifer, and Godfrey Hounsfield.

Meanwhile, the awards continued, so he made extra long-haul flights that he might have preferred to avoid. John recalls a trip to Brazil in October 1977 for Godfrey to receive the Order of the Southern Cross, and to meet the Minister of Health and other senior people: *he arrived at the airport worried that his best shirt was damp, in a plastic bag in his luggage. I told him to give it to the hotel laundry service as soon as we checked in. On the return flight I found out that he had forgotten all about the shirt until packing for our return, when it was so mouldy that he had to throw it away.* Godfrey overslept and missed one of the events, probably owing to his watch being set to UK time. With so much long-haul travel it is hardly surprising that he tried to keep to UK time as much as possible. However,

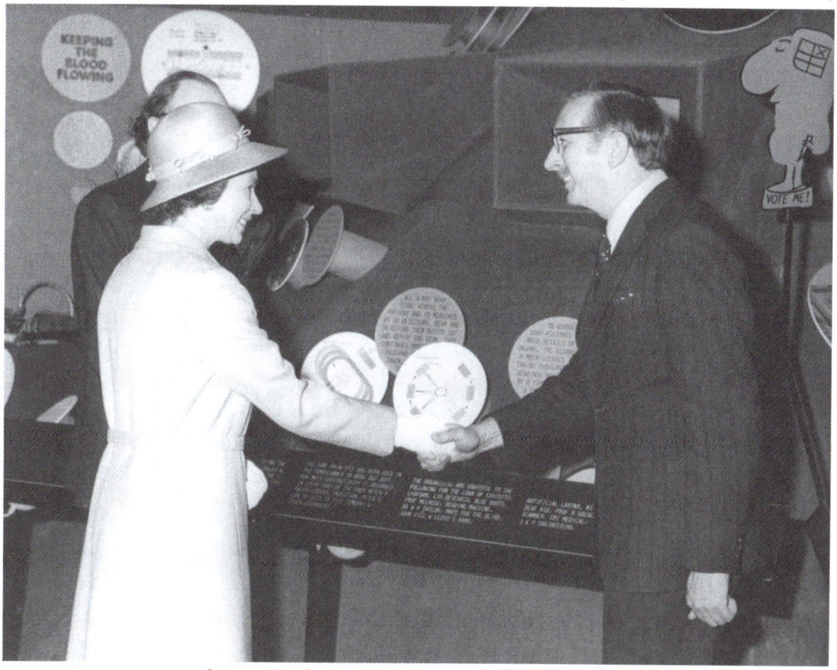

At the British Genius Exhibition, June 1977
(Photo: Desmond O'Neill Features for The John Player Foundation)

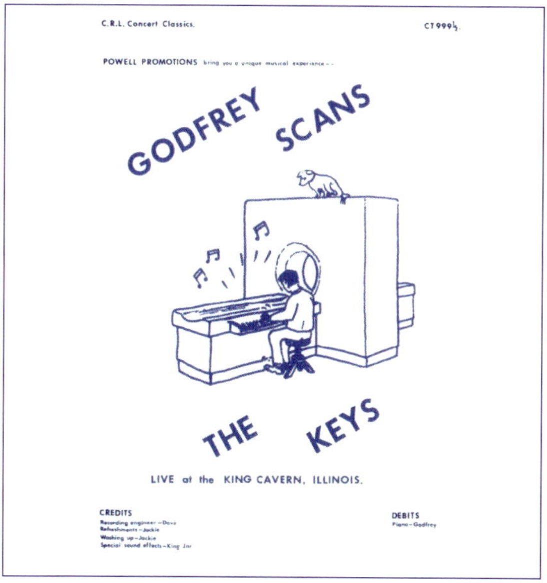

Album artwork: Godfrey scans the keys
(Courtesy of Tony Williams)

he also had the unusual habit of not altering his watch for daylight-saving time. Thus his watch was an hour out of step with all other people in the UK for six months in each year.

The British Genius Exhibition was rather closer to home, in London's Battersea Park, where the photo of Godfrey and Her Majesty The Queen was taken on 30 June 1977.

The album artwork was for a recording of Godfrey playing piano at Dave King's house. Godfrey plays a keyboard attached to the patient's table, while "Nipper" the dog from the "His Master's Voice" record label watches. Near the end of the recording Dave says, *When I was in New York last Saturday night with Bob Froggatt he gave me very strict instructions that I should give you lots to drink and tape record you playing the piano. This is going to be a record!* Godfrey replies, *Oh no, it's not!* But he continues playing.

The recording was made soon after the birth of Matt King, and probably while Godfrey was working on the 7070 scanner. The words on the artwork are difficult to read when reduced to this size. They are:

CRL Concert Classics CT999½

Powell Promotions bring you a unique musical experience

Godfrey scans the keys

Live at the King Cavern, Illinois

Credits:	**Debits:**
Recording engineer – Dave, Refreshments – Jackie, Washing up – Jackie, Special sound effects – King jnr.	Piano – Godfrey

Godfrey said that the 7070 design was an evolutionary dead end. It needed three times as many detectors as were needed by a rotate-only design of the same spatial resolution, although the design did eliminate ring artefacts. These extra detectors meant that the 7070 could not compete on cost with rotate-only designs such as Topaz or the three- to five-second scanners offered at that time by suppliers such as General Electric. There was no possibility of having a higher-resolution central region of the detector array to make a zoom image. Godfrey disliked the fact that the detectors could not be properly collimated to reduce scatter. The prototypes had defects in the CT scans due to off-focal radiation from the X-ray tube. The 7070 used a rotating anode X-ray tube that needed time to cool down after a scan, and this impeded his vision of rapidly acquired volume-scan data. When Godfrey first saw the 7070 in July 1977 it was too late to change the basic design. His main role was to work out what was causing defects in the CT scan pictures and try to patch up the design to cure them. Eventually, the defects were brought under adequate control, but it took too long. With hindsight it might have been better to begin again from scratch in July 1977 rather than to apply a patchwork of fixes.

Bill Ingham recalls an episode in March 1978: *A key event in which Godfrey Hounsfield was involved has never been disclosed. As the situation in the US got worse and worse, and Corporate became increasingly concerned about the delay and the ever increasing costs which already greatly exceeded budget, I was called to the Boardroom to meet the Chairman and three senior members of the EMI Board. After some discussion I was asked to carry out what was called by one 'a technical audit' of the situation at Medical Inc in Northbrook and to report back. And I was informed that in view of the grave importance of the matter I could, as a Divisional Director of EMI as well as the Director of CRL, take anyone I wanted, whether in CRL or not.*

The team I selected included Godfrey Hounsfield and Steve Bates from CRL, three senior managers from EMI Medical Ltd in the UK, and one from EMI Electronics. In addition I took someone from McKinsey International Consultants [...] So there were eight people, covering all aspects from software to drawings.

We were in Northbrook for several days and we then put together a bound report in the McKinsey offices in Chicago. It was quite clear to us that the US scanner would not be available in anything like the time or at the cost expected by EMI, and this was spelled out in our report.

On my return overnight to the UK I reported within hours to Head Office, and was then asked to attend the next meeting of the EMI Board to report on the results of the investigation. I prepared my notes with great care and waited in the lobby outside the boardroom to be called in for the discussion of the medical situation when this came up on the agenda. Time passed and eventually Lord Shawcross came out and expressed surprise to see me waiting there, saying that the meeting was nearly at an end. I was never called.

Our report and advice turned out to be all too correct, and the consequences of EMI Medical having to continue in a difficult market without the promised new scanner, trying to sell the obsolete system, was to prove disastrous.

EMI Medical Ltd in the UK, with all the experience that had been laboriously built up, was now virtually out of the picture as Northbrook went its own way. And the work of Godfrey and his team was now seriously disrupted by the need to try to correct the problems in the US.

On video, Godfrey says that the problem at Northbrook was strategy. The management took decisions that were unreliable because they did not have adequate experience in scanners. There were excellent working-level people at Northbrook, but the management did not listen closely enough to them, or to Godfrey. Stephen Bates rightly points out that anyone can get some kind of picture from a newly developed CT scanner, but producing a good picture requires a lot more skill and work.

Anne Sivers worked in Chicago and got to know Godfrey well while she wrote software to implement some of his ideas for improving the performance of the scanner. She recalls first meeting him in 1977: *Godfrey Hounsfield visited our facility as a consultant. Of course we were all in awe of the inventor of the CT scanner, but I observed that his entourage treated him like a favorite uncle.*

Two years later, Godfrey was awarded a Nobel Prize, but there was no obvious change in his personality. By that time we had built several working prototypes and Godfrey began to spend several months each year in Illinois helping us to perfect our images. Godfrey shared his knowledge with us without reservation and generated new ideas faster than we could evaluate or implement them. Some of these ideas were unprofitable, but many were brilliant.

While I never overcame my awe of Godfrey, I too came to view him as a favorite uncle. There are numerous stories about Godfrey's tunnel vision. When he broke the bridge of his black glasses, he really did put them back together with white adhesive tape and continue to wear them. On one occasion he volunteered to bring us coffee from the cafeteria. Unfortunately, he put the coffee into waxed-paper cups which had disintegrated by the time he reached the computer room. Such unconventional behavior was considered perfectly normal by all who knew him.

As he became more familiar with our staff, he sometimes came alone to work in Northbrook. Since he was uncomfortable driving on the right side of the road, we took turns accompanying Godfrey to dinner. When it was my turn, I was somewhat surprised to find him a charming conversationalist. I don't remember much of what we discussed that evening, but at some point he wondered aloud if he had chosen the right direction for his life. He was about 60 by then and had never married nor had any children. I said, 'Godfrey, how can you even think that? You gave the world the CT scanner and you've just won a Nobel Prize.' 'Well yes', he said, 'but I did that work several years ago. I haven't done anything very noteworthy lately'. That statement summarizes Godfrey's character better than any amount of exposition. He was wrong, of course. He proceeded to conduct research for at least another 20 years and while he never won another Nobel Prize, he never ceased to generate new ideas. And, although he has no biological children, he has many nieces and nephews, both biological and otherwise.

Chuck Smith was part of the same team, and also remembers Godfrey well: *He avoided jet lag by working at night (the systems were always available then and there were fewer distractions). I would operate the system so he could do experiments and collect data. To record the data, he used a #2 lead pencil that he sharpened with his teeth (there was really never a point on the lead). Instead of using equations and math, he would plot data on a piece of graph paper and find the integral of the function by counting the squares under the curve. He liked to refer to the 'false zero' phenomena as a cause of artefacts. This was a nice practical way to describe the problems caused by scatter and afterglow.*

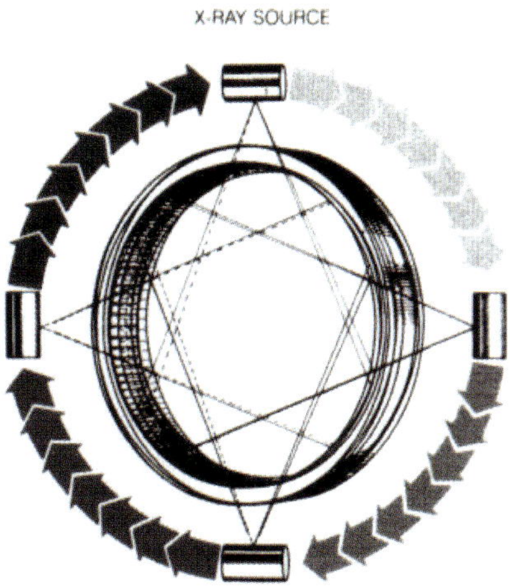

The 7070 scanner
(Copyright EMI Music)
The detectors are in the inner ring, all the way round the scanner. The X-ray tube rotates outside the detector ring. The ring pivots slightly, taking the detectors out of the way when the X-ray tube is behind them. In the final design the tube was closer to the patient than in this early drawing.

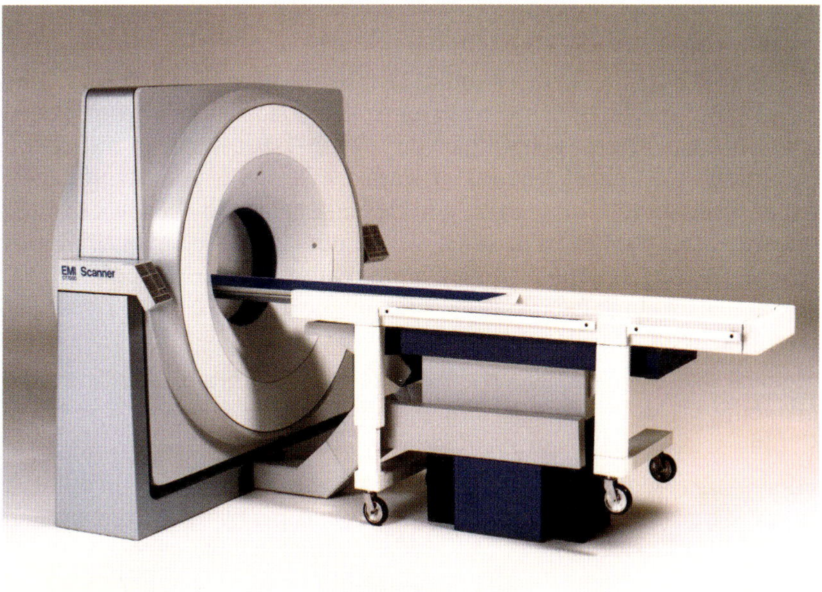

A scale model of the 7070 scanner
(Copyright EMI Music)

The prime aim of the 7070 was to compete with three- to five-second rotate-only scanners being prepared by competitors in 1976, which at the time were based on Xenon gas detectors. (Xenon was not the best choice for efficient use of the X-ray dose, but its performance was stable over time, which reduced ring artefacts.) Bill and Godfrey thought, with hindsight, that Northbrook could have copied that design, but did not do so in 1976 to avoid loss of face. By 1978, the delays on the 7070 caused this path to be taken by purchasing a design and installed base of scanners from the G.D. Searle company. It was too late, and it made little commercial impact.

Chuck Smith remembers Godfrey being invited to evaluate the Searle CT scanner prior to EMI acquiring the design. *With a roll of electrical tape, a few bits of lead, and a couple of water cylinders, he found all the faults and shortcomings of the system in about 30 minutes of experimentation.*

Godfrey continued to go to IVC events, and David Bosomworth knew him there over many years: *I remember he wanted to talk about railways and he tackled me as a life long enthusiast. Godfrey insisted there must be a way of improving on the present system of steel flanged wheel on steel rail and wanted to know what I thought. So I trotted out the arguments in favour of the present system, how it had evolved despite many an engineer over the last 150 years asking the same question, and trying different arrangements and how difficult it would be to change now especially if we had to maintain through running and compatibility between adjacent systems. But Godfrey was not convinced so I was left wondering if this tenacity to an idea or the need to challenge the status quo was the road to winning a Nobel Prize.* Tenacity was indeed one of the ingredients of Godfrey's intuitive genius.

In a 1992 BBC film, Walter Robb of General Electric says that during the mid-1970s General Electric was desperate to stop orders being placed with EMI, which was "gobbling up the market". He also says that General Electric was delighted when EMI started a design team at Northbrook without using the UK research and development lead. Insiders at EMI suspected that the tactics of some competitors included announcing fast scanners a long time before they were ready, to deter customers from buying the available but slower EMI equipment.

Product development was not the only drain of cash: by 1978 EMI Medical had expanded greatly and was spending heavily on sales and marketing as well as on developing scanners and viewers. Worldwide staffing peaked at 4000 in 1977 and was 2500 in 1979.

Everything reached a crisis in 1979 as EMI was also facing difficulties in the music business. EMI merged with Thorn (effectively a takeover) and embarked on a sad and rapid exit from the medical market in 1979–80. Most of the operating divisions outside the USA were sold to General Electric, Toshiba manufactured the 7070, and Topaz was completed and transferred to Philips.

The installed base of CT scanners continued to grow, benefiting millions of patients around the world. Godfrey remained active and interested in medical imaging and in many other technical areas. Long after normal retirement age, he continued to work both in hospitals and at EMI's research labs, ceasing only when breathing problems associated with his final illness became acute. Investigation and experimentation were what he had always done, he enjoyed them, and it was a relief to be able to go back to his roots now that he was less in the public eye.

Godfrey labelled the next photo "Knighthood 1981", but it is possible that it was taken on a different day. The photo on page 178, which shows

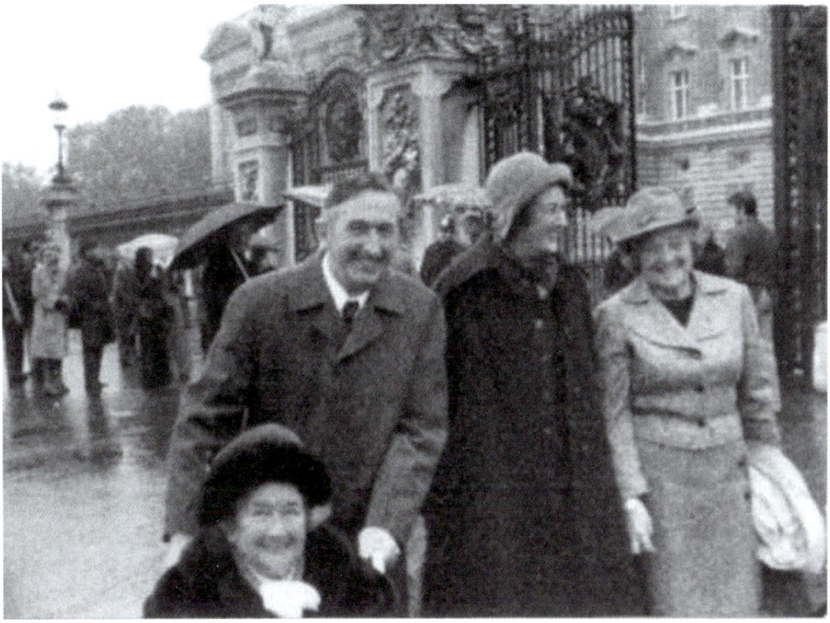

At Buckingham Palace with his mother, Joan, and Mary
(Courtesy of Andrew Hounsfield)

Godfrey with his two brothers outside the palace, is definitely from the knighthood ceremony on 15 July 1981, for which Godfrey wore a white tie in dry weather. His niece Ruth says that there were two guest tickets for the knighthood, and Godfrey took his brothers. After the ceremony, he took them and their wives to the theatre, possibly to see Barnum at the London Palladium, and other family members may have joined them. So the photo of Godfrey pushing his mother's wheelchair may have been taken the day after the Knighthood photo, or at the CBE award in 1976.

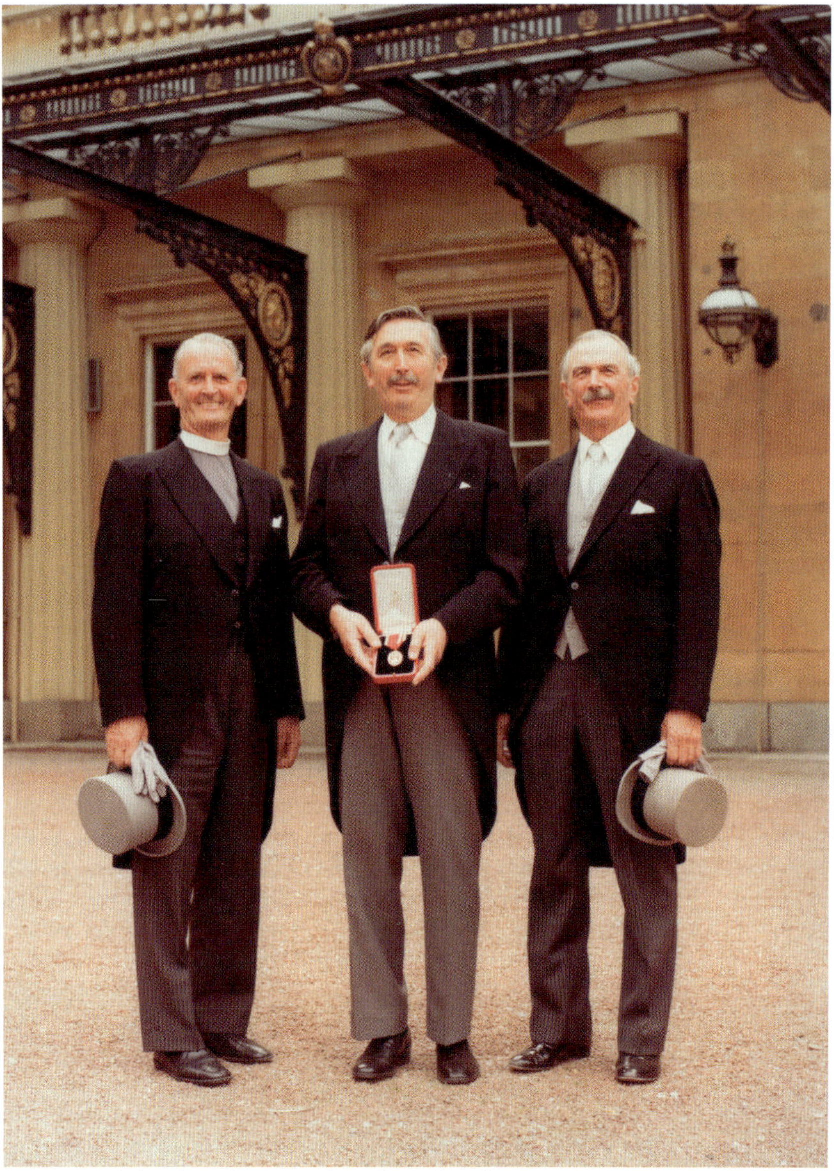

With his brothers Paul and Michael at Buckingham Palace
(Courtesy of Studio D Photography)

Chapter 11
Getting older, but still a child at heart

What does a retired bachelor do all day?

Godfrey was three years short of normal retiring age when he read about the invention of a "scanning tunnelling microscope" at IBM in Zürich in 1981. This ingenious device could see individual atoms and move them about, and it wrote the letters "IBM" using about fifty atoms. Godfrey was fascinated, and set about trying to make an improved version at lower cost. The fact that he failed seems less interesting than the magnitude of the leap that he was attempting, and, typically, the extent of his improvisation.

Godfrey's starting point was cable TV which at that time was big in the USA but not in the UK. (This was partly because the cables had to be buried under the street in the UK, because of urban planning rules, whereas they were strung on poles in the USA at significantly lower cost.) In 1981, cable TV was a hot topic in England, and the government encouraged it as part of moves towards modernising and liberalising the telephone and communications services. Godfrey was sceptical and thought that there might be a better solution.

The UK had four terrestrial TV channels, which concentrated their mass-market programmes into peak viewing hours because few people had video recorders. The midnight hours included niche programmes such as the Open University. There was no other television option for the ordinary person: satellite, DVDs, and internet TV all arrived after this period.

Godfrey said that if you had a 100-hour four-channel video recorder then it could automatically record everything that had been broadcast over the last twenty-four hours and you could take your pick when you sat down to watch TV. If you watch four hours a day, then you have the equivalent of a 100-channel cable TV system, without having to bury any cables. Ideally you extend this to record a week or more of programmes. So you broadcast on the existing four TV channels for the full twenty-four-hour day, rather than shutting them down overnight. This needs a large capacity video recorder with the ability to instantly replay any item (without waiting for a tape to rewind) at a mass market price. This eventually arrived on the market as TiVo in 1999 and Sky+ in 2001, so Godfrey was a long way ahead of his time.

Ian Green shared an office with Godfrey in the later 1980s and he recalls the equipment sitting in a corner of their room: *it was based on the famous IBM microscope from the early 1980s; the one that won them the Nobel Prize, and that operated at cryogenic temperatures. Well, Godfrey's room temperature version, which was constructed with much help from Stuart Best, was the most Heath Robinson-ish thing you ever saw. When working, it was suspended from dangly springs in a vacuum chamber to isolate it from vibration, with electrical connections via thin coiled wires for the same reason.*

Heath Robinson was an English cartoonist who drew improvised machines and eccentric inventors. The IBM team needed very low "cryogenic" temperatures to isolate the sample from vibration by superconducting levitation at about -269ºC (-452ºF).

Godfrey eventually produced an atomic plot on graph paper with a regular pattern, that looked as if it might be an image of about 10 by 10 atoms. It took a long time to scan, and wasn't repeatable, I suspect because even the slightest thermal expansion or contraction would have moved the scanning point more than that distance. It couldn't (intentionally) deposit or remove atoms, so it couldn't write a pattern, let alone do so at any speed.

And Godfrey's motivation? He was fed up with having to look up the Radio Times and program his VCR in advance. What he wanted was a little box to sit in a corner and record a week's worth of all the channels, so he could decide what to watch after the programmes had been transmitted. He had worked out how much data needed to be stored (this was before MPEG changed the rules on video compression) and decided that atomic resolution would fit the bill. What he achieved with the lash-up was remarkable. But what he wanted to achieve was mind-boggling. Intrepid doesn't begin to describe it. I don't know what this proves, but it was certainly extraordinary.

Stuart Best remembers, *I was asked to assist him with his idea for a Scanning Tunnelling Microscope. He had retired, and was working for what I think was just two days a week. He had already built the mechanical part of the device, and Ian Green is right when he says it was a Heath Robinson affair! My job was to construct the electronics which drove the piezo actuators, controlled the tunnelling current and drove the analogue storage oscilloscope on which we hoped to see a recognisable atomic image. I used to operate the vacuum pump, and kept it topped up with liquid nitrogen. I had to repair the 'dangly' springs and connecting wires when they dropped off, on a regular basis! I often suggested to Godfrey it would be better if we started again and constructed a more robust version, but he insisted this one was fine!*

Several times, after waiting ages for the vacuum in the bell jar covering the device to reach a high enough level, something would come adrift and we would have to stop the pump, bring the bell jar up to atmospheric pressure, make repairs and then start the pumping process again! As I remember we only once saw and photographed an image on the oscilloscope screen that could possibly show atoms. It was an exciting moment, I had always thought it would be a miracle if the contraption actually worked!

Godfrey was a pleasure to work with, but could be a little frustrating at times. To me he was the typical 'absent minded professor' type. Often we would work past 5pm and Godfrey would say 'Look at the time! We must go home now, but let's just try this first ...', this would be repeated many times until it was 9.30 or 10pm and we really had to leave. The first time this happened I had to walk two and a half miles home with my bicycle, as not expecting to leave so late I hadn't brought any lights with me!

I certainly remember Godfrey's ideas on the storage of data at the atomic level. He told me several times about his calculation that you could fit at least 10 years worth of full bandwidth video into a volume of 1 cubic centimetre!

Godfrey did not need to work: he could have taken early retirement. He worked because he was interested in it, and enjoyed the challenge. At this stage his employer would be likely to back his ideas in the hope of striking gold again. He did not have to economise, but if he thought of a quick and improvised way of testing something, then he preferred to follow that route rather than build expensive equipment for his experiment.

He continued painting, although the example below is unlike the earlier landscape watercolours that he painted with the IVC.

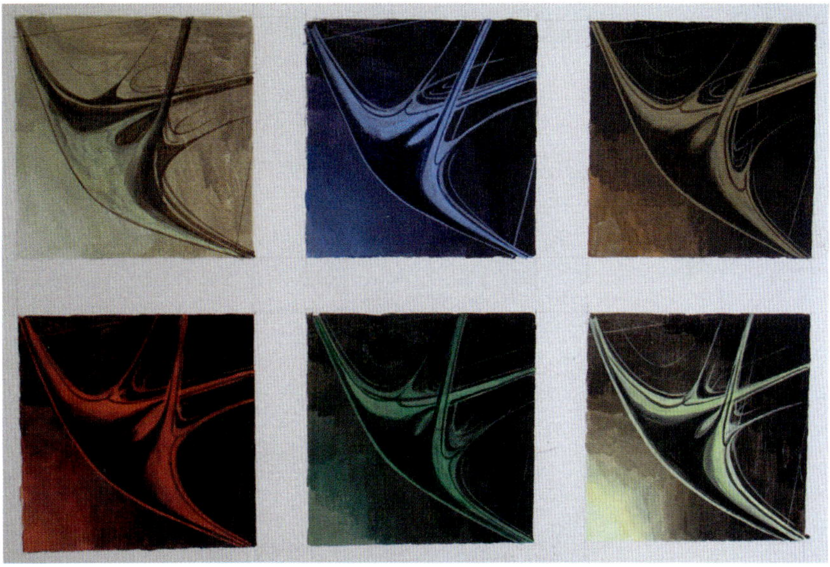

Painting by Godfrey
(Courtesy of Lynda Hounsfield)

He never took himself too seriously. Pete Walters says that the following photo dates from the early 1980s when he worked with Godfrey, Ian Green, and Bob Froggatt.

Peter Walters says, *We were on our way to the canteen and Godders walked into the old car park, presumably as a short cut. I pulled my camera out, which I happened to have in my pocket, thinking I'll take a 'beware of the Godfrey' photo. He saw me, and understood my unspoken idea, and played along superbly. When the prints came back I gave him one which he photocopied and drew over.*

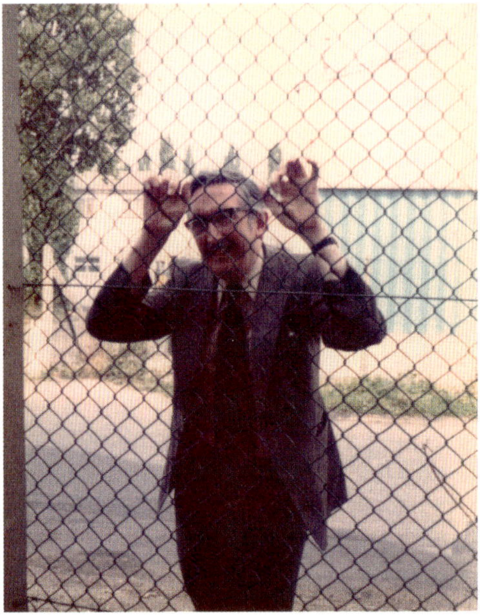

Caged Godfrey
(Photo courtesy of Peter Walters)
Godfrey drew a cartoon cage around this, complete with a banana and a car tyre, perhaps so that he could play like a monkey

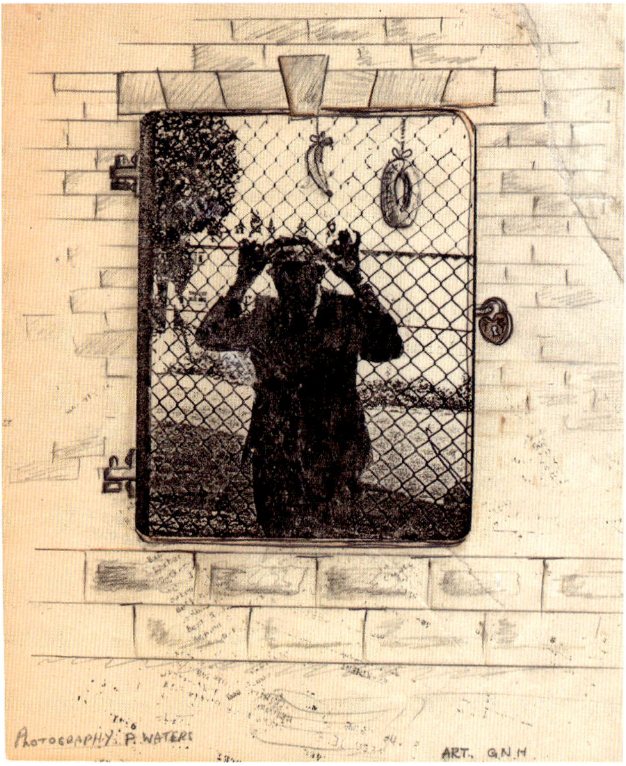

(Drawing by Godfrey courtesy of Andrew Hounsfield)

Andrew Hounsfield says, *I was down in London with a couple of friends, I think we had been to a rugby match, and I rang up Godfrey and said I'm in London, can we meet up? He said 'where do you want to go?' and I thought it would be good to go to the Science Museum with Godfrey. He was famous by then, so my friends were very proud to meet Sir Godfrey Hounsfield. He said 'I'll treat you out for the day' and it was funny when we got to the computer bit of the Science Museum and he turned round and said 'we don't want to go in there, we know all about that don't we', and he walked on. Then he treated us to lunch at the local Wimpy Bar!* Godfrey probably had fond memories of Wimpy as an early British burger bar in the otherwise rather bleak London of the 1950s. At the time of this story they were not the most fashionable of London restaurants, but those present would have been pleased to see each other in any setting. Andrew's daughter Kate says, *when we went to see him we were in a little room with all of the computers which he had taken apart, all of the disks on the floor. He took us all on the London Eye, and he had a pet fox which he fed in his garden. Because we were dyslexic and we think that he was dyslexic, he said that he didn't understand dyslexia at all, but he said that the brain isn't wired normally. He was quite keen on dyslexia because of that, because it created original thinking, or an original angle on things. He wasn't the best at reading or writing, and he didn't progress far at school.* What he achieved with those drawbacks is stunning.

The CT scanner was no longer a major factor in Godfrey's life, although he took an interest in developments in radiology. He liked to go to meetings at the BIR, where people soon realised that he simply wanted to blend in with everyone else. He wanted to hear about the future, rather than have people "making a fuss" about his role in the history.

His employer stopped making CT scanners in 1980, soon after EMI was taken over by Thorn. Initially Thorn expected that the medical business would be a liability, but it was wrong. S. A. Pandit says that the net profit from the medical business, *taking into account both the patent income and all the costs incurred in withdrawing from the business was in the region of £70 million, and since the costs were largely the writing off in the accounts against assets inherited from EMI, and, therefore, absorbed no cash, the cash benefit was closer to £100 million. The medical business turned out to be a net asset to THORN EMI, rather than a net liability as many had feared.* Of course the money went to the company rather than to Godfrey, but it was good to know that his invention had been a great benefit to the company as well as benefiting medical science and improving the health of so many patients.

Godfrey hated speaking in public, but in February 1983 he agreed to speak at Magnus school, forty-seven years after he left it. He wanted to encourage young people to work in science and engineering and to be bold and creative in their work. He finished by saying, *Well I hope I haven't spoken too long about what is after all, history, past and done with. My purpose in telling my story is to impress on those of you who are about to leave school, especially those who are going into science and technology, that a career in this field can be an extremely rewarding experience, particularly if you can carry through an idea of your own making, as I did.*

Remember, too, that each new discovery brings with it the seeds of other, future, inventions. There are many discoveries, probably just around the corner, waiting for someone to bring them to life. Could this possibly be you?

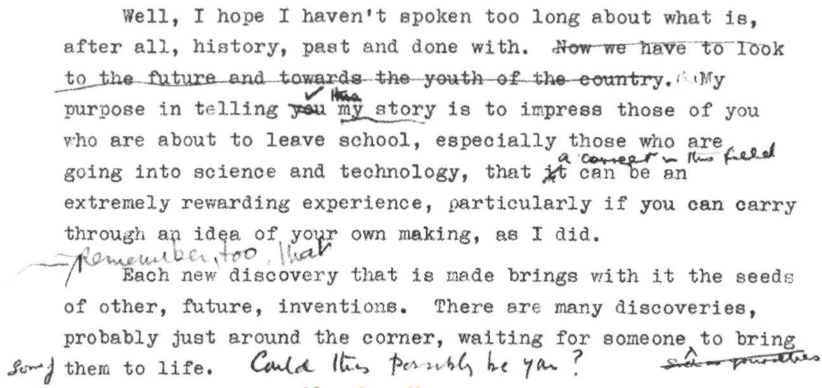

Well, I hope I haven't spoken too long about what is, after all, history, past and done with. ~~Now we have to look to the future and towards the youth of the country.~~ My purpose in telling ~~you~~ my story is to impress those of you who are about to leave school, especially those who are going into science and technology, that ~~it~~ can be an extremely rewarding experience, particularly if you can carry through an idea of your own making, as I did.

Each new discovery that is made brings with it the seeds of other, future, inventions. There are many discoveries, probably just around the corner, waiting for someone to bring them to life. Could this possibly be you?

Godfrey's talk at Magnus
(Courtesy of Andrew Hounsfield)

You can see from Godfrey's handwritten notes (above) how hard he tried to make his message clear and vivid. He wanted to reach across the age gap to the young people, and he tried to remember how he felt about things at their age. The full text can be found in Chapter 12.

Godfrey's assistant Audrey got entangled in his legendary car problems, as Monica Johnson recalls, *on one occasion she had a call from the police saying it was about the car which Godfrey had reported stolen and she took a note into the meeting where he was, asking him to come and speak to the police. When he came out he looked a bit embarrassed and he said 'Oh, I've just remembered I've actually put the car into the garage for servicing today and it hasn't been stolen at all'. So he then went back into the meeting and left Audrey to ring the police back and say, in rather embarrassed fashion, that actually the car was in the garage. The policeman wanted to know whether they were being funny and were they wasting police time but she assured him that, no, this was just one of Godfrey's memory problems and that he genuinely hadn't meant to be a nuisance.*

He joined the MGR (Merry Go Round) social club in Maidenhead for discussion meetings and outings. Jeannette Lemon says, *I knew Godfrey from about 1984 when he joined the MGR group. We all loved him. He was a very humble man and never ever said that he was knighted, or talked about what he had developed. I had a friend who had been working in Israel on the CT scanner and who talked about it at one of our meetings, but Godfrey never mentioned his involvement, he just let my friend have the floor.*

I worked for 15 years with ICL from 1968 onwards and we had debates at MGR about computers but I thought that perhaps he wasn't very computer literate. Godfrey had not told Jeanette that he was in charge of the team which designed the EMIDEC 1100 computer! However, it is true that after he stopped designing computers he learnt only about what would help him, rather than learning everything about computers for their own sake.

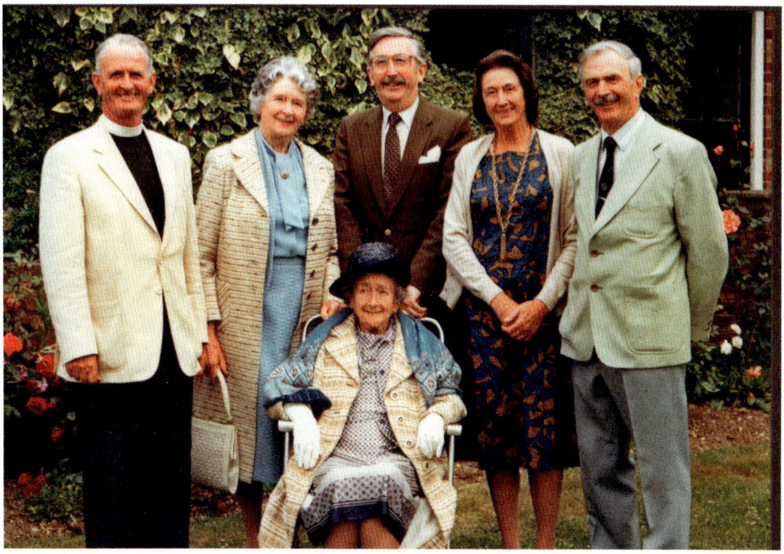

At his mother's ninety-ninth birthday with Paul, Molly, Joan, and Michael

(Courtesy of the Newark Advertiser)

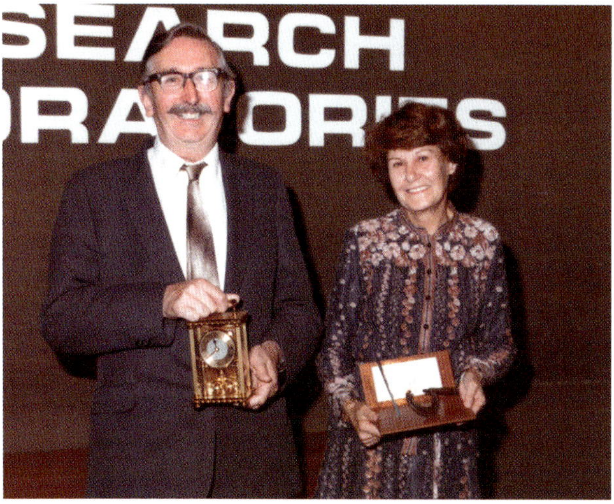

"Retirement" in August 1984

(Copyright EMI Music)

1984 was also the year of his mother's ninety-ninth birthday and his own sixty-fifth birthday, which triggered his official retirement.

In the "retirement" photo, Godfrey is holding the traditional present of a clock, while his long-serving assistant Audrey Lester holds a micrometer and hacksaw blade, which hark back to his 1977 remark and the cartoon by Tony Williams.

Godfrey's retirement did not make much difference. He still came to work at CRL regularly. He spent one day each week helping in a hospital and one or two days at CRL, and the other days he worked at home. Perhaps he took a few more holidays than in the 1960s. Gordon Hopewell describes a holiday episode: *On an outing to Pompeii in Italy, Godfrey broke away from the group because he wanted to see the tracks of the carriages to measure them and photograph them with his old Box Brownie camera. He was particularly interested because they were the same gauge as the first railway tracks. He was such a likeable person, very uncomplicated and friendly, and interested in lively discussion of all sorts of issues from nuclear power to art and music.*

Many people have stories of Godfrey from MGR events. Jean Robertson remembers him *on a visit to a stately home, looking at an 18th century sewing machine, unwilling to join the rest of us for tea until he had understood how it operated, which of course he worked out. Godfrey was a modest humorous man who we shall miss greatly.*

Roger Garstang says, *One day in July we gathered for a barbeque in Cookham on a rather cloudy evening. The barbeque was lit but the fire was not progressing very well. A couple of men were trying to fan it with plates. Godfrey appeared with a vacuum cleaner borrowed from the lady of the house. Somehow he had reversed the air flow so that it blew rather than sucked, and he soon had the fire roaring like a blacksmith's forge.* This was absolutely typical of Godfrey's improvisation.

Sally Radford was at a dinner party with Godfrey *and a new member started a reasonably heated discussion about religion. After a while Godfrey put his two-pennyworth in saying something including 'from the scientific point of view', to which the new member said 'You must be a scientist then.' Godfrey paused and then replied 'Yes, well, some people call me that.' He was always very understated.*

We all went out on a boat trip on the Thames in the late 1990s. Godfrey arrived late and a bit flustered. We went on the boat trip and when we got off the boat three or four hours later he found his car door open, with the keys in the ignition and the engine still running! He told me about this when we were on another outing a few weeks later. He had no qualms about telling people things like that, about his weaknesses. He saw the funny side of it and shared the joke. Godfrey was not simply an absent-minded professor: he was very sociable and able to laugh about himself.

He still went on IVC outings, as Kathleen Dix describes, *in Provence in 1985, the hotel in Arles was new, but the plumbing and electrics left much to be desired. Godfrey was often up until the early hours sorting out problems in various rooms, for example a loo that flushed continually. One morning at breakfast he told us that he had rewired his room overnight!*

In the Loire Valley in 1986 we stopped for our mid morning coffee en route to visit a chateau. Godfrey went in to order four coffees. I followed him in a few minutes later and heard him asking for quatorze café au lait. I imagined that had he been given fourteen, he would have paid up and nonchalantly asked if anyone wanted a second.

When in Amboise we visited Le Clos-Luce, home of Leonardo da Vinci. There was an exhibition of models of Leonardo's inventions. I remember Godfrey touring the exhibition with us and shaking his head and pronouncing them all unworkable.

While in Blois we discovered the Poulain chocolate factory, mainly by following the wonderful smell from the factory, that was near the hotel. We arranged a tour and the photo shows some of us immediately after the visit, wearing the hats we had worn in the factory and clutching our samples.

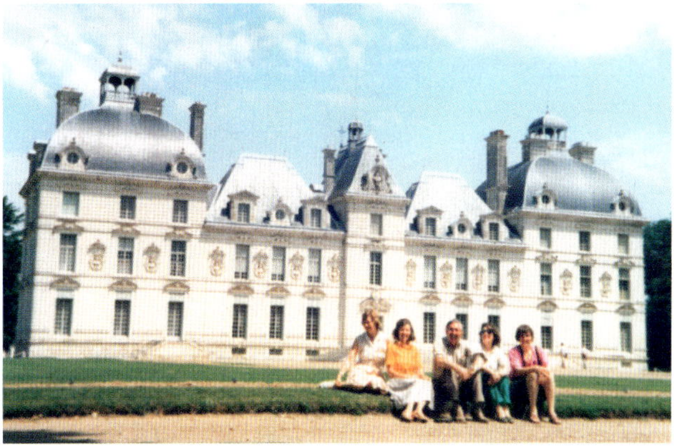

Godfrey and friends at Cheverny, Loire Valley, France

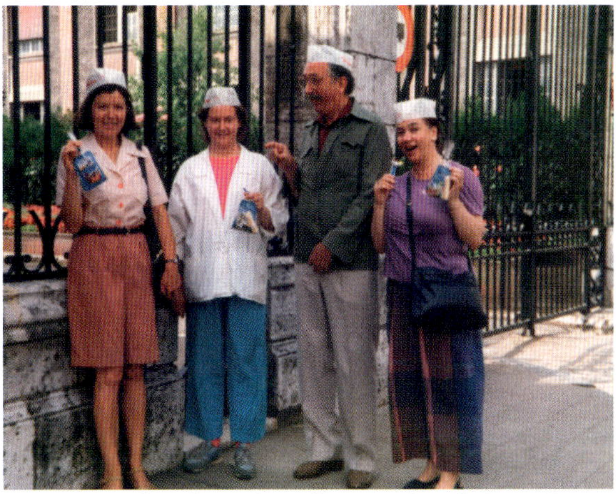

After visiting the chocolate factory in Blois, Loire Valley
(Both photos courtesy of Dr Kathleen Dix)

Pauline Figgins was on the same tour: *We collected rental cars in Paris and set off to the Loire Valley. I shared some of the driving with Godfrey. I enclose a photograph taken at a relaxing break for lunch. I think it is Anne Routledge who is expecting the cherries.*

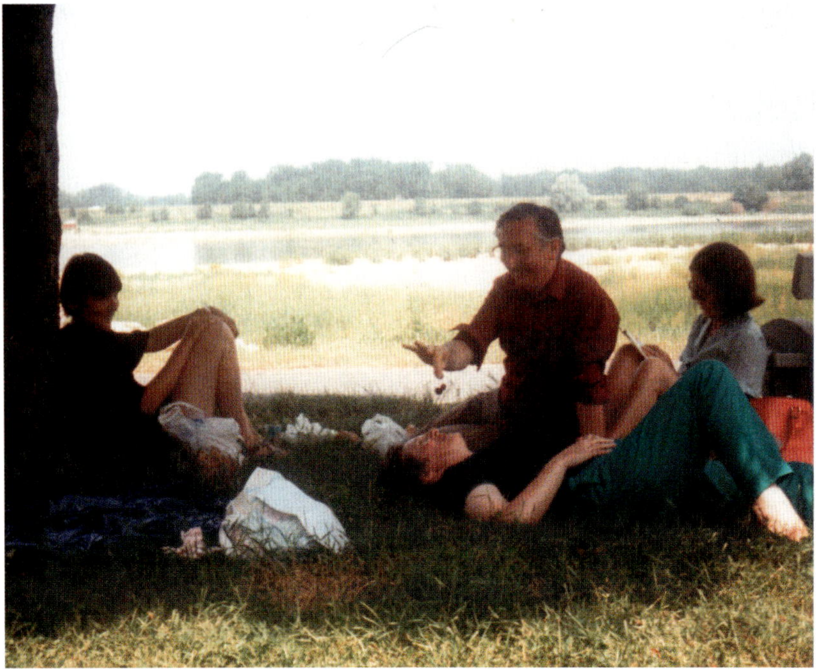

Loire valley 1986
(Courtesy of Pauline Figgins)

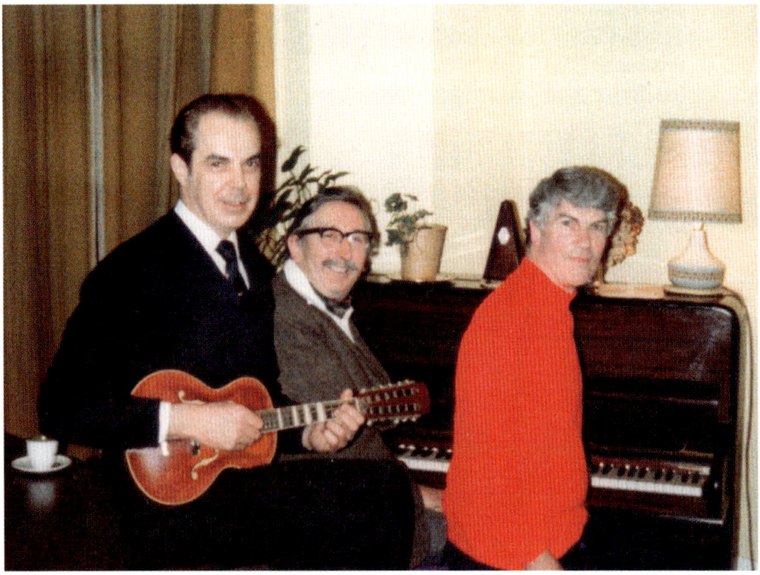

With John Douglas, who is on the right
(Courtesy of Rosemary Douglas)

The weather was unseasonably hot and some of us were more energetic than others. The more active group reckoned on seeing 6-8 chateaux a day and was nicknamed the 'chateau group'. The rest of us, including Godfrey, became the 'gateau group' and reckoned on seeing about 4–5 chateaux a day and have time to enjoy the coffee and cakes, and make the day more leisurely. I met him several times since then and noticed that on any discussion relating to physics he took off as it were on cloud nine and beyond most people's understanding. He also played the organ very well one evening at John Douglas's home. In spite of his talent he was always unassuming and said he preferred to relate to 'ordinary' people.

Jean Sichel says, *We knew Godfrey particularly through his love of jazz. Did you know that he had his own jazz group in the RAF? We often attended events organised by him, particularly at the Runnymede hotel, which were part of his commitment to MGR. I often attended discussion evenings at MGR when Godfrey was present and you can imagine how stimulating and interesting they were. He also had a lovely, gentle sense of humour when prompted.*

In Godfrey's papers there are some handwritten notes that may give a snapshot of one of the discussion meetings. One topic was *Can democracy work in the long term? Will society learn to beat the system as it did in Russia, where everyone demanded a meal ticket and nobody worked? Should there be a third house, not so democratic, which generates a purpose for society? Will people get dispirited by governments not taking unpopular decisions in order to keep the votes of mindless and destructive pressure groups, by governments selling off the family silver, and by them allowing the decline of science and industry?* Other topics included the morality of executive pay versus winning money on a lottery, and how to properly control genetic engineering, leaving the emotion on one side and weighing up the risks and benefits.

Doug Jackson says that Godfrey joined a University of Oxford philosophy course. *It was mainly for undergraduates and post graduates so he was by far the oldest. The lectures took a good deal longer that normal because whilst the younger members accepted the overall concepts but challenged on all the usual fronts Godfrey was at pains (for him and the lecturer) to get to the very fundamentals of philosophy, with his usual tenacity. He continued questioning until satisfied or the lecturer was exhausted. As his attendance was a concession, it only lasted one term.*

He became interested in "artificial neural networks", which are computer programs that try to learn from experience in a similar way to how people learn. This is radically different from the traditional way in which computers have been taught (or programmed), which involves telling the computer exactly what steps to follow. This work forced Godfrey to learn a relatively modern computer programming language. Ian Green says, *Long after the EMI-scanner he started to learn Microsoft Visual Basic, and was frequently on the phone to Microsoft support for explanations. I remember him appearing one day, saying that the books on Visual Basic had 'got it all wrong', but that he understood it now and was going to write his own book on the subject.* It sounds as if Godfrey had eventually translated the topic into his own internal mental pictures. Whether or not he ever wrote the book is not known. It is tempting to speculate on whether his book would have helped many other students of Visual Basic, or only those who shared his unusual ways of thinking.

Stuart Best says: *Godfrey knew that I had been using other forms of Basic for some time, so he would come and ask questions on programming and complain about the 'poorly written' and 'confusing' Visual Basic manuals. Around this time Godfrey, who was sharing an office with Reg Willard, would tell Reg and me that he was suffering from pains in his legs and backside. He later mentioned that he was sitting up at home nearly every night, until very late, writing software! We suggested that this could be the cause of his pains and he agreed. His answer to the problem was to begin to sketch out the plans for adapting his chair using a water filled cushion, pipes and I think controlling the temperature of the water! I don't know whether he ever got around to making anything. We just suggested he spent less time in the chair!*

Anthony Strong saw the resulting massaging chair and tried it out! *I visited Godfrey at his house and he demonstrated a pneumatically driven massaging machine he had invented to relieve the pain he got in his legs. It consisted on a number of rubber tubes and levers which he sat on. I tried it and found it a rather alarming contraption.*

During his retirement, Godfrey contributed enthusiastically to work on magnetic resonance imaging of the heart at the Royal Brompton Hospital. He usually went there on Wednesdays, and worked with David Firmin: *He was continuously thinking and questioning [...] he thought differently. He would always take everything back to absolute basics, so you'd have something that you would just take as read from what you had been taught, and of course Godfrey wouldn't believe it. He would want to go back to basics and work it all out in his own way. He spoke in a different language, so we would have these conversations, he would talk in terms of, you know, rotation, phase rotation. He would always go clockwise while we would think anticlockwise, and everything would be the other way round. And terminology: he wouldn't talk about excitation, he would call it something else. So his terminology was very different and that made it hard work.*

Jenny Keegan was part of the same team: *Godfrey was just remarkably persistent so there was no idea of time or getting to the end, he would just keep going, keep going, keep going.*

David Firmin continues, *We have still got the same problem with magnetic resonance, which is motion correction, and he was really interested in trying to solve it. All of his time here was spent trying to come up with different ideas to solve motion problems.*

He drew out how it all works in the way he thinks: phase encoding and slice selection and everything else. But because of the way the slice was

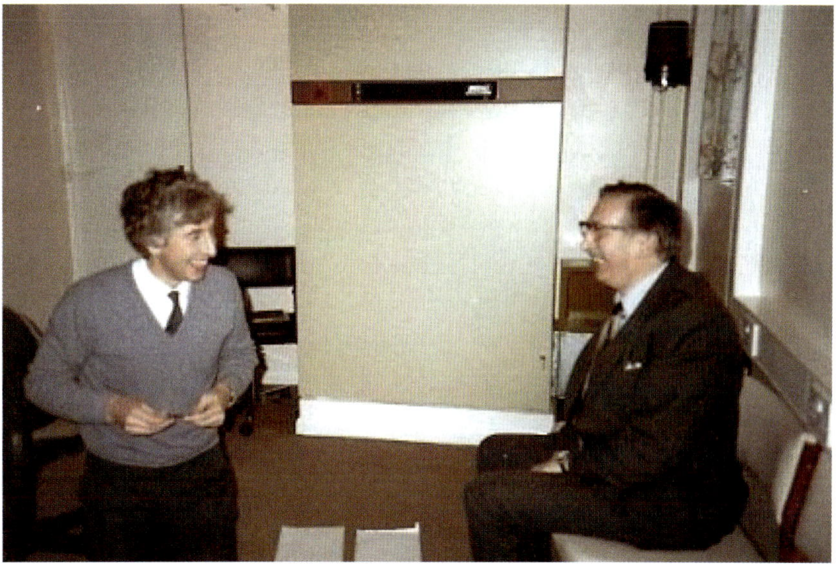

David Firmin and Godfrey
(Courtesy of Lizzy Burman)

formed, on this particular diagram, the person had to be upside down! Anyone else drawing this picture would have put the person the right way up. I'm sure he was correct that the way it worked out this person had to be upside down to get the image the right way.

He wrote a programme on an Archimedes computer (an early alternative to an IBM PC) and this took about two hours to run. He took the data home from here, and he used to set his alarm clock through the night to wake up when the programme was going to be finished to keep it going. This was how persistent he was [...] we found it amazing.

We used to get lunch from Waitrose, always the prawn sandwich with Marie Rose dressing. When they didn't have it, it was a real problem, we stood there for about 10 minutes trying to work out what he was going to have. I remember him telling me once on the way to Waitrose 'I could have married you know'. In practice I don't think he could, I don't think any woman could have coped. I don't think he would be able to concentrate on the marriage very much.

Lizzy Burman was a nurse at Brompton Hospital and has happy memories of Godfrey. While David and Lizzy shared an office, *David said 'Godfrey that is absolutely impossible, that's rubbish' and Godfrey burst out laughing. I said 'you can't say that to Godfrey' but he found it hysterically funny! He liked David challenging him and saying he was wrong. It was a kind of banter which I loved to watch, and he had such a hearty laugh.*

It was on the table for ages with coffee cup stains and the task of restoring it fell to me, but when it was finished it was very hard to persuade him to sign this beautiful masterpiece.

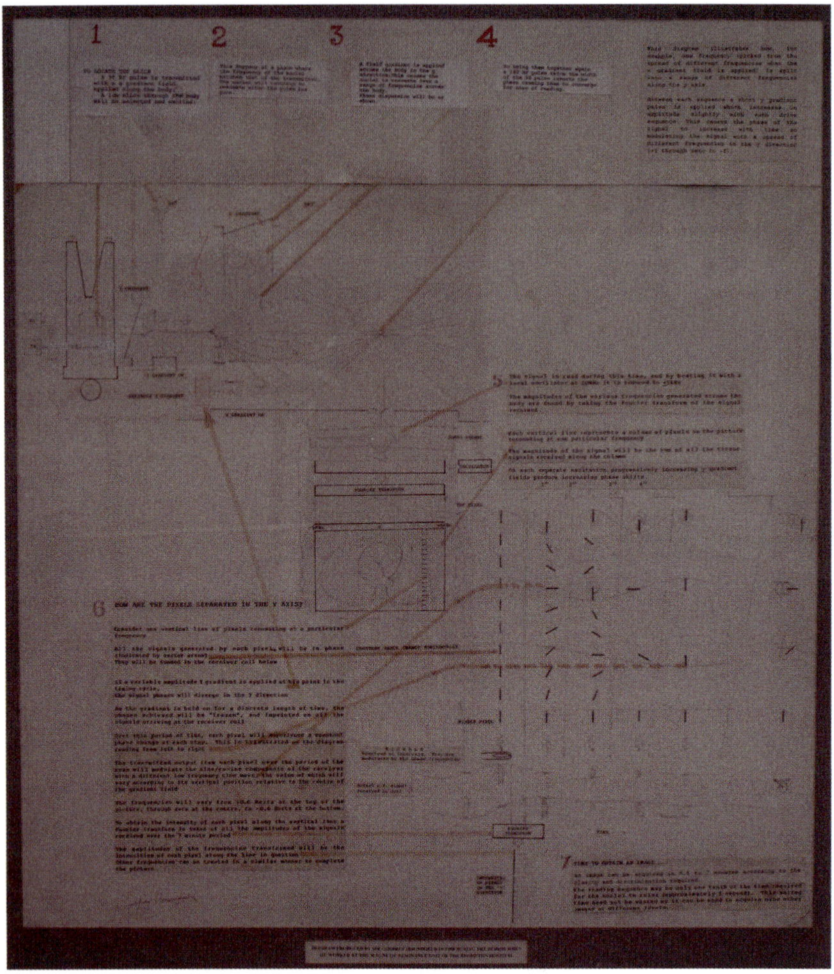

Description of MRI by Godfrey
(Courtesy of Liz Beckmann)
This is on display at the Royal Brompton Hospital.

He was a humble, self-effacing, seemingly ordinary sort of person. He was a kind man rather like a grandfather. No one called him Sir Godfrey, just Godfrey. He came to Brompton for nearly twenty years, from about 1984. He would often talk to me, maybe because I wasn't a scientist, and he was just like an ordinary person. At an event in Birmingham where he was manning a stall, he said 'come and talk to me'. I said 'people are waiting to see you, and they look important'. 'Oh just let them wait' he said, it was really nice of him.

You could never leave anything around: I left my lunch box out and the next day there were holes drilled through the sides and a tube running through it, it was one of their phantoms! [A "phantom" is used in place of the patient when testing scanners.] *They made such a mess and I often had to move their phantoms out of the way before I could use the scanner.*

If I had left a patient in the scanner before their tests they would not have been best pleased!

On Valentine's Day we were in the kitchen making coffee and I said 'Godfrey where is my big padded card and my flowers and chocolates?' As quick as anything he said 'they're in the post'.

He had this dreadful car, a brown Toyota. You'd think he was driving a brand new 6 Litre Bentley, the way he very carefully edged out of the drive in that old rust bucket. It was always breaking down. He used to come to the unit on a Wednesday, and the phone rang and it was Godfrey 'I'm in a fire station and I have broken down, I wonder if you can come and jump-start me?' A few Wednesdays later he was on the phone again 'I'm in a spot of bother I'm broken down and I'm facing the wrong way down a one way street.' 'Oh Godfrey that sounds terrible, no doubt you've got the whole of the rush hour traffic backed up behind you!' but I don't remember him getting particularly uptight at the honking of irate drivers. The good thing was that I'd be facing the right way to jump start his car! I asked one of the doctors to come with me as moral support, and in case I needed some muscle to move Godfrey's car.

We were worried about Godfrey at one stage: he didn't feel well and had a headache and it went on for weeks. It transpired that he had made an enormous pot of stew and re-heated it every evening for about two weeks it to save cooking every night. He had given himself food poisoning!

Our Christmas party started about 11 o'clock with cake and mince pies, nibbles and cocktails about 12, and one of the doctors made such lethal cocktails that by the time I served lunch people probably weren't bothered if I had burned the turkey!

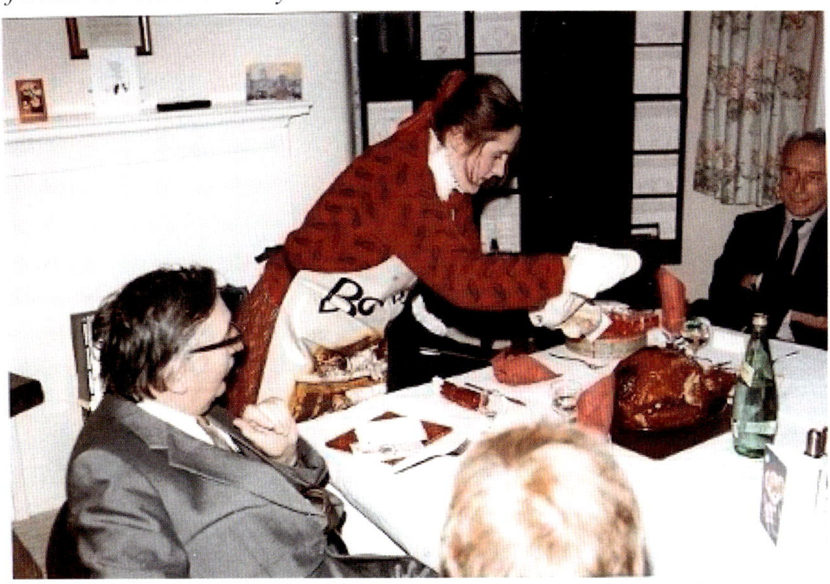

Christmas 1985: Godfrey, Lizzy Burman, and John Plant
(Courtesy of Lizzy Burman)

No one quite understood his mind scientifically or on a personal level but Godfrey was a hundred percent genuine and what you saw was what you got, he had no hidden agendas.

Someone was giving a lecture and said 'Sir Godfrey Hounsfield is in the audience' and listed a whole load of things that Godfrey had done. I have never seen Godfrey cross before, but he popped up like a jack-in-a-box in the middle of the talk and said I did not do this! I looked at David and we just said 'Wow that's quite something – he would never take credit for a thing he hadn't done.'

Alexis Wiltshire met Godfrey at the MGR club. *I remember when we arranged a museum visit at Windsor Station (now full of designer shops) in about 1986. I had taken my sons then aged 14 and 15 and they were talking science and genetic engineering with Godfrey. We came across a glass cabinet with old Victorian items of clothing and underwear – bloomers, thick lisle stockings and liberty bodice etc. Godfrey didn't know what a Liberty Bodice was so I had to explain to him that it was an undergarment with rubber buttons used instead of a brassier to keep the wearer warm. He was very intrigued and continued to ask about the various pieces of underwear on display.*

He had such a wonderful innocence about him even though he had such magnificent brain. One of my sons went on to study Genetic Engineering and Bio Technology at Swansea University. Godfrey was a lovely man and greatly missed.

In October 1991, Godfrey and Bill Ingham were asked by William Cavendish to take part in a filmed interview. This was at the suggestion of Sir Joseph Lockwood, who had recently died, leaving William as his executor. William explains Sir Joseph's motive at the beginning of the film: *Sir Joseph Lockwood, who I worked for, was chairman of Electric and Musical Industries (EMI) for twenty years from 1954 to 1974. Many years later looking back on the success of the company, he felt it could be attributed directly to three great inventions: the gramophone, invented by Berliner, which formed the Gramophone Company from which EMI developed, secondly, television which was developed in EMI's Central Research Laboratories in the 1930s under Sir Isaac Shoenberg's direction by a team including Blumlein, and thirdly the brain scanner invented by Sir Godfrey Hounsfield in the same research laboratories in Sir Joseph's time as chairman.*

The gramophone is sometimes credited to Edison and television to Baird and that worried Sir Joseph, that people should still be misinformed. In the case of Hounsfield no one could take away his great achievement because he has been honoured with a Nobel Prize and a knighthood. Nevertheless Sir Joseph felt that as he was a modest retiring person, that his achievement may be taken away from him unless it was stamped indelibly, and that is the purpose of this film.

The resulting film is a valuable part of the historical record, and extracts from it have been quoted in this book wherever they fit into the story. The participants agreed in advance that the film should be a true picture of the history, which diverged somewhat from previously published versions. Bill Ingham arrived for the filming with detailed notes that he could use in his role as an informal interviewer, and also as an important participant in the birth of the CT scanner in his own right. Godfrey was not so well-prepared, and the film shows that he really only warmed up after lunch and its associated glass of sherry or wine. Several topics that had been filmed in the morning were reshot after lunch, usually with better results. At the end of the afternoon the film crew departed, and all that was left to do was the editing.

The editing hit a snag. The transcripts and a videotape arrived, and William sent copies to Bill and Godfrey asking for their views on how to edit the film. Godfrey replied with an annotated version of the transcript, but this gave William a knotty problem. Godfrey suggested some changes in the words that he had used, which would have been easy to do if the end result was going to be a written transcript. But Godfrey had overlooked the fact that he was suggesting changes that actually required him and Bill to put on the same clothes, go and sit in the same room in the same chairs, and be filmed again according to the revised script that he was now proposing. This was rather a lot of work, but on the other hand the film was being made to record Godfrey's work, so his views on its content were important. It was a dilemma: the editing paused, and the issue was not resolved until John Ryan completed it in 2006.

Godfrey's copy of the videotape turned up after his death, and John became involved in editing it into a set of video clips, which were shown at lunch at the Royal Society after Godfrey's memorial service at St Clement Dane's church on 25 May 2005. Sadly, William was not present because at that stage his contact details were unknown to the organisers, but contact was established soon afterwards. William asked if John might be interested in completing the editing process, which John volunteered to do, helped by his wife Chip who retyped the annotated transcript. At this stage, of course, it was impossible to film any of the sequences again. The task now was to edit the film in line with Godfrey's requests, as far as that was possible with the existing video footage, and with advice from Bill Ingham. After the editing was finished, William assigned the copyright to the BIR, so the film is now available as Sir Joseph wished, and it includes some good quotes from both Godfrey and Bill Ingham. It also includes the photos and freehand sketches that Godfrey had lent to William for use as illustrations in the film. This made Bill remember Godfrey watching the video in 1991 and saying, *I wish I had sat up straighter so that you could not see so much of my double chin!* (He was slightly overweight at the time.)

Godfrey acted as a consultant to Imatron, a company that developed ultra-fast CT scanners and that Dave King was involved with. Matt King remembers his father saying that *all he ever did was filter Godfrey's ideas, 99% of which were barmy but 1% of which were sheer genius.* This is typical of Godfrey: he had a lot of ideas, and talked about them until they were shot down or survived. Matt remembers, *riding a tandem bicycle around Kew Gardens with him and my mother-in-law, and Godfrey telling me that I should forget physics and go into genetic engineering!*

Andrew Hounsfield has some stories about Godfrey's attitude to money: *He did some work in America for some company, I can't remember the name of the company, and rather than being paid for it he was given a share option which he stuffed in a draw and forgot about. Father* [Godfrey's brother Michael] *was down in Twickenham helping him to sort out his papers and came across this share option: I think it was worth two million pounds, and it had just run out! But it didn't worry Godfrey, he didn't worry about money at all. In the mid 1970s he was offered seven figure salaries to work for competitors of EMI in the USA, but he wasn't interested. I thought he was absolutely mad not to take it, but if he had enough money he didn't care.*

Jean Waltham found an exchange of letters while she was sorting through Godfrey's photos and documents at Andrew Hounsfield's house. *There was a letter from a man who had written to ask Godfrey's permission to leave some money to him in his Testament – I suppose that he meant his Will. He wanted to leave money to Godfrey. Next there was a rather grumpy letter from the same person, saying that some time ago he had written this letter and had had no reply. He was surprised and disappointed, but the offer still stood and he would like Godfrey's permission to do this. Then there was a page with various scribbled notes as Godfrey composed a reply. Then a typed letter saying sorry to be late in replying but your letter had been sent to the wrong building. Thank you very much for the very kind thought, but I am now retired and do not need the money. It would be much better if the money went to a more deserving cause. 'If I might make a suggestion, genetic research into cancer.'*

Godfrey grew interested in ball lightning in the early 1990s, as Ian Green remembers. *I had been working with low pressure gas plasmas for lighting. Even under quite favourable conditions, the plasma decays within a few milliseconds without an external energy input. Small amounts of oxygen greatly speed up the decay, as does an increase in gas pressure. So you can imagine how hard it is to maintain a plasma in air at atmospheric pressure.*

The only mention I had seen of air plasmas came from a fascinating Russian paper written in the 1940s. A huge amount of energy was coupled into a low pressure discharge inside a glass capsule, and when the capsule broke the discharge continued in the surrounding air. It produced a brown gas, which would have been nitrogen dioxide due to the high energies involved. The same paper made the fanciful suggestion that they could see their way to striking plasmas at a distance of a kilometre, which was no doubt a way of getting funding from Stalin, but that's by the by.

Anyway, Godfrey would come into the office, saying that he thought that ball lighting might be a form of plasma, and ask my opinion on the matter.

I would say that the path of a lighting strike is indeed a plasma, but that from all I knew of the physics it should decay very rapidly indeed. Then there was the question of the movement of ball lighting. A plasma consists of gas ions and electrons, so should move with the surrounding gas, whereas what I had read of ball lighting in the popular press suggested that it could move through walls, sit on the wing tips of aeroplanes, and so on. Even if many of the descriptions were mistaken, it did seem to be a phenomenon that didn't just follow the air flow.

Perhaps the most puzzling aspect was that the reports described a ball of localised energy that didn't spread out, and didn't decay for at least a few seconds, and no physics that I knew could even vaguely account for it.

So we would have this conversation, and a week later he would come back with what seemed to me exactly the same question. I suppose that if I had had an inkling of a solution, Godfrey would eventually have got it out of me. Except I hadn't.

It was typical of Godfrey to just keep "leaning" on a problem for weeks, and to keep thinking about it long after others might give up. Often he was on the wrong track, but sometimes he produced excellent results. Perhaps he had an inkling of the solution, and was trying to get it out of himself? Ian was a good person to talk to, because he knew a lot about plasmas. The fact that Godfrey came back a week later with the same questions fits with his patchy memory. Perhaps he was imposing his own way of thinking on Ian, but the load on Ian was not as heavy as the load that Godfrey imposed on himself. This is all speculation, but certainly he liked to discuss his ideas, and would do so with anyone who seemed interested, or who did not actually walk away.

Godfrey mentioned two other subjects on which he was working when chatting to Alastair Sibbald in the research labs in Hayes: *He went on a*

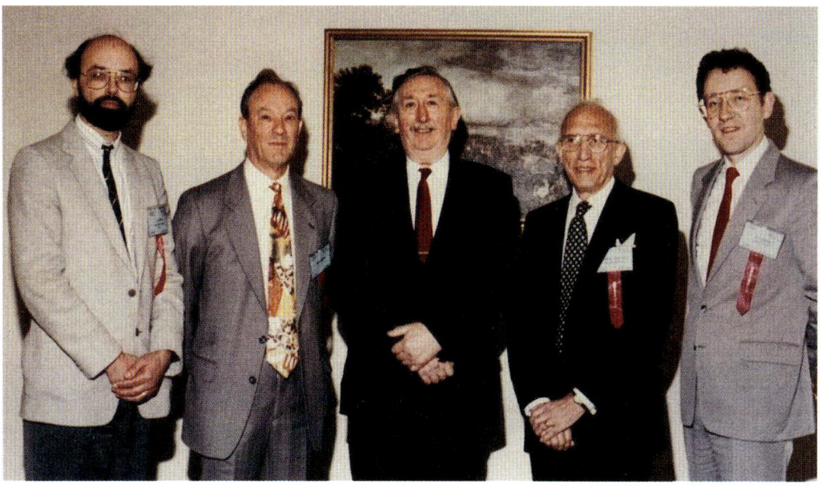

Twenty-first year of CT: Steve Webb, Gordon Higson, Godfrey, Ian Isherwood, and Stephen Golding at the 1993 BIR Congress
(Copyright RAD Magazine)

short course somewhere in Oxford about DNA amplification processes and chemistry, and he was interested in what might be achieved in this area. He was keen to help his sister, who was becoming increasingly deaf, especially at higher frequencies, and had the idea that if you could detect sibilants ('s'-sounding sounds), and then convert them to sounds at a lower frequency, then this might allow a person to detect the 's' sounds again, making speech more intelligible.

Lynda Hounsfield says, *Joan, Godfrey and Dad used to go to Oxford, to the university, and go to seminars on space and astronomy, and they used to spend a lot of time doing that together. They used to do that at least once or twice a year, the three of them. Dad and Godfrey went to Mexico, and all over on holiday together, this was the time after Dad lost Mum.* [During the 1990s.] *They went on cruises and they went over to study the Aztec and the pyramids over there, and they went to Russia together and they had a lot of fun.*

I remember having problems with my water pipes for the horses. We talked through all the things it could be, and he was absolutely right! They are metal pipes, and the nitrates in the water had helped to cause a chemical reaction with the pipes, which had turned the nitrates into nitrites and was poisoning the horses. He was the one who helped me to sort it out.

He met an old friend at the Röntgen Centenary exhibition at Birmingham, UK, in 1995.

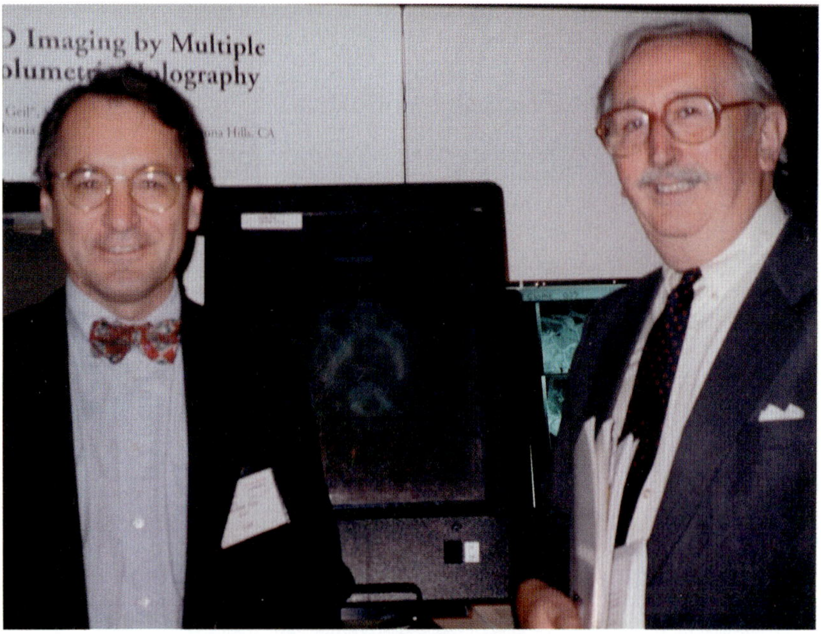

Raymond and Godfrey
(Courtesy of Raymond Schulz)

Raymond Schulz had worked with Godfrey on the 7070 scanner eighteen years before, and they recognised each other: *Godfrey was walking by and of course I engaged him in a conversation. He remembered me and was intrigued with our technology, Digital Holography and it's application in CT and MR imaging. I won the prize for the best scientific exhibit.*

A different example of Godfrey's curiosity and eagerness to get involved in new things comes from Ian Dadley of the MGR social club, who says, *Godfrey rang me up one day, probably about 1996. He was going to Poppham and he asked me if I'd like to come, and I said yes. So we got to this place where they were flying microlights, and off we went, taking it in turns to fly up to about 5000 feet, hanging next to an experienced person, with nothing between us and the ground. Farm tractors looked about the size a box of Swan Vesta matches! Godfrey enjoyed it tremendously: he was just like a schoolboy.* This was quite an adventure, as Godfrey was about age 75.

He gave a lecture about black holes at an MGR meeting in a member's house in Maidenhead, I sat through it but it went completely over my head, like casting pearls before swine.

He told me that while he was walking in Crane Park, near his home, he was surrounded by half a dozen hooligans who were threatening him. He didn't run away, he just faced them quietly and they didn't do anything, they just went away.

Sally Radford says, *Two or three years before he died we were at a pub I asked him 'what are you up to Godfrey'. He said 'We are working on a 3D camera to be used in keyhole surgery. Do you know, I've got so many young people working with me in my lab, and they are so inspirational to work with.' I thought: how wonderful that a man who is so accomplished, and absolutely at the top his field, can look on young people in that way, whereas other older people sometimes act as if young people are a waste of space.*

I was very fond of Godfrey. When my two sons were small I was on an outing to Clivden with the MGR group. There were huge carp in the lake. Godfrey lay on his front and showed my boys how to dangle blades of grass in the water to tempt the fish. He pulled a big carp up out of the water with the grass! He was a big kid himself in some ways.

In 1992 and 2002, Godfrey was again involved in filmed interviews about his work on CT scanning, which were broadcast in the BBC2 programmes "Great British Inventions" and "EMI and me". The authors have placed copies (derived from contemporary recordings on videotape) at the Royal Society and BIR, just in case the BBC archives are lost. The 1992 programme included Gordon Higson, Godfrey, Sir John Read, and Walter Robb. The focus was mainly on what EMI could have done better, with the benefit of hindsight. This is the only video footage of Gordon Higson that the authors are aware of, so the film is interesting for that, as well as for the quotes that are included in this book at the appropriate places. The 2002 programme included Bill Ingham and Sir John Read, with a little about the scanner and a lot more about EMI Music.

Godfrey's eightieth birthday was in 1999, and Jeannette Lemon was at the party. *We booked a boat on the river at Hungerford for his birthday. We did a supper on this boat, about 50 of us, and he had no idea what he was coming to and was very surprised to see the balloons, and there was marvellous conversation on that evening.* Alexis Wiltshire adds, *He was kept away from the boat yard so that we could decorate the boat. We hung up a large banner saying Happy 80th Birthday. When he arrived we all sang Happy Birthday and he joined in. Then he asked whose birthday was it. He hadn't realised it was his!* Iris Glass recalls a birthday in a different year, when IVC members surprised Godfrey by saying *Happy Birthday!*, and he whispered to her, *How do they know?*, to which she replied, *It is printed in today's Daily Telegraph!*

Monica Leggett lived next door to Godfrey for many years. When she did not have a computer Godfrey invited her to use his. She often visited to use email on his "laboratory" computer, or to have a chat, and frequently for both of these reasons. She says, *Every time we had a gathering, you know, family or friends, we always invited Godfrey and he always came. He was very sociable and very pleasant, he was delightful. He'd put his hand out and say 'My name's Godfrey and I live next door.' People would say 'What a lovely chap, who is he?' and be very surprised when I told them. Everyone in the road still thinks of it as Godfrey's house although the new people there are very pleasant. He was very welcoming, I sometimes said 'I must not chat too long' but he said that he liked talking. We had a street party, we had all been living here for about 25 years, and he said 'Now come along, let's have a dance'. He was actually quite a good dancer, you can't imagine it but he was!*

David Stanbury knew Godfrey through the MGR club, and he recalls, *Godfrey was such a lovely chap, and very humble. He liked to go on long walks. On one of the walks we were chatting to one another and I asked him 'What are you doing this evening?' and he said he was going to the pub night. Well the pub happened to be just opposite where I live. So I asked him what he was going to do in between – about three hours – and he said 'Well, I'll just sit in the car'. I said 'no you're not, you come home with me, I've made a casserole: come and eat with me'. I had made the casserole that morning, and there was more than enough for two. So we're sitting eating and chatting, a Nobel Prize winner, a man of great distinction, and he said 'this is nice David, I couldn't do anything like this', and I said 'well, I couldn't invent an EMI-scanner!' He would come out with little things like that: he was very humble. Once when I was chairman I introduced him as Sir Godfrey and he said 'please don't ever say that, just say Godfrey': little things like that represent the man that he was: very modest and a lovely chap, very nice. Godfrey organised some of the visits to country houses. We went to Highclere Abbey, near Newbury, where they have Egyptian artefacts and where Downton Abbey was filmed later, and had a pub lunch and then visited the gardens, although the house was closed for some reason.*

Liz Beckmann went to Manchester with her late partner Neil Ridyard and Godfrey in 2002: *Neil was driving, Godfrey was sitting next to him and I was sitting in the back of the car thinking how can Neil be arguing avidly with a Nobel Prize winner for three hours there and three hours back? We were going to one of the big hotels where the meeting was the BIR AGM, and they had booked Godfrey a room in this 4 or 5 star hotel. When we spoke to Godfrey about the trip he asked where we were staying and we said in a Travelodge, and Godfrey said 'oh I'll come and stay with you then' because he wanted to be with people he would know.*

Early in 2003 he went to see his doctor because he was increasingly breathless. He was diagnosed with fibrosis, was told it was incurable, and that if he wanted to know any more he should look on the internet. This sounds very abrupt, and it may have been said more sympathetically than it sounds. If not, it was a pity that anyone should be treated that way, even if they had not made such a great contribution to medicine, and indeed to the funds of the Department of Health. Godfrey gradually became more unwell and depressed.

Richard Waltham recalls, *in April 2003 Dave King alerted me to the fact that our old friend Godfrey was unwell. Dave was unwell himself throughout this period, and sadly died in April 2004, but he was very keen to support Godfrey in spite of his own illness and of being based in Florida, many thousands of miles away. I noticed at the time that he signed his emails 'David;' but it wasn't until I read his obituary in The Independent that I learnt that the semi-colon at the end of his signature was dark humour for the fact that cancer had taken half of his colon, and it was, although he did not yet know it, en route to his liver.*

Dave persuaded me to visit Godfrey at home and I turned up unannounced because I knew that he would decline any offer to visit if I phoned first. So I called him from my mobile phone, while standing in Crane Park Road. He said that he didn't feel up to seeing me, but we chatted for a while about Dave and other topics from the past. Then he said 'John wants to speak to you' and this was John Roburn, who said 'Godfrey may not want to see you but I do' and he came out of the house to have a chat with me in the road outside. Thus I met John, who was worried about what to do for Godfrey, and we exchanged phone numbers. John went back into the house to ask again if Godfrey would have a brief word with me, and he agreed.

Godfrey lived in an ordinary suburban house which was pleasant, comfortable, and considerably tidier than his office at work. He had a cleaning lady who visited once or twice a week and helped him with anything which he was finding difficult. The house had a through-lounge which looked out on the street on the front and a garden and parkland behind. He chose it because he could walk in the park, which had a river running through it. His piano was in the lounge, along with books, pictures and all the usual things.

An April 2003 email from Dave King said, *He is of course terribly private and I think I may be one of the few people that have ever crossed the threshold, let alone stayed the night there!*

This form of lung disease has no cure, but is frequently quite responsive to steroids. Godfrey, rightly, is spooked by this powerful drug with all its attendant problems – but at this stage I think it may give him some real relief. He may have to go on oxygen otherwise – and at that stage I am not sure that he will be able to continue looking after himself. All very depressing. I must say that having gone through a fairly major scare myself, I start looking at others who are less fortunate through somewhat different eyes. His primary pain is violent headaches which he has experienced on and off for many years – greatly aggravated by any coughing.

Thanks so much for jumping on this. I feel a very long way away – although if there was a crisis I could and would be there in a few hours (and Godfrey knows that).

Over the next two months Godfrey went through a very difficult period, trying to fight on many fronts: infections in his kidneys and urinary tract, pneumonia on top of his underlying lung problem, polymyalgia rheumatica, serious depression, and a gradual acceptance that he was not going to be able to manage at home at Crane Park. He started to talk about Dignitas, which was a clear signal of how bad he was feeling. Dave and Richard recruited other ex-colleagues such as Reg Willard, Mac Gollifer, Ken Charles, Tony Williams, and Stephen Bates into an informal "support group" to phone or visit and try to cheer him up, but it did not make much difference. His family, friends, and neighbours were all working along similar lines, but everyone faced the same difficulties. For example, Godfrey's dogged determination meant that if he made his mind up not to take a particular medicine it could be difficult to convince him to do so. There was nothing to be done beyond talking things through with him, trying to lift his spirits, and letting him make his own decisions in his own time.

He spent some time in hospital in Kingston and he had CT scans at Brompton Hospital, where he knew and trusted the consultant. The CT scan showed that Godfrey had more lung left than the "postage stamp" that he previously imagined. He had sixty-two per cent of his lung, and it is good to think that his own invention helped to cheer him up a bit, although the underlying illness remained progressive and incurable. In June he moved into Arbrook House care home in Esher: a pleasant place with a large garden, and Godfrey's room had French windows leading directly outside. The depression lifted and he gradually recovered enough strength to get out into the garden, and to join the other residents at the regular sherry parties on Tuesday mornings.

He was still the same: he took a scientific interest in how his legs were recovering after a long time in bed. He found a length of wire that he converted into a tape measure. He calibrated this against the length of his shoe, which according to him was exactly twelve inches. Using this improvised tape measure he could keep track of how his thigh muscles were growing back. He could easily have asked someone to bring in a tape measure, but he enjoyed making his own.

Richard Waltham says, *on 10th June I picked up Reg Willard in Hayes and took him over to Esher to see Godfrey. Reg was about as old as Godfrey, and a longstanding friend and colleague. He could still drive himself for short distances, but driving to Esher was beyond him. When we arrived we found that Godfrey was settling in well and the staff were clearly getting to know him. He could take a few steps with a zimmer frame, if he was first lifted out of bed by a miniature crane. He was feeling a bit sorry for himself, so Reg told him that he looked pretty fit, and he should pull himself together and do as much exercise as possible. Hard work is the answer, not curling up in comfort! Reg was never one to mince his words, but Godfrey seemed to have expected Reg to say something like this, and I think he took more notice of Reg than the opinion of someone who did not yet feel the pains of old age, or someone who spoke more tactfully. Reg calling for hard work may have been like a seed falling on fertile ground, and perhaps that idea stayed and grew in Godfrey's mind.*

Reg handed Godfrey some letters which had arrived for him at CRL, and one of these was from a boy in Africa asking for money. Godfrey was not surprised, so I guess he received many such letters as a result of his name and awards being easy to find on the internet. He could not decide what to do with this letter, and he asked us to write 'begging boy' on it and put it on his growing pending pile. Reg was in no doubt: the letter was most likely a scam, from someone who was neither a child nor poor, and in any case Godfrey was going to need his money to look after himself. I'm not sure what to make of this: in the 1970s Godfrey often mentioned the letters of thanks, but I was unaware of the begging letters or that they continued long after the thanks had tailed off. It seemed strange that Godfrey didn't have a set way of dealing with them, but perhaps it related to his tendency to always reinvent, rather than to stick to previous paths.

In July he had a fall which did not injure him, but he could not get up while waiting for help to arrive. He could roll from his back onto his side but then could not get his arm out from under his body to push himself up. This set him thinking of a gadget that could be inflated to lift him enough to free his arm. This was an excellent thing to keep his mind occupied, and visitors were now likely to be asked if they could produce an air-inflatable panel about eight inches square and able to inflate to give about three inches of lift, or to discuss other solutions to the problem.

The irrepressible inventor was back to his old ways, but at age eighty-three, in poor health, and in a care home. By August he was able to make visits home to Crane Park, being driven there by John Roburn, with some hope of being able to return there to live and to be able to drive a car himself again.

Looking back reflectively at this point we can take stock of Godfrey's life so far, which includes several paradoxes:

- He failed to gain any qualifications at school, and his diploma was neither mathematical nor related to electronic signal processing. Yet he made breakthroughs in both computing and CT scanning, in which electronics and mathematics played a significant role.
- He was largely self-taught and hated public speaking, yet he felt it important to try to encourage the next generation to follow a career in science or engineering.
- He was a mild-mannered and peaceful person, yet his time in the RAF was a turning point in his life and the assistance that Air Vice-Marshal Cassidy gave him was exceptionally important.
- He was not domineering or ambitious, or skilled in the internal company politics that is usually needed to get funding, nor was he keen to manage a department. Instead he got things done by inspiring loyalty and trust from his colleagues and collaborators, who admired his hard work, and who wanted to follow him on interesting and exciting new paths.
- He avoided the limelight yet he gained the highest awards in science. But still he felt that he had not done enough. He said, *I did that work several years ago, I haven't done anything very noteworthy lately,* and after he had "retired" he set his alarm clock to wake him every two hours through the night so that he could keep his experiments going as fast as possible.
- He never married although he wistfully regretted this. He was exceptionally dedicated to his work, and to helping science to make the world a better place. Yet he was not the archetypal scientific bachelor. He enjoyed the company of women and children, and they liked him. Even when almost every other waking hour was filled with work, he placed a high priority on attending social occasions.
- He could be very absent minded and forgetful, yet he never forgot what he was trying to do. His persistence and determination were amongst the most important contributors to his genius. He is one of the strongest examples of the fact that anyone can have an idea, but only a genius can put in all of the hard work to bring it to fruition.
- He was not very interested in money, yet he developed the CT scanner at zero cost to his employer, and the development funds were about half the price of a single CT scanner! He had a remarkable talent for improvisation and economy.
- Godfrey and his employer were not experts in medicine, yet they launched not just a new product, but a whole new era in medical imaging, and a whole new industry.
- Countless grateful patients wrote to Godfrey thanking him for inventing equipment that had saved their lives. Some thanked him

for saving them from risky and painful examinations. Yet his own invention did not save Godfrey from the violent migraines from which he suffered throughout his life.

- And finally there was his car. How could anyone with such mechanical aptitude have so many bizarre motoring episodes? Who else would leave his car unlocked with the engine running while he took a three-hour boat trip on the river Thames? Who else would deliberately run their car with no water in the radiator?

Godfrey would not have taken stock in this way. He always preferred to look forwards, not back, although he was now an old man.

A 28 August 2003 email from Dave King said:

GNH's 84th

I just spoke to Godfrey who was surprised and pleased to get 'royal' greetings from the USA for his birthday. He said he wasn't up to going out to the pub, but that at the home they had given him a cake, albeit with only one candle on it! I think that any attempt to blow out 84 of them might have singed his moustache! David;

Dave King kept finding one or two more old photos and posting them to Godfrey, and phoning him regularly from Florida, in spite of the fact that Dave was now being badly mauled by the chemotherapy for liver cancer. He continued phoning almost until his death on 24 April 2004. Bruce Friedman and others raised funds for memorials to Dave at both Nottingham University in the UK where he studied, and at the Mayo Clinic where he installed the first EMI-scanner in the USA. This was a tribute to Dave's work for over twenty years on coronary heart imaging to enable early detection of heart disease, and of course Godfrey wanted to contribute to this memorial fund.

Keena Millar and the staff at Arbrook House remember Godfrey very well (and that he loved mince pies). *During his stay one of our ladies died, and she had loved the home. In her Will she left some money for improving the home for the enjoyment of the residents. As the Manager I did not get involved, but a couple of residents, relatives and our Activities Organiser decided what the money was to be spent on. Sir Godfrey was on this committee and suggested that we extend the garden path closer to the lake by running it deeper into the wood. Sadly he died before it was finished. We had a grand opening for the path, and a sign post 'Sir Godfrey's Walk'.*

In his enthusiasm for improving the world, and his attitude that there was nothing which could not be done, he was an inspiration to us all.

Godfrey got gradually less well through the summer of 2004, but was still able to walk (with difficulty) when Reg and Richard visited him in Arbrook House on 15 July. Soon after that he went into New Victoria Hospital, in Kingston, where he was breathing oxygen and sleeping most of the time. He died on 12 August.

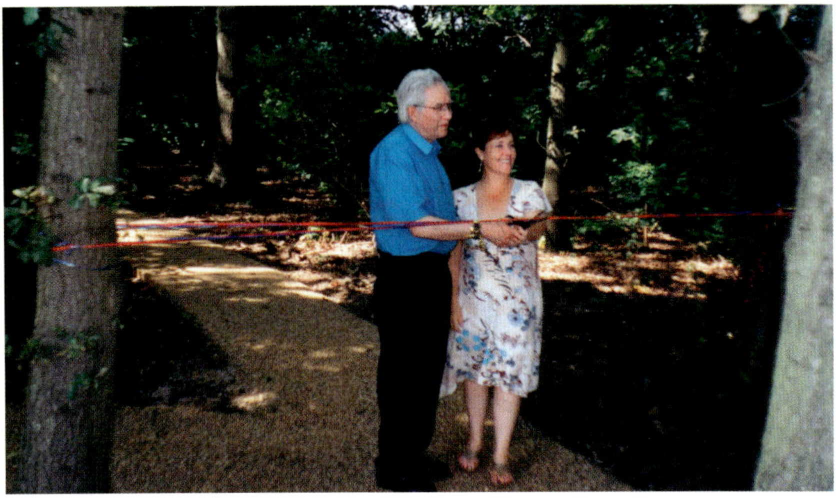

The opening of Sir Godfrey's walk at Arbrook House
(Courtesy of Keena Millar)

Ken Charles sent a message from California, which Andrew Hounsfield read out at Godfrey's funeral: *I am so sorry to hear about Godfrey. He was the nicest and most genuinely good person you could ever hope to meet. It is rare to have met and worked with someone who was so creative and knowledgeable but who had so little interest in power, position or possessions. I feel very privileged to have known him and he was an inspiration to everyone he worked with. The world is a poorer place for his loss.*

The last words should be left to John Roburn, who did so much to help Godfrey in the eighteen months before his death. At the funeral, John said, *I am not going to talk about Sir Godfrey Hounsfield as the brilliant scientist, whose work did so much to save lives and reduce suffering, and received world-wide recognition. Instead, I should like to say a few words about the man whom I knew as a friend.*

I first met Godfrey 42 years ago on a skiing holiday. I had a heavy cold and he had some other health problem, so that for three days, while the rest of the party went skiing, we both stayed in the attic of a Swiss chalet. Luckily we both recovered in time to get in a few days of skiing before returning home.

For many years afterwards we used to meet on country walks, mainly in Surrey and Hampshire, and on group sightseeing weekends all over England. Those weekends were enjoyable social occasions, but their main purpose was to visit cathedrals, country churches, castles, gardens and stately homes. Not everything went always according to plan. One amusing incident was when Godfrey's car got stuck in a ford. I was not there, but I remember seeing a photograph of him and his passengers with rolled up trousers trying to push the car out of the river. On other occasions his car found its way to places not on the arranged itinerary, but no doubt of considerable scientific interest!

About 15 years ago we started going together on fairly long walks usually exploring the Surrey countryside, observing what was around us and talking about science and other things. More recently and until his illness those walks became shorter and less ambitious, sometimes in small nearby commons or more often in the big parks that we are fortunate to have in the SW London area.

Godfrey's house backed on to a long and narrow park along the River Crane where he used to jog or walk nearly every morning. He was well informed about its history, especially that of the gun powder factory which used to be there and traces of which still remain.

He liked visiting gardens, especially when in full flower and he introduced me and other people to the beautiful Savill and Valley gardens near Windsor Park.

Godfrey was fond of music. He taught himself to play the piano and sometimes relaxed playing it. Though not interested in art, he had some artistic ability and I have seen a few of his imaginative drawings, which showed his slightly mischievous sense of humour.

His main interests were in science and engineering. He could identify any machine or other mechanical device and explain how they worked, often suggesting possible improvements. He was also interested in industrial archaeology and astronomy. Until his illness he kept well informed about all these subjects and whenever I mentioned what I thought was a new development or discovery it was not news to him.

He had a passionate belief in scientific progress and believed that it could be of great benefit to mankind, leading to a brighter future.

Like many prominent scientists Godfrey could be absent-minded and was known for usually being late, though he always did get there. Being a bachelor and not being bothered about his surroundings he lived for a long time in hostels and lodgings. When eventually he bought a house it was a suburban semi, where one room was occupied by computers and where, after retirement, he spent a lot of time writing programmes elaborating his scientific ideas.

He liked discussions and meeting people in an informal setting but disliked formal occasions.

He was very modest and tried to avoid the limelight. When asked what his job was he would usually say that it was in medical physics. Many people whom he met socially did not learn about his distinguished career and achievements for a long time, or even not at all.

Godfrey Hounsfield was a soft-spoken, kind and considerate person, very interesting to be with and very likeable, liked by all who met him. I feel privileged to have been his friend and to have been able to get to know him so well. I shall miss him greatly, as I am sure will all his friends.

Chapter 12
Historic documents

October 1968 project proposal
(Copyright EMI Music)

<u>Proposed Project:</u>

AN
IMPROVED FORM
OF
X-RADIOGRAPHY

RESEARCH — Electric & Musical Industries Ltd

1967

RESEARCH LABORATORIES OF ELECTRIC & MUSICAL INDUSTRIES, LTD.,
HAYES, MIDDLESEX.

PROPOSED PROJECT: AN IMPROVED FORM OF X-RADIOGRAPHY

1. INTRODUCTION

The purpose of the study is to investigate the employment of a computer to make better use of the information obtained when an object is examined by gamma rays or X-rays.

It is well known that when an X-ray picture is taken through an object the three dimensional interior must be shown as a two dimentional picture. Hence all details from front to rear appear superimposed one upon another and a confused picture results; indeed, any 'submerged' ~~object~~ tissue usually has to be comparatively thick to be seen at all. As an illustration, if the object to be studied was one such as a book, normal methods of X-ray pictures would reveal little of the content, because the information on, say, a middle page could not be extracted from the confusion caused by all the other pages in front of and behind it. However, it is hoped that the system under investigation would be capable of extracting the information from one page (or slice) only, thus presenting a map of all the information contained in that slice only, irrespective of that on the pages on either side of it. This concept is illustrated in Figures 1 and 2 ~~on page~~ .

In Figure 1 the normal X-ray technique is shown producing a confused and fuzzy picture of all the objects in the path of the X-ray beam AB, whereas in Figure 2 the proposed system produces a clear outline of all submerged objects within the body.

- 1 -

- 2 -

2. DESCRIPTION OF THE SYSTEM

Figure 3 illustrates the scanning system. The object to be examined would be scanned in one plane only by a very narrow beam of gamma rays* emitted by source A not only linearly across the plane in a direction X, but at all angles as illustrated by the 2nd, 3rd, etc. scans.

The gamma rays* which penetrate the object would be detected by an accurately aligned collimator and sensing device, B, which would always be pointing towards the source of the gamma rays. The readings from the detector taken "round the edge" of the object would be digitised and fed to a computer for processing. If sufficient scans and angles of scan are made there should be enough information from the 'edge' readings in the detector to produce sufficient equations to calculate by computer the value of transmission of each cubic millimetre of material within the slice (i.e. there would be more equations than variables). A crude picture could, therefore, be built up in matrix form of the absorption of the material within the 'slice'.

* or any other rays used for diagnosis.

3. ADVANTAGES OVER THE CONVENTIONAL X-RAY EQUIPMENT IN THE MEDICAL FIELD

The principal application would be for detecting tumours and suchlike tissues which are likely to vary from a minimum of 1 cubic centimetre to a maximum of 60 cubic centimetres in volume. A high definition would therefore not be called for and it is accordingly possible to concentrate on accurate absorption readings.

The importance of this new system lies in the fact that the calculated absorption values are 100% due to the material constituting the tumour, whereas in the conventional X-ray picture they represent the mean absorption of all the material along the line of the penetrating rays (line AB in Figure 1) of which only a very small percentage will be due

In the first line, Godfrey has altered Figure 3 to Figure 2 in faint pencil. Godfrey hand wrote on the back of the previous page *If the slice is divided into a mesh of say 20 thousand 1mm cubes* with an arrow to insert those words in line 6 of paragraph 2 above.

to the tumour. This is very important since tumours may only absorb 5% more gamma rays or X-rays than the normal healthy tissue round them, and therefore higher accuracies of detection are very much in demand.

Further advantages of such a system would be:

(1) In general the system makes better use of available information which is presented in the form of more accurate absorption readings and an increased number of pictures for the same dose of radiation to the patient. The tones and detail of the picture would not be obscured as in normal X-ray pictures by other confusing information being printed on top (equivalent to, say, 40 superimposed pictures).

(2) Absolute values of absorption could be plotted accurately for each cubic centimetre of material within the slice (if necessary these could be plotted as numbers for comparison with each other). The 'contrast' of the picture could be arranged so that the full black to white range represents a window of very small ranges of absorption.

4. COMPARISON WITH TOMOGRAPHY

The following paragraphs describe how a simple comparison can be drawn between the proposed system and tomography, and indicate that it must be possible to obtain more information and better accuracy, for a given dosage, by means of the system proposed.

Figure 4A illustrates the usual movement of the plate and source in tomography. The line A B is on a row of elements through the slice to be viewed, which would be perpendicular to the paper. The shadow of these elements would be kept stationary on the photographic plate whereas areas at O and P would move and blur; and information concerning these areas is therefore lost. For convenience, the beam from the X-ray source is shown as a multiplicity of beams 1 cm in diameter and the elements to be measured 1 cm^3. If the body is 40 cm thick, then 1 cm^3 of material in the slice would influence only a small proportion of the X-rays arriving at the plate - approximately 3%; the rest of the rays arriving produce fogging or blurred images superimposed upon the picture.

It is possible to replace the plate with a series of detectors (at a, b, c ...) approximately 1 cm apart and to take readings at a number of angles (representing say 1 cm of movement of the source) as the source is rotated around the body. The sum of the readings on each detector during one partial rotation of the source would then produce a tomograph of AB equivalent to the normal method, and with no extra radiation required. The two systems are therefore comparable. However, it can be seen in Fig. 4A that there is a whole series of lines above and below the line AB, e.g. CD and EF, which, if the readings from the detectors are chosen in a certain order and added, would produce a different section through the body. The whole body therefore can be covered by a series of calculated tomograms with the dose required only for one tomogram produced in the normal way. A possible method of removing blur might be as follows -

(a) Produce tomogram of line AB.

(b) Calculate the blurring of this tomogram from the information contained in all the other tomograms on either side of it, i.e. areas O and P.

(c) Subtract (b) from (a).

This method of producing a more accurate tomogram is however impractical. It only serves to show in a simple way that information is avalable for obtaining:-

(1) Considerably more pictures for the same dose.

- 5 -

(2) More accurate absorption readings with "blurring" and "fogging" removed.

In practice, it is easier and more accurate to calculate the picture from the readings as described in paragraph 2 above , as it can be seen that Fig. 4A is only a special case of Fig. 3, the scan in the latter being shown as parallel lines rotated through 180° whereas the former scans over approximately 90° with slightly converging lines. The proposed system is therefore a method of producing an idealised type of tomogram.

Note

Methods of producing a number of pictures at the same time in tomography by using more than one plate must result in an overall reduction of information on each plate as the available photons must be shared by the plates.

5. TECHNICAL CONSIDERATIONS

The method described at the beginning of this paper illustrates a simple system. A study has been made of the practical problems of this system and the following conclusions have been drawn.

5.1 Choice of Source

(1) Low energy gamma sources (such as Americium 60 keV) produce an ideal single line spectrum at the correct energy level, but have insufficient intensity of radiation. It would take many hours to produce a picture from these sources.

(2) Higher energy sources (such as Caesium 137 - 600 keV) are a considerable improvement; the production of a picture would take less than one hour but the separation and detection of the various tissues of the body is not as good as the low energy X-rays or gamma rays.

(3) X-rays. There is theoretically sufficient intensity to produce a series of 40 pictures in less than one minute, but to handle this rate of information a special array of linear detectors would have to be developed (described later). However, using a bank of 10 scintillation counters at present obtainable, a useful picture could be obtained in 3 minutes. A picture with the maximum possible information would take 1 hour. or using a linear detector 3 minutes.

It is well known that X-ray sources have considerable spread over the energy spectrum and this could complicate the computer program. It may be possible that the source would have to be calibrated by means of a "phantom" wedge and the results fed into the computer for reference. Experiments would have to be conducted to deduce the limits of accuracy of such a system.

5.2 Detectors

For most laboratory and prototype machines scintillation counters would be adequate. However, their use is restricted by an upper limit of the rate of counting; they are costly and the number used per equipment must therefore be restricted. Both these factors must increase the time taken to obtain a picture. It can be shown that the accuracy of the detector need be no greater than 1 part in 1000 to produce approximately 2% accuracy of absorption reading on the picture. The range of accuracy need cover only 1/3 of the full range of the detector. It may be possible therefore in the future to use analogue methods of proportional detection from a bank of semiconductors*(see Fig. 4B). The output of each detector could be integrated and electronically scanned sequentially to reduce the complexity of equipment (variations of d.c. levels and gain could be corrected by the computer).

One half rotation of 180° would be required (Fig. 4B) to produce 40 "slices" in considerably less than 1 minute. Such a device must be considered as a possible future solution to the problem of excessive time to obtain a picture. Picture time approx 3 mins

* As an interim measure one scintillator and photomultiplier could be used in a linear mode of operation but later semiconductors may be developed to fit this application.

- 7 -

5.3 Definition

If a one centimetre wide beam is chosen, a resolution better than 1 cm could be obtained; for example, if the shape of the cross-section of the beam is known, at least three extra values may be computed from this information. Hence it may be possible to build up a picture with a 120 x 120 matrix instead of 40 x 40. However, the most accurate readings would only be produced in areas greater than 1 cm^2.

5.4 Compton Scatter

Compton scatter presents no problem with a simple system using a single detector and collimator. However, should multiple detectors be used (above 10) it would be necessary to correct for this effect, and a system to achieve this has been worked out.

6. RESEARCH PROPOSALS

A simple test jig could be made in which the object is rotated in front of a fixed radioactive source and collimator, and detected by a fixed scintillation counter and collimator. Blocks of material of known absorption could be arranged in various patterns within the beam and readings taken through them at known angles. These could be compared with the calculated values of absorption and accuracy assessed of the picture that would have been obtained. If the assessments are favourable, readings could be fed into a paper tape punch. A program for accepting the information and reconstructing the picture could be written and used on the 1905 computer. This being only a practical experiment, the time taken to form a picture would be very much slower than would be the case in normal use. Phantoms of tumours of varying size and density could be presented to the machine and the pictures produced compared with normal X-ray photographs and tomograms of the same phantom.

A theoretical study to overcome the computing problems associated with the broad spectrum produced by an X-ray tube could also be included.

7. APPLICATIONS

There are two main applications for the equipment:

(1) In Hospitals, Clinics and Medical Centres for the early detection of tumours when symptoms indicate that such may be present.

(2) For fitting in static and mobile Mass Radiography Units used for "screening". In this case a bank of detectors used side by side so that many picture slices may be taken through the patient at the same time would be essential. The digital information presented is in a form such as can be compared in a computer with other pictures by pattern recognition techniques, and by this means it could deal with the large amount of information that would come from Mass Radiography Units of this type.

8. CONCLUSIONS

The theoretical studies conducted so far have indicated that present methods of tomography do not use the majority of information available to the detector (film). It is theoretically possible to improve the accuracy of detection of absorption within the body by at least an order. At the same time at least 20 times as many pictures for the same amount of radiation through the body could be obtained.

Although scintillation counters are very time consuming they would be quite suitable for accurate systems where the 'rate' of taking a picture is of low importance. They could also be used in cases where a minimum radiation dose is necessary, when a smaller number of counts would be taken for each reading (which would also increase the picture rate). This would reduce the accuracy of detection but it could still be kept as good as a conventional tomogram. However, scintillation counters are not suitable for faster systems in which 40 "slices" would be required in one minute. In this case it is hoped that in the future a bank of linear detectors could be developed to fit this requirement.

At the moment it is necessary to prove that the theory works in practice with currently available components, irrespective of how long it takes to produce a picture.

If the proposed system can be proved successfully, it would be a very considerable incentive for the component manufacturers to produce components capable of speeding up the process.

9. ESTIMATED COST

It is estimated that £10,000 would be required to cover the work involved in proving the system.

B.653/2
08314/R/GNH/JPC
7.10.68.

<u>APPENDIX</u> Table of Comparisons between existing Systems and Proposed System of Radiography

	Normal X-Ray Picture	Tomography	Proposed System
<u>Accuracy</u> of absorption reading 1 cu cm of material	High accuracies of detection impossible. 1 cubic cm of material controls only 3% of radiation received through the body. A random distribution of material in line with it varying ±1% could obliterate all possibility of detection.	Picture obscurred by "blurring" and fog, e.g. if readings through the body vary randomly by 5% then the "blurring" produced by this would allow the tumour to be detected to an accuracy of 30%.	Accuracy of detection is theoretically better than 1%. The accuracy of these readings is practically independent of the nature of the material which surrounds a given element.
<u>Definition</u> minimum size of picture elements.	Better than 0.1 mm	Approx. 1 sq. cm.	1 sq. cm detected accurately. 1/9th sq. cm would be defined less accurately. Picture matrix 120 x 120
Ability to deduce absolute values of absorption.	Impossible to deduce absolute values.	Vague comparison of absorption with the mean value of the rest of the body.	Absolute values of absorption can be plotted for each cubic cm of material.
Number of pictures produced for a given radiation dose.	One	One (or 3 less accurate pictures).	Theoretically between 20 and 40 pictures.

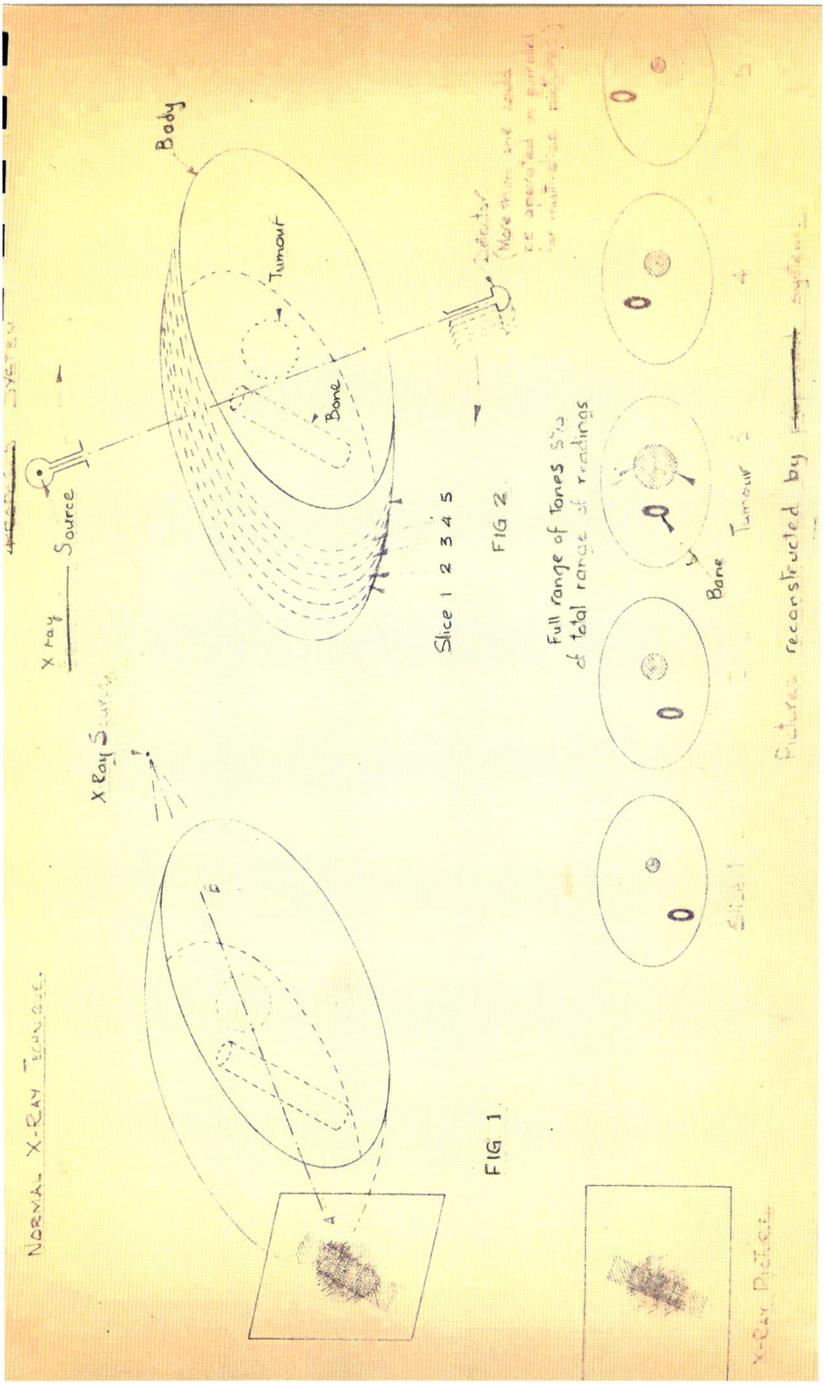
NORMAL X-RAY
X Ray
FIG 1
X ray
Source
Body
Tumour
Bone
Slice 1 2 3 4 5
FIG 2
Full range of tones 5%
of total range of readings
Bone
Tumour

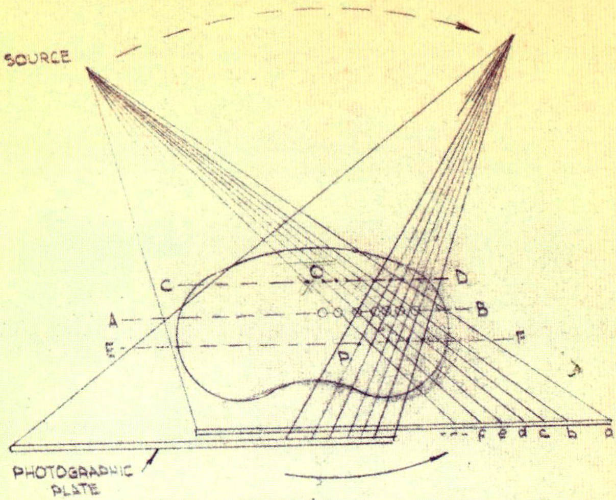
SOURCE
C
O
D
A
B
E
F
P
f e d c b a
PHOTOGRAPHIC PLATE

FIG.4A

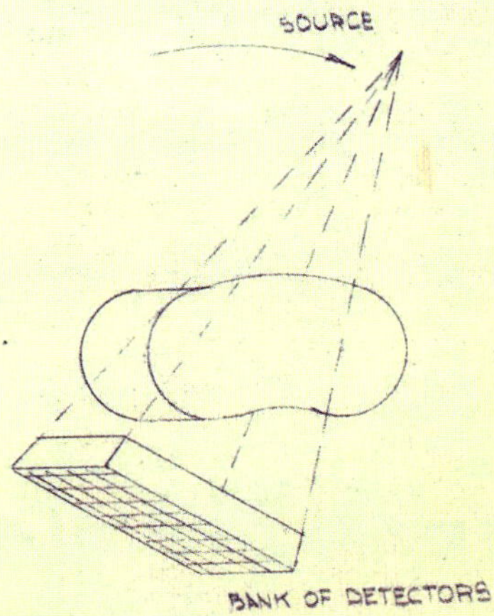
SOURCE
BANK OF DETECTORS

FIG.4B

Speech at Magnus school
(Courtesy of Andrew Hounsfield)

I was very pleased to receive you

~~It was with great pleasure that I~~ accepted the kind invitation to open this new Library, and I do appreciate the great honour of having it named after me. ~~There are not many things I'd rather~~ be associated with ~~than~~ a building designed to help young people with their studies.

DAYS AT MAGNUS

As an old Magnusian, now more than "Forty Years On", I am naturally delighted to visit my old school again and to see how it has grown. How different it looks now! I can still remember my first years at Magnus when I was taught for a while in a temporary classroom that was an ex-Army hut with a ~~coke~~ stove in the middle. ~~It was quite a cosy place.~~

Mr Carswell and Mr Vernon, two of the staff who patiently tried to teach this rather reluctant student, are happily with us today, and so some of my thanks must also go to them and to all the other teachers who tried hard to educate me. I'm particularly grateful for the grounding in physics and maths that I received at Magnus, and sincerely wish the school as much success in the future as it has had in the past.

THE IDEA OF THE SCANNER

I have been asked to say a few brief words, particularly to the students present here, about the work I did in developing the system of the medical scanner which I ~~had the fortune~~ to invent. It now has the sophisticated name of Computed Tomography. I don't want to burden you with detail, ~~but I'd~~ like to remind you that it is a machine using X-rays that examine the body as a series of slices, much as you would get using a bacon slicer. It has the advantage of being very much more sensitive than conventional X-ray ~~techniques~~. ~~This helps~~ medical diagnosis, ~~as soft tissue organs can be clearly seen.~~

Many people have asked me how I got the idea of this invention. They are very disappointed, I assure you, when I tell them that I didn't jump out of a bath, rather like Archimedes, shouting, "Eureka! I have found it!" No, the idea came much more slowly than that.

-2-

PATTERN RECOGNITION - THE BLACK BOX

At that time I was busily engaged in what was then called "Pattern Recognition". This meant, in my case, trying to teach a rather stupid computer, with a camera coupled to it, how to recognize objects placed in front of the camera. ~~This~~ required a certain amount of complicated information processing.

~~It was one day, probably in my spare time at home, that~~ the idea occurred to me that, if there were a box with an unknown object in it, and if an X-ray beam and detector were to take accurate absorption measurements through the box at a multitude of different angles, then a computer should be able to work out in detail exactly what was inside the box and present it in picture form. You see, each measurement would be interrelated with other measurements in the form of hundreds of thousands of simultaneous equasions. ~~This~~ could be handled by a computer, which would be good at solving ~~this~~ vast amount of data. All of this information could be transposed into pictures in three dimensions.

~~It~~ was a very exciting moment when I realized, ~~after further study, that this system~~ was indeed capable of producing pictures which were very much more sensitive than the conventional X-ray pictures that we know at present.

APPLICATION TO THE HUMAN BODY

I wondered ~~whether~~ this method could be ~~used~~ to look inside the human body, ~~as I had theoretical evidence that~~ it ~~should~~ be able to see soft organs such as liver and pancreas. ~~This~~ challenge was far from easy for me because I had no particular medical experience and the firm I was working for had only little medical interest.

~~I first tested the theory~~ by simulating ~~objects~~ within the computer and attempting to reconstruct them, ~~using the~~ mathematical procedure that ~~I hoped to~~ use in practice.

~~This worked so well, that I knocked~~ on the door of the Department of Health and Social Security ~~to show them~~ that it

-3-

~~would work~~, clutching my only evidence -- a piece of paper with rows and rows of numbers on ~~it to~~ represent ~~the~~ picture. ~~This~~ must have impressed them to some extent, as they gave the firm some money to help ~~with the building of~~ a laboratory machine which I set out, wi~~thout delay, to build~~.

SOME BIZARRE EVENTS - LEADING TO SUCCESS

~~This was~~ a rather Heath Robinson ~~connection~~, made up of old equipment that happened to be lying around, but it triggered off a very bizarre series of events: my crossing London carrying a paper bag full of bullocks' brains; or fetching pigs' carcases, bought from a local slaughterhouse; or grisly specimens of human remains from the local hospital. These were all tried out on the machine. Because this was only an experimental machine, it took as long as nine hours to produce a picture, and on a hot day there was a constant battle to compose a picture before the specimen decomposed.

Looking back now on this period, I know I found it all tremendous fun. When the machine began to display very startling pictures of the interiors of the specimens, we ~~knew~~ that we had to design and build a proper clinical scanner. This task had its moments of hard work ~~and~~ frustration -- it was a field completely new to me. The machine was eventually installed in a London hospital, and you can imagine what a great day it was for me when the first patient was scanned. A tumour in the head was clearly seen, in detail sufficient for a successful operation to be performed.

GROWING MOMENTUM

From then on, events moved very rapidly. ~~We~~ built hundreds ~~more~~ machines, which were sent all over the world. ~~We were seeing many abnormalities in the body which could not be seen by any other means.~~

Meanwhile, I was rushing around the world, introducing the system to hospitals and studying the findings of the many doctors who were using the scanner.

APPEAL TO YOUTH

Well, I hope I haven't spoken too long about what is, after all, history, past and done with. ~~Now we have to look to the future and towards the youth of the country.~~ My purpose in telling ~~you~~ this story is to impress those of you who are about to leave school, especially those who are going into science and technology, that ~~it~~ a career in this field can be an extremely rewarding experience, particularly if you can carry through an idea of your own making, as I did.

Remember, too, that each new discovery that is made brings with it the seeds of other, future, inventions. There are many discoveries, probably just around the corner, waiting for someone to bring them to life. Could this possibly be you?

It is possible that many of these ideas will come out in the straight forward way by one saying "I have a problem; I am going to find a solution" but by saying "I have a potential solution; let us find a problem that fits it".

It is apparent that this happened to me.

Cinematography too only came about because of Celluloid not because of Photography as it was by then a well known art.

In the same way Celluloid was the solution to cinematography.

or the same way as the laser is the solution to many problems of the past & will be to many unknown problems of the future.

Appendix 1
Publications of Sir Godfrey Hounsfield

Hounsfield GN. "Computerised Transverse Axial Scanning." 2nd Conference of European Association of Radiology, Amsterdam, 1971.

Hounsfield GN. "Computerised transverse axial scanning (tomography), Part 1, description of the system." *British Journal of Radiology* 1973;46:1016–22.

Ambrose J, Hounsfield GN. "Computerized Transverse Axial Tomography." *British Journal of Radiology* 1973;46:148–9.

Hounsfield GN. "Historical notes on computerized axial tomography." *Journal of the Canadian Association of Radiology* 1976;27:135–42.

Sagel S, Weiss E, Gillard R, Hounsfield G, Jost G, Stanley R, Ter-pogossian M. "Gated computer tomography of the human heart." *Investigative Radiology* 1977;12:563–6.

Hounsfield GN. "Picture quality in computer tomography." *American Journal of Roentgenology* 1976;127:3–9.

Hounsfield GN. "Potential uses of more accurate CT absorption values by filtering." *American Journal of Roentgenology* 1978;131:103–6.

Hounsfield GN. "Computed medical imaging (Nobel Prize lecture)." *Science* 1980;210:22–8.

Hounsfield GN. "Computer reconstructed X-ray imaging." *Philosophical Transactions of The Royal Society A* 1979;292:223–32.

Nobel Foundation. "Autobiography." 1979. Available at: www.nobelprize.org/nobel_prizes/medicine/laureates/1979/hounsfield-autobio.html

Appendix 2
Other publications including film and TV

Ambrose J. "Computerised X-ray scanning of the brain." *Journal of Neurosurgery* 1974;40(6):697–5.

Ambrose J. "CT scanning, a backward look." *Seminars in Roentgenology* 1977;XII:7–11.

Ambrose J, Lloyd G, Wright J. "A preliminary examination of fine matrix computerized transverse axial tomography (EMI-scanner) in the diagnosis of orbital space-occupying lesions." *British Journal of Radiology* 1974;47:747–51.

Bull J. The history of computed tomography. In: "Radiology of the skull and brain". Newton TH, Potts DG, editors. New York: NY: Elsevier; 1981. pp. 3835–49.

Hendry J. "Innovating for failure: Government policy and the early british computer industry." Cambridge, MA, and London: MIT Press; 1989.

Higson G. "The beginning of CT scanning, a personal recollection." *Bulletin of British Institute of Radiology* 1979;5:3–4.

Lodge JA. "THORN EMI Central Research Laboratories: an anecdotal history." *Physics Technology* 1987;18:258–68.

Oldendorf WH. US Patent 3106640. "Radiant energy apparatus for investigating selected areas of the interior of objects obscured by dense material." 8 October 1963.

Pandit SA. "From making to music – The history of THORN EMI." London: Hodder & Stoughton; 1996.

Paxton R, Ambrose J. "The EMI Scanner: a brief review of the first 650 patients." *British Journal of Radiology* 1974;47:530–65.

Süsskind C. The invention of computed tomography. In: "History of technology 1981." Hall AR, Smith N, editors. London: Mansell Publishing; 1981. pp. 39–80.

Webb S. "From the watching of shadows: origins of radiological tomography." Bristol: Adam Hilger (IOP Publishing); 1990.

Wells PNT. "Sir Godfrey Newbold Hounsfield KT CBE. 28 August 1919–12 August 2004: Elected F.R.S. 1975". *Biographical Memoirs of Fellows of the Royal Society* 2005;51:221. doi:10.1098/rsbm.2005.0014.

Information about the EMIDEC 1100 computer is available at: www.emidec.org.uk

Many other documents describe Godfrey and the development of the CT scanner, but most add little to what EMI published at the time. The information from EMI's publications in the 1970s is collected in "The Scanner Story" document by Colin Woodley, which was not published but can be found in EMI's archives.

Several video segments show Godfrey and others discussing the history of the CT scanner, as summarised below:

Title and owner	Description
"The Scanner Story" EMI	A 1978 film which includes Dr James Ambrose, Professor Ian Isherwood and others talking about the introduction of the scanner. Dr Ron Evans describes why a CT scan is better than pumping air into the spine and brain.
"Bill and Godfrey" BIR	Recorded in 1991 by William Cavendish as executor of Sir Joseph Lockwood, this shows Godfrey in conversation with Bill Ingham. It gives an unvarnished history. Two versions exist: one was edited and broadly agreed between the participants in 1992, and the second was re-edited in 2006 by John Ryan to implement, as far as was then possible, Godfrey's annotations on a transcript.
Nobel Prize BBC	A short clip of the award ceremony, once shown on the BBC.
Dr Forrest Clore Drs Clore and Klioze	In a recording by Dr Scott Klioze, Dr Clore recalls Godfrey's talk in New York on 15 May 1972, and the impact on diagnostic procedures. Previous procedures relied on inference from displacement of small blood vessels.
"Early days" EMI	Godfrey filmed in about 1992 with the lathe bed and an Mk1 brain scanner.
"Multiplanar and reconstruction" EMI	These show navigation through Topaz volume scans on the CRL image processor and how the cross-sectional image is reconstructed by the "filtered back-projection" method.
"Great British Inventions" BBC	A 1992 BBC2 programme including Gordon Higson (DHSS), Godfrey, Professor Ian Young, Sir John Read (EMI), Sir Peter Laister (Thorn), and Walter Robb (General Electric). The focus is mainly on what EMI could have done better, with the benefit of hindsight.

"EMI and me" BBC	A 2002 BBC2 programme including Bill Ingham and Sir John Read. The CT part includes Bill Ingham and John Read.
Faraday lecture EMI	"The Diagnostic Electron", presented by Dr J. A. Powell at the IEE, Savoy Place, London. 1978/79.

The BIR holds copies of some of these items. Appropriate permission should be sought from the relevant copyright holder before making public or commercial use of them.

Appendix 3
Some awards

Colin Woodley of EMI kept a list of awards and honours, which is probably reasonably complete for the years from 1972 to the start of 1978. After that date the list below is based on "Who's Who", and recollections of the authors, and is probably incomplete. Unless noted otherwise, all awards were presented to Godfrey.

1972

MacRobert Award
(Awarded to Godfrey Hounsfield and EMI Limited)

1973

Queen's Award to Industry for Technological Achievement
(Awarded to the Central Research Laboratories of EMI)

1974

IR 100 Award
(Awarded to Central Research Laboratories of EMI)

Barclay Prize (BIR)
(Awarded to Dr James Ambrose and Godfrey Hounsfield)

Wilhelm Exner Medal (Austrian Industrial Association)

Ziedses des Plantes Medal
(Awarded to Godfrey Hounsfield and William Oldendorf by the Physikalisch-Medizinische Gesellschaft of Wurzburg and the Deutschen Gesellschaft fur Neuroradiologie)

1975

Godfrey Hounsfield elected Fellow of the Royal Society

Prince Philip Medal Award for 1974
(Presented by City & Guilds, the award ceremony was 28 March 1975)

Achievement Award of the Worshipful Company of Scientific Instrument Makers
(Presented to W. E. Ingham on behalf of EMI Central Research Laboratories)

Doctor of Medicine Honoris Causa of the Universitat Basel

ANS Radiation Industry Award (Georgia Institute of Technology)

Lasker Award
(Presented by The Lasker Foundation to Godfrey Hounsfield and Dr William Oldendorf)

1976

Honorary Membership of Spanish Radiological and Neuroradiological Societies and of Spanish Society of Physical Science

Duddell Bronze Medal and Prize
(Awarded by the Institute of Physics)

Honorary Doctorate of Science
(Awarded by City University)

Honorary Fellowship
(Awarded by the Royal College of Physicians)

Golden Plate Award
(Awarded by the American Academy of Achievement)

Honorary Doctorate of Technology
(Awarded by Loughborough University)

Reginald Mitchell Gold Medal
(Awarded by the Stoke-on-Trent Association of Engineers)

Churchill Gold Medal
(Awarded by the Society of Engineers)

Honorary Doctorate of Science
(Awarded by the Council for National Academic Awards and presented by HRH The Prince of Wales)

Gairdner Founder Award of Merit and Prize
(Awarded by the Gairdner Foundation of Canada)

Radiation Industry Award
(Awarded by the American Nuclear society)

Invested with the CBE at Buckingham Palace

Honorary Fellowship
(Awarded by the Royal College of Radiologists)

Honorary Doctorate of Science
(Awarded by the University of London and presented by HM Queen Elizabeth, The Queen Mother)

1977

Silvanus Thompson Bronze Medal
(Awarded by the BIR)

Honorary Fellowship
(University of Manchester Institute of Science and Technology)

Honorary Doctorate of Science
(University of Manchester)

Caldwell Medal
(Awarded by the American Roentgen Ray Society)

John Scott Award
(Awarded by City of Philadelphia Trustee)

Order of the Southern Cross
(Awarded by the Brazilian Minister of Health on behalf of the President of Brazil)

Howard N. Potts Medal
(Awarded by the Franklin Institute of Philadelphia)

Royal Society Mullard Award

The Royal Society of Medicine Diploma

1978

The Harold Laufman Award
(Presented by the Association for the Advancement of Medical Instrumentation Foundation, USA)

The list prepared by Colin Woodley stops here, but the awards continued. The remainder of this list is probably incomplete. We apologise for any awards omitted.

1979

Nobel Prize for Physiology or Medicine (jointly)
(Presented by King Carl XVI Gustaf of Sweden)

Ambrogino d'Oro Award, City of Milan

Premio Internazionale "La Madonnina"

1980

Deutsche Roentgen Plakette (Deutsche Roentgen Museum)

RSNA Gold Medal (Radiological Society of North America)

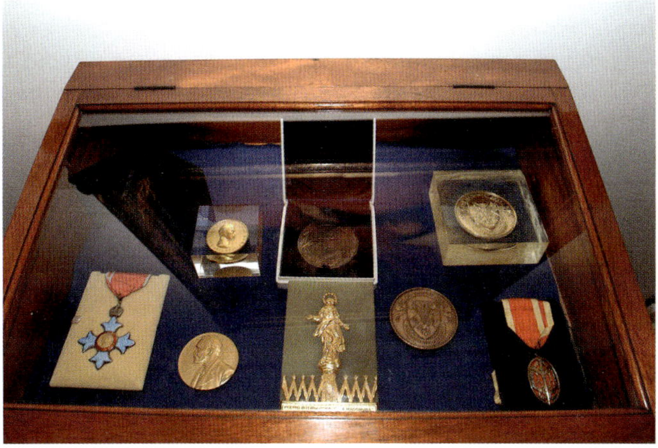

Awards on display
(Courtesy of the BIR)
Clockwise from the top left: Prince Philip Medal, Photographic Society of America, MacRobert (encased), Knighthood, MacRobert, Premio Internazionale "La Madonnina", Nobel Prize, and CBE.

In 1976–77 Godfrey was receiving an award every month!

Appendix 4
Bill Ingham's views on the years 1975–82

EMI Medical Ltd in the UK, under John Willsher, had done an amazing job in building up from nothing a capability for manufacture and sales, including the recruiting and training of technical staff for design and servicing.

As most of the sales were in the US EMI decided to form EMI Medical Inc as a marketing and service organization in USA. I subscribe to the view that it would probably have been better to have acquired a medical supplier with an established name in the US, (which could have been planned earlier, if there had been a plan).

A committee was formed which met monthly, in the UK and US alternately. The committee was not a board, nor even a management group, and it merely reviewed progress. It was chaired by John Powell, and members included the Chairman of EMI Medical Ltd, the President of EMI Medical Inc, the Director of CRL, and the Finance Director of Medical.

The Medical Ltd/Medical Inc arrangement was to be changed disastrously following the arrival of Normand Provost. The Chief Executive of Medical Inc was replaced and soon the balance of the whole operation was altered as the US division started to form a design team in addition to a manufacturing unit. Normand Provost came to see me to seek advice on the staffing levels and costs, which I gave him, but my queries about the role of the proposed group did not elucidate any clear response. It soon became obvious however that the objective was a virtually autonomous company.

Medical Inc soon started to design new scanners itself, without close links with the UK. This was of course crazy; it threw away EMI's main advantage and was to have the gravest possible consequences.

Godfrey Hounsfield and his team were now working in CRL (though greatly interrupted by assisting EMI Medical) on an idea of Godfrey for a much faster scanner, which was given the code name Topaz.

Before long EMI Medical Inc, having by now established their own design team, came up with a counter proposal for a body scanner to follow the one then being sold. Dates and costs were quoted and it was claimed that their work on the scanner would be completed in 90 days.

The Medical Inc proposal was the subject of an efficient presentation in the US, with some members of the EMI board present, and in spite of warnings was approved and the project commenced. The Medical Inc proposal was a bit like the market ploy by an American company which offered a 5 sec scanner long before it was available, just to stop the competition.

The 90 days quickly passed and of course no scanner appeared. As the delay got longer and longer the position became more and more serious. [So Godfrey and others made a "technical audit" as Bill Ingham describes in Chapter 10.]

Special review meetings, attended by EMI board members, were held in US and UK at which the priority of the Northbrook program was emphasised, culminating in a meeting in the board room at EMI House at which, with US pressure, the support of everyone was required for the US project. All present agreed because it was by then simply too late to reverse the US project with which the company was now inextricably linked. There was a great feeling of despondency in the CRL teams, and in EMI Medical Ltd, after the meeting. What would have been more useful was a strategic planning meeting, recognising the true position and considering possible links and deals, strengths and weaknesses, technical leads such as Topaz and NMR, to address the serious situation and assess the options for the future. But this overall planning was not an EMI strength. [NMR is now known as MRI.]

As the position, inevitably, got worse, just as we had predicted, Central Research Labs gave more and more help to the US company. Godfrey and his key colleagues spent long periods at Northbrook correcting the mistakes of the inexperienced US team. The severe software / processor problems that had been identified by Godfrey and Steve Bates in our earlier assessment of the Northbrook project were confirmed just as predicted. So Godfrey made available to Medical Inc the special processor that had been devised and constructed in CRL for Topaz (it was a very powerful unit of dedicated electronics which CRL had realised would be needed to replace the mini computers used previously).

But it was all far too late. Nothing now could stop the bleeding in time.

Eventually an MD was appointed to take charge of both US and UK Medical companies. But instead of appointing one of the very experienced MD's of Medical Ltd, who had been giving sound advice all along, someone was brought in from outside and the learning process began again. This finally put paid to any chance of salvaging the medical business.

One of the great benefits to the company of Godfrey Hounsfield's invention was the massive royalties received by EMI over many years from the patents that had been filed.

We attached great importance in CRL to the filing of patents. This is not a popular activity for creative people keen to avoid paper chores and get on with their work. So a system was set up in the research lab, covering all departments, to review the ideas that were generated and ensure that they were considered, filtered by the CRL Directorate and passed to the patent department. The key patents were Godfrey's main patent and LeMay's reconstruction patent, but the objective, as identified by patent department, was to build up what was referred to as a minefield around the scanner on which other companies would be caught in more than one violation. The success of this is clear from the many millions of pounds which were provided annually in royalties for the company over more than a decade.

It is a pleasure here to record the support received from Allan Logan and his patent department, not only in discussing and filing the patents in the first place, but also in the licensing and litigation later on. But the litigation undertaken by the patent department involved Godfrey and key CRL staff and took much of their time for a long period, time which they gave without complaint. It was inevitably disruptive for CRL, but the disruption would have been much worse without the magnificent help of patent department.

Following the collapse of EMI and the take over of the company by Thorn, the medical business was reviewed. I drew attention to the Topaz project in CRL and to the pioneering work on NMR imaging in the lab, but the losses of EMI Medical following the fatal delay of the US system were high and the decision was taken to dispose of the Medical interests.

In addition to the scanner research (project Topaz) in Central Research Labs, there were also departments in CRL working on ultra sound scanner technology and the NMR scanner. The ultrasound and NMR activities have not been covered in this note, but the NMR research had led to an NMR scanner being placed in the Hammersmith hospital.

It was decided that the research in CRL was to be disposed of separately from the EMI Medical activities. Our negotiations were complicated by the involvement of DHSS, and another complication was the need to negotiate arrangements for the sale of the technology without losing all the key people as well.

Discussions were held with a number of interested companies in USA and Europe and eventually the Topaz X-ray scanner technology was sold to Phillips in the Netherlands without the X ray team being lost. Negotiations with General Electric in US for the sale of the NMR technology were going well, but then DHSS brought pressure to bear for the sale to be to a UK company; that meant to GEC. This gave GEC a buyer's market and, worse, enabled them to press to take the whole NMR team, which they did.

It was a sad time for Godfrey and those who had created the X-ray scanner and the great opportunity that it gave to EMI. Morale was of course already low following the collapse of EMI, and now all the medical research was to be sold. The difficulty of holding staff and getting them to be enthusiastic about whole new fields for Thorn has never been understood. But apart from the NMR team very few were lost in spite of the offers made to Godfrey Hounsfield and key members of the team; their loyalty to the Lab was outstanding in this very difficult time.

Various reasons have been given for the failure of EMI Medical, and some are suggested in the official Thorn EMI book. [Bill means the book by S.A. Pandit as listed in Appendix 2.] *John Powell has unfairly taken much of the blame whilst others have professed, after the event, to have been supporters of licensing rather than go it alone. The problems of the body scanner have even been cited as one of the major causes of the failure, but the body scanner problem was the result, not the cause, of the failure and criticism of Godfrey Hounsfield and his team for the delay, made in ignorance of the facts, is grossly misleading. It is important therefore to record this and the real reasons for the commercial failure.*

The general problem was of course the lack of any overriding business mission, correctly identified in the Thorn EMI book as a weakness of EMI. This weakness was not confined just to the medical business.

Within the Medical business there were two main reasons for the failure to turn the invention of the scanner into a successful international business. The first and prime cause for the failure was the lack of any preparation to follow up the research. This jeopardized any subsequent action. Even after John Powell was brought in to take the lead there was, inevitably, further delay before EMI could get into gear, which of course allowed other companies a breathing space to get started. But the damage was not confined to this serious initial delay: the lack of a commercial plan travelled with the medical business for years, with the gravest effect on the venture and was the prime cause of subsequent problems of EMI Medical. For example, as recorded earlier there was no real commercial design for the head scanner (there was no commercial division to do it) so EMI Medical, whilst building up from nothing, was forced to try to cope with sales by making and marketing copies of the CRL experimental scanner. This was not a temporary situation as the machine was marketed for years. And the on-going research in CRL by Godfrey and his team was disrupted because the lab had to act first as an EMI factory making scanners and, for some time after that, as trouble shooter for the new EMI Medical which was in the learning stage. The lack of any commercial plan to follow the research was disastrous.

Another main cause of the failure was the decision to allow Medical Inc to break away and start to design scanners itself, without close links with EMI Medical Ltd in the UK. One of the main advantages that EMI had over its competitors was, of course, its lead and the experience that had been built up by CRL and then Medical Ltd in the UK. But, after having got EMI Medical Ltd established in the UK, this experience was thrown away when Northbrook, with completely inexperienced staff, started to build up from scratch on its own, ignoring the UK. This resulted in a critical loss of EMI's main advantage, as well as a split of resources.

In fact this did not just throw away the 'experience' advantage which had been one of EMI's greatest strengths, it reversed the position because by then GE had already got somewhere down the road of scanner experience and Medical Inc had not. So now, in the critical US market, GE had the experience advantage over EMI. I know from subsequent contacts with very senior people in General Electric that they watched in amazement, and with some gratitude, when an embryo EMI unit in the US started up to establish its own operation. They told me that they could hardly believe their good fortune.

Other factors also contributed to the collapse of the EMI Medical business, for example the EMI decision to require an up front non returnable deposit on sales. The notion of an up front non returnable deposit was unheard of in the medical business, and it was seen in the US as a foreign company greedily exploiting the hospitals and was greatly resented. Customers paid up because it was the only way to secure a scanner in the early days when EMI was the only source, but when other systems became available it was not forgotten. The insistence on a non returnable deposit in the early days later resulted in a loss of sales just at the critical time when the company was struggling to cope with the problems noted above, trying to sell obsolete systems when every sale was of vital importance to keep the business alive. The reaction, against the earlier demand for a non returnable deposit, was fatal.

These notes record some of the key events in the research by Godfrey Hounsfield and his team leading to the creation of the first scanner, and reveal the difficult climate in which Hounsfield worked. The lack of support in the early stages of the scanner research is reminiscent of Whittle and his jet engine, one of the other great inventions of the century.

The notes also record some of the key events following the invention of the scanner, including the real reasons for the commercial failure. It is important that the tremendous achievement of Godfrey Hounsfield and his team should not be overshadowed by the commercial disaster when, in fact, the problems in the commercial business led to disruption of Godfrey's work and an enormously increased burden on him and his staff, and make their achievements even greater.

Appendix 5
City & Guilds and Faraday House qualifications

The City & Guilds Radio Communication Examination could be taken at three levels. Godfrey sat and passed Grade 2 in 1944 while he was based at RAF Cranwell. His self-taught work for this exam covered more small-signal electronics than his subsequent course at Faraday House. The 1941 syllabus is shown below.

50 C.—RADIO-COMMUNICATION.

Grade I.

Questions may be set with the object of testing the candidate's knowledge of the elementary electrical principles applied at this stage of radio-communication, and his ability to deal with problems and calculations based on these principles, in addition to the questions more directly concerned with the following subject-matter:—

1. Construction of transmitting and receiving inductors.
2. Capacitance; construction of fixed and variable condensers for low voltage, fixed condensors for high voltage.
3. Qualitative treatment of eddy current loss including skin effect in conductors, and of dielectric loss in condensers.
4. Construction of two electrode and three electrode thermionic valves; principles of action and characteristic curves with application to non-reactive load.
5. Detecting devices for small alternating potentials; contact rectifiers and valves.
6. Construction and action of telephone receivers and electromagnetic loud speakers.
7. High frequency and low frequency thermionic amplifiers, essential principles of action. Causes of distortion.
8. Simple circuits of radio receivers including use of retroaction. Qualitative ideas of selectivity.
9. Simple omni-directional aerials for reception purposes.
10. Use of a loop aerial for reception and direction finding.
11. Qualitative treatment of simple valve oscillator.
12. Simple wavemeter.
13. General principles of heterodyne reception.

Grade II.

More difficult questions on the subject-matter of the Grade I. Syllabus may be set in this examination, in addition to questions on such subjects as the following:—

50 *C.—Radio-Communication.* 15

1. Elementary ideas of the radiation and propagation of electromagnetic waves and of the properties of transmitting and receiving antennæ; simple computations neglecting absorption and reflexion.
2. The theory of coupled circuits and their application to the problem of selectivity.
3. The generation of oscillations in a valve circuit. Self-oscillating and master-controlled valve transmitters for C.W. and I.C.W. Neutralizing circuits; Simple spark transmitter.
4. The modulation of valve transmitters by keying, tone and speech. Sidebands. Frequency bands necessary for various modulation systems.
5. Construction and action of devices for rectifying alternating current for H.T. supply. Smoothing circuits.
6. Transmitting valves including cooled anode and demountable type valves.
7. Omni-directional aerials for transmitting and reception, effective height and radiation resistance.
8. The reception of C.W. and I.C.W. telegraphy and of radio telephony signals. Superheterodyne and super-regenerative receivers. Methods of minimizing interference from atmospherics and unwanted stations.
9. Multi-electrode valves and their uses, including the cathode ray tube.
10. Schematic arrangements and principles of operation of radio telephone channels connected to land line circuits.
11. High frequency measurements of current, voltage, resistance, inductance, capacitance, frequency and field strength.
12. Decibel and neper. Simple computations, T and H type of attenuators and their applications, design of simple sections.
13. Interference with radio reception by industrial and domestic electric plant. Devices and circuits for preventing or minimizing such interference.

Radio Communications, Grade 2
(Courtesy of City & Guilds)

Details of Godfrey's course at Faraday House are stored in the IET archives. This includes the lecture notes of Douglas Foster, who was a student on the same course as Godfrey, doing (we believe) the same design projects at the same time. It was an engineering course, but surprisingly little was relevant to his subsequent work. The electrical content mainly covered motors and generators. Mechanical design and magnetism were studied at a very detailed level in the three design projects that Douglas Foster completed:

> "Design of a 925 KVA Alternator" (December 1947).
> "Design of a 16 H.P. D.C. Motor" (February 1948).
> "Design of a 37½ H.P. Induction Motor" (February 1948).

The course hardly covered small-signal electronics at all. For example, it did not mention radio, and valves (vacuum tubes) were mentioned in only one lecture, on the design of an oscilloscope. Radar was not mentioned, and computers and transistors were not sufficiently mainstream to appear in a course in 1946-49.

The course often included two ways of solving the same problem, one by drawing a diagram, and the other by a mathematical formula. Probably Godfrey preferred to draw. An example of this is shown in the beautifully neat student notes below.

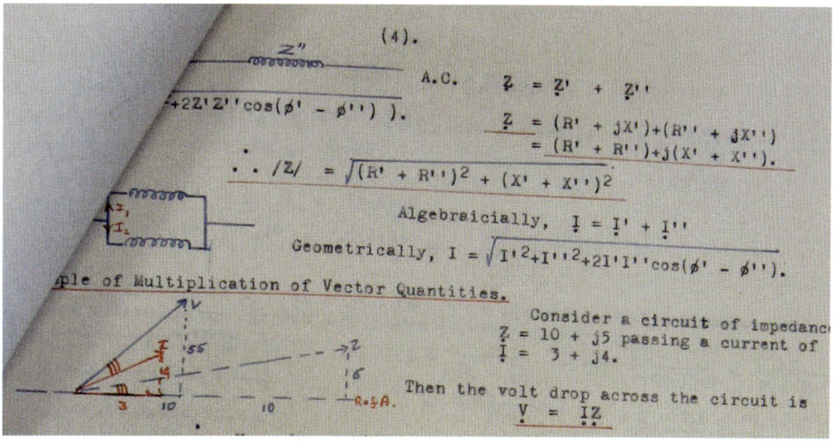

Douglas Foster's student notes
(Courtesy of Ian Green)

Overall, the course used little more maths than would be familiar to someone who studied maths at school to age eighteen.

The IET archives' website shows a summary of the lecture notes. The course covered many non-electrical topics including hydraulics, strength and elasticity of materials, tensile testing, hardness testing, theory of structures, deflection of beams, torsion of shafts, fluid flow, steam tables, and heat engines.

The IET archive reference for this is UK 108 NAEST 098.

Appendix 6
Main patents

This annex contains Godfrey's main patents, and a few other patents that were closely linked to his work.

Often the same invention results in patents in several countries. In that case the table below includes only the US patent or the GB patent if it was not filed in the USA. GB is the prefix for UK patents. Where two patent numbers are shown, the patent was divided into two because the patent office thought it was two separate inventions (a "divisional" patent for which they could charge a separate set of fees). Sometimes EMI initiated a "continuation in part", which allowed subsequent material to be added to an earlier patent to produce a new variant.

In the table below, GNH means Godfrey Newbold Hounsfield. The date is when the patent application was received by the patent office. The topic column links the patent with a phase of Godfrey's work. The title omits phrases such as "Improvements relating to".

Patents can be viewed online free of charge. Go to http://ep.espacenet.com/numberSearch, type in the patent number, click on the title and follow the link to see the original document.

Patent and date	**Inventor(s)**	**Title**	**Topic**
GB 707,450 27 September 1950	GNH	Electron discharge tube amplifiers	Amplifier for analogue computer
GB 893,355 30 April 1957	GNH	Pulse transfer devices	Digital computers, Austin and EMIDEC 1100
US3,120,661 20 October 1957	GNH, Eric White	Radar apparatus	"Interscan" radar displays
US3,230,388 17 September 1960	GNH	Integrated structure forming shift register from reactively coupled elements	Digital computers

GB 996,171 22 February 1961	GNH	Electrical apparatus	A configurable logic array
US3,257,581 17 October 1961	GNH, James Alec Lodge	Electron discharge device with tunnel effect cathode and selectively scanned target	A digital store different from the subsequent large thin-film store
GB1,045,571 GB1,045,572 4 November 1961	GNH	Data storage devices	Early ideas leading towards thin film store
GB1,103,871 16 April 1963	GNH, Patrick Harold Brown	Magnetic thin film elements for magnetic stores	Large thin-film store
GB1,103,871 11 March 1964	GNH	Magnetic matrix stores	Large thin-film store
GB1,164,122 25 August 1965	GNH, Patrick Brown	Data Storage Devices and Methods of Manufacturing	Large thin-film store
GB1,255,626 24 January 1968	GNH, Peter Langstone, Patrick Brown	Magnetic Matrix Data Storage Arrangements	Large thin-film store
GB1,255,629 25 March 1968	GNH	Data Storage Arrangements	Large thin-film store
US3,778,614 27 December 1971	GNH (litigated)	Measuring X- or gamma radiation at plural angles	CT including iterative reconstruction
US3,866,047 9 April 1973	GNH (litigated)	Apparatus having a scanning collimator	CT – scanning collimator

US3,919,552 9 May 1974	GNH (litigated)	(ditto)	CT using a water box
US3,924,131 9 May 1974	GNH (litigated)	Examining a body by radiation such as X or gamma radiation	CT using a translate-rotate motion
US3,944,833 7 May 1974	GNH (litigated)	Examining a body by radiation such as X or gamma radiation	CT stacking photomultipliers efficiently
US3,946,234 30 August 1974	GNH (litigated)	Examining bodies by means of penetrating radiation	CT using translate-rotate of a fan of detectors
US3,956,633 29 April 1975	GNH (litigated)	Radiology method and apparatus	CT control of detector gains
US3,965,357 1st March 1974	GNH (litigated)	Examining a body by means of penetrating radiation	CT lead and water detector calibration
US4,035,647 20 June 1974	GNH (litigated), David Gibbons	Radiography	CT rotate only
US4,052,618 12 February 1976	GNH (litigated)	Examining a body by radiation such as X or gamma radiation	CT using scanning collimator
US4,052,619 5 February 1975	GNH (litigated)	Measuring & analysing radiation at plural angles	CT using more than 180 degrees to reduce motion artefact

US4,069,422 18 February 1976	GNH (litigated)	Examining objects by means of penetrating radiation	CT – wedge controls beam hardness
US3,924,129 18 April 1974	Christopher LeMay	Constructing a representation of a planar slice of body	CT – "circle method" convolution
US3,940,599 23 May 1974	Paul Beaven, Brian Lill, GNH	Data processing arrangements	CT – fast mapping
US4,066,903 26 October 1976	Christopher LeMay	Radiology	CT – third difference interpolation
US4,010,370 11 November 1975	Christopher LeMay	CT with periodically displaced radiation source	CT – Topaz with parallel beams
US4,125,858 25 March 1977	GNH, Donald McLean	Video display arrangements	Filtered image colour overlay
US4,178,511 17 August 1978	GNH, Richard Waltham	Radiography	CT – Topaz with fan beams
US4,250,387 12 October 1979	GNH, Daniel J Pisano, Erlvada Anne Olson, Richard Waltham	Medical radiological apparatus and method	Correction for off-focal radiation

Appendix 7
Some notes on Godfrey's predecessors

Many books describe people who worked before Godfrey on the problem of how to reconstruct what is inside a box by looking at it from all possible directions. Steve Webb gives a thorough and readable description in his book "From the watching of shadows".

The list starts with Johann Radon in Austria in 1917, who approached the problem as pure maths. Next comes Gabriel Frank in Budapest in a patent in 1940 which includes most of modern CT, albeit in analog form and with no "filtration" before the back projection. The list includes Bracewell in 1956, Tetel'Baum and Korenblyum in Russia in 1957, Oldendorf in 1960, Cormack and Kuhl and Edwards in 1963, and Bracewell and Riddle in 1967. (Many others published after Godfrey filed his patent in 1968.)

It is clear from this list that it was not sufficient merely to have ideas about solving the image reconstruction problem in order to make the breakthrough to practical CT scanning. What else was needed, and why was it Godfrey who made the breakthrough?

Our aim is to give our opinion of some of the differences between Godfrey and his predecessors. This is not to be taken as a statement of fact, nor as a criticism of their excellent work, nor as adding anything to the detailed descriptions of their work that are already available elsewhere.

The first requirement is having an interest in the medical application (CT scanning). It seems clear that Radon was interested in mathematics but not in the medical application. Bracewell and Riddle were interested in astronomy and radio-astronomy. Bracewell's 1956 work was both early and successful.

A second requirement is adequate computer power. Gabriel Frank was interested the medical application in 1940, but adequate computing power was not available until the 1960s, long after his remarkable work. His analogue method recorded the X-ray projection data on film and back projected it optically. This is intriguing but unsuitable for widespread use.

Oldendorf was also interested in the medical application. He made a prototype in which the object that is being scanned was rotated many times, with a small movement of the centre of rotation between each scan, to build up a picture without using a computer.

In Oldendorf's technique each X-ray beam contributes only to the pixel that is currently at the centre of rotation. His method needs more than 5,000 rotations to match Godfrey's 80×80 CT scan (or 80,000 rotations for a 320×320 scan), so it would be very slow. More importantly, the method was inefficient because the X-ray dose contributes to only one pixel, and the remainder of the length of the X-ray beam is wasted. However, Oldendorf's method is impressive: it is simple and elegant engineering, and it shows that he understood the need for a cross-sectional X-ray of the brain when few other people did.

Another drawback in Oldendorf's method, and in Gabriel Frank's, is lack of "filtration". Each object in a picture without filtration has a shadow around it, a bit like a skirt. These shadows fade away at pixels that are at increasing distance from the object, but they blur the picture and interfere with diagnosis. In filtered back-projection these shadows are removed by a filter, which boosts the strength of the higher frequencies in the scan.

These drawbacks were not the reason why Oldendorf did not make the breakthrough. He fell at a different hurdle: he could not obtain backing to develop his ideas. This was not his fault: he tried hard, but he kept encountering people who did not believe that a cross-sectional X-ray was worth having.

Oldendorf met all of the first three requirements, and he met a fourth, which is to have the engineering skill to build a prototype.

Oldendorf's experience shows that recognising the need for a solution and inventing a method is not enough. A fifth (and crucial) requirement is a level of determination and persistence which is obsessive. A sixth requirement is to prove medical and commercial viability, and a seventh is to find a manufacturer, or to set up in manufacturing yourself.

When the UK patent examiner found Odendorf's patent, he asked Allan Logan to explain why it was not "prior art" that undermined Godfrey's patent. Logan was easily able to do so.

Allan Cormack published papers in 1963–64 showing pictures without the shadows caused by lack of "filtration" (as does Ronald Bracewell's 1956 work, which he was unaware of at that stage). But Cormack's method has disadvantages that mean that it has as far as we know never been used in medical CT scanners. The 1963–64 papers contained complex maths that Godfrey would have rejected as taking too long to process on the computers of that day. (For mathematicians only, Cormack used Fourier transforms, Hankel transforms, Hermite polynomials, Jacobi polynomials, Lageurre polynomials, Tsechebycheff polynomials, and Zerneike polynomials. These are beyond the maths that Godfrey studied at college.) The papers showed a method that is adequate for planning radiation therapy, which was the aim, but they did not show suitability for diagnosis in soft tissue. Diagnosis within the brain needs an accuracy of better than half a per cent, whereas the 1963–64 papers showed inaccuracies that exceed that by an order of magnitude. Areas of the scan that should be as flat as a mill pond look like rough seas. That drawback was not the reason why Cormack did not make the breakthrough: the cause may have been a combination of items five, six, and seven in our list.

Cormack, as an academic, was more interested in publishing papers than Godfrey, and less interested than Godfrey in producing a practical scanner to keep his employer's factories busy.

Two points that Cormack made are worth mentioning. He complained about EMI's approach to patenting and patent litigation, and he mentioned that his name had been found in Godfrey's daybook.

The point about patenting seems to be a simple misunderstanding of differences between the academic and industrial worlds. Industrial companies routinely patent new inventions. In the rare cases in which these patents come to court there is a "full disclosure" in which each side sees all of the evidence held by the other. Cormack suspected that EMI had in some way pulled the wool over the eyes of their opponents, and then bound them to secrecy. The fact is that the opponents saw absolutely every piece of evidence and that they would not have conceded and paid royalties unless they realised that they could not win the litigation.

Godfrey wrote Cormack's name in his daybook at one of his meetings with the DHSS in the summer of 1968. This seems to have made Cormack suspicious, although he later wrote that he had studied Godfrey's patents and found nothing based on his own methods. There was a little flurry of interest in about 1977 when the following was found in Godfrey's daybook during the "full disclosure": *Dr Dennis Rutovitz 278 2890 recommends A Cormack 56-60 Physics Review Abstract*. Cliff Gregory had suggested that Godfrey should phone Rutovitz, on that phone number in London, about Cormack's work between 1956 and 1960. The excitement faded when it was seen that this meeting with Cliff Gregory was after Godfrey had developed his own method of reconstructing the picture and applied for a patent. Godfrey ignored Cliff Gregory's suggestion: he did not phone Rutovitz or study the 1963–64 papers by Cormack at this stage. Godfrey looked at those papers in 1973 during discussions with the US patent examiner about possible prior art. Allan Logan was able to show the examiner that Godfrey's method was a new invention beyond Cormack's earlier work.

David Kuhl set his own work and Godfrey's in context in a 2009 speech in Japan which is (at the time of writing) available on YouTube. Kuhl modestly says that his 1965 work generated a "first approximation to CT scanning". Kuhl's main focus was on positron emission scanning, in which a small amount of radioactive material is inserted into the patient and tracked as it interacts with parts of the body. Often the radioactive material is in a glucose-like molecule and is used to track the spread of cancer. He used a very low-dose CT scan to locate his positron image on to the anatomy of the patient. His 1965 CT scan used too few photons to find tumours or blood clots, but the positron image aimed to find those.

We had reached number seven in a list of things that are needed, beyond ideas about image reconstruction, in order to make the breakthrough. An eighth requirement is described by Stephen Bates: one of the problems of CT was its apparent simplicity. *It was very easy to describe the basic scanning and reconstruction process but achieving the necessary numerical accuracy and picture quality required attention to detail and an appreciation of the subtleties involved. Anyone could produce some sort of picture in a short time but producing a good picture required a lot more work.* We could add many more, but the list is already long enough to show that having good ideas about reconstructing an image from X-ray beams is only a small part of what is needed. This helps to explain why Godfrey had so many predecessors, and why he was unique in actually making the breakthrough.

The facts are that before Godfrey there were a few predecessors and they often worked independently of each other. At that stage the medical and industrial spheres were largely unaware of the potential of CT scanning. After Godfrey showed his results all of this changed. He showed that CT could detect tumours and blood clots at an acceptable X-ray dose, saving lives and preserving the quality of life in a commercially available product for cost-effective use in hospitals. That was his breakthrough.

Appendix 8
Shortcuts in reconstruction

For technically inclined people only….

The process of mapping X-ray beams into a picture matrix needs a lot of arithmetic. For example, a circular picture with a diameter of 320 pixels contains about 81,000 pixels. Multiplying this by 540 different angles gives 44 million operations, which was quite a challenge for the computers that were available to Godfrey.

Iterative system

The main speed-up techniques for the iterative system of reconstruction are described in Chapters 5 and 6: stepping through the angles in large steps such as thirty-seven degrees rather than one degree gives a twelve-fold increase in the speed of convergence. The use of assembler code rather than the high-level language Fortran and removing any non-essential code from the inner loops gave about another six-fold increase in speed. It is important to select the right feedback factor to ensure fast convergence.

The iterative system used a "beam path data table", which was a pre-computed look-up table for mapping the beams into the picture matrix. This was implemented like a linked list. It defined what proportion of a particular beam to add into a pixel. The beam path data implemented Godfrey's "jacked-up-sine wave" method of interpolating between the beams. It worked efficiently on the ICL 1905, but less so on the Nova minicomputer.

Faster back-projection

Brian Lill and Paul Beaven's method eliminated the "beam path data" look-up-table. They found a fast way of calculating the beam path. Chris LeMay added a fast way of calculating the required weighting factors.

$P_{1,1}$ and $P_{1,2}$ are pixels in following image. $P_{1,1}$ receives a signal from beam r at roughly half-weighting on the sine wave curve, whereas $P_{1,2}$ receives a signal from beam r+1 at full weight. Lill and Beaven realised that as you step from one pixel to the next pixel, you must step a constant length along the set of edge readings.

In EMI's implementation, all of the weighting calculations were made once before starting to map these beams into the picture, rather than many times during the mapping process. They "expanded" the projection data by putting nineteen new beams in between the existing beams, making the values in this enlarged set of beams follow a smooth curve using the sine wave interpolation. The mapping process simply calculates the correct expanded edge reading to map into the first pixel, and then steps a constant length along the edge readings to find the correct address in

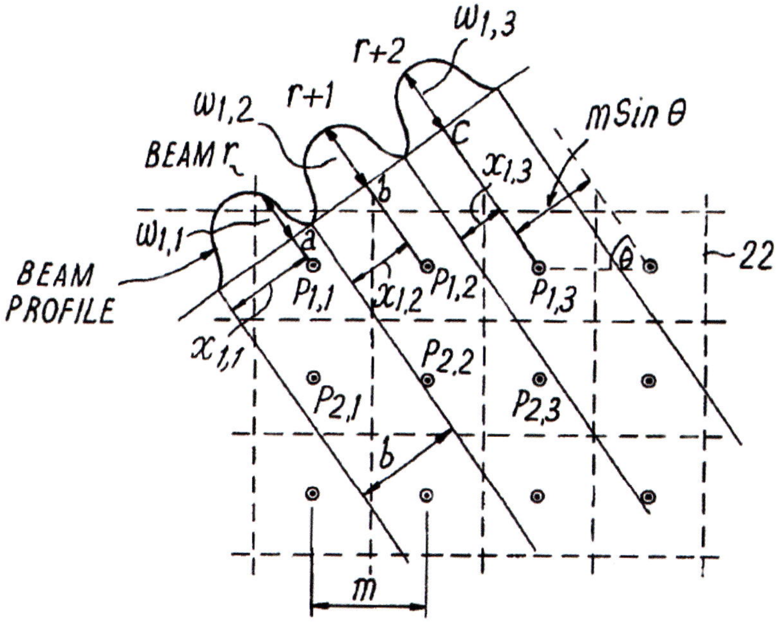

The Lill and Beaven mapping process

the expanded edge readings to map into each of the remaining pixels in that row of the picture matrix. The step is not a whole number, and the fractional part has to be preserved. In EMI's case this was done by using a double-length integer, which was faster on its hardware than using floating point numbers.

In the Super Opal scanner the interpolation was a true sine wave, whereas Emerald and later scanners used Christopher LeMay's "third difference" method of approximating the sine wave, which needed no multiplications.

Convolution (the filter in filtered back-projection)

Christopher LeMay's circle method (also known as convolution) avoided the successive approximations of the iterative method. It got the answer right first time. In principle, this made it about four times faster than the iterative system, but only if the time to run the convolution is small compared with the time needed for back-projection. Initially, the convolution time was the dominant factor, because it involved many multiplications, which were much slower than additions. LeMay found a way of reducing the number of multiplications by a factor of about thirty. He did this by implementing the long, smooth tail of the convolution function by a few exponentials, and by exploiting the fact that each exponential can be implemented with a single multiplication per data point, whereas the full convolution required 480 multiplications per data point. The early implementation used three exponentials, but this was found to be barely adequate. Moving to four exponentials gave a much more accurate result.

Fan beams

Godfrey's early CT scanners produced parallel beams. The Topaz and 7070 scanners produced fan beams. Initially this seemed likely to slow down the reconstruction process because it required several functions that were slow on the available hardware. (It needed a cosine weighting across the fan, a $1/D^2$ weighting down the fan, and an arctan function in the mapping loop.) Ways of ameliorating all of these were found, with the most significant improvement coming from a process called stretching, which moved the trigonometry out of the inner loop of the back-projection. Stretching started by expanding the readings within the fan in the normal way, but then remapped them onto a straight line that was parallel with one of the axes of the picture matrix or a diagonal in the matrix.

Microcode in the Eclipse and image processor

The remaining problem to be solved was how to implement the back-projection and whether special hardware needed to be built. There followed what can only be described as an incredible piece of luck. In 1974 Data General announced the Eclipse to replace the Nova minicomputer. The Eclipse was a micro-coded machine that emulated the Nova instruction set. The microcode comprised a limited instruction set that controlled the operations and data paths. The microcode was fifty-six-bits long and the firmware that defined the machine-code instructions was held in a 'control store' ROM with a cycle-time of 200 nanoseconds. The preliminary publicity material mentioned an option to add additional control store RAM. This option was called Writable Control Store, or WCS, which enabled the programmer to add customised instructions. Data General had not expected early customers to order this option, in fact it was not intended to be available in the first release. However, Stephen Bates and John Ryan were interested in whether any useful instructions could be customised and integrated into the back-projection operation.

In May 1974, Stephen Bates and John Ryan went to the Data General plant in Southborough, Massachusetts, to receive a technical presentation on the Eclipse and a course on how to use the WCS. It soon became apparent that the back-projection operation of indexing to the next expanded edge reading and adding this to the next pixel could be micro coded. Even better, by overlapping the code to produce a pipelining effect, two pixels could be mapped, thus doubling the speed. This solved the back-projection problem for Emerald as the WCS allowed the Eclipse to be used as the back-projector, operating at a similar speed to a hardware solution.

Later scanners (Topaz and the CT7070) used an image processor mentioned in Chapter 10. This contained many separate processing units that could all operate at the same time.

The image processor had six arithmetic processors, two multipliers, a shifter, and some scratch pads. Each of these had two inputs: one from the bus that linked all of the cards together, and one from the "special connections" that allowed data to be passed between processing units in an efficient pipeline for CT image reconstruction. This left the bus free for other uses, such as disk transfers.

The processor included a video output card, which could display thirty slices as three dimensions, giving axial, coronal, sagittal, and oblique views, and allowing real-time manipulation of the images.

The image processor did the mapping of an Emerald 320×320 CT scan in three seconds. Topaz and CT7070 used more data and fan beams, which took slightly longer.

These techniques show that getting the reconstruction to run fast on early, simple minicomputers and the image processor was an interesting challenge.

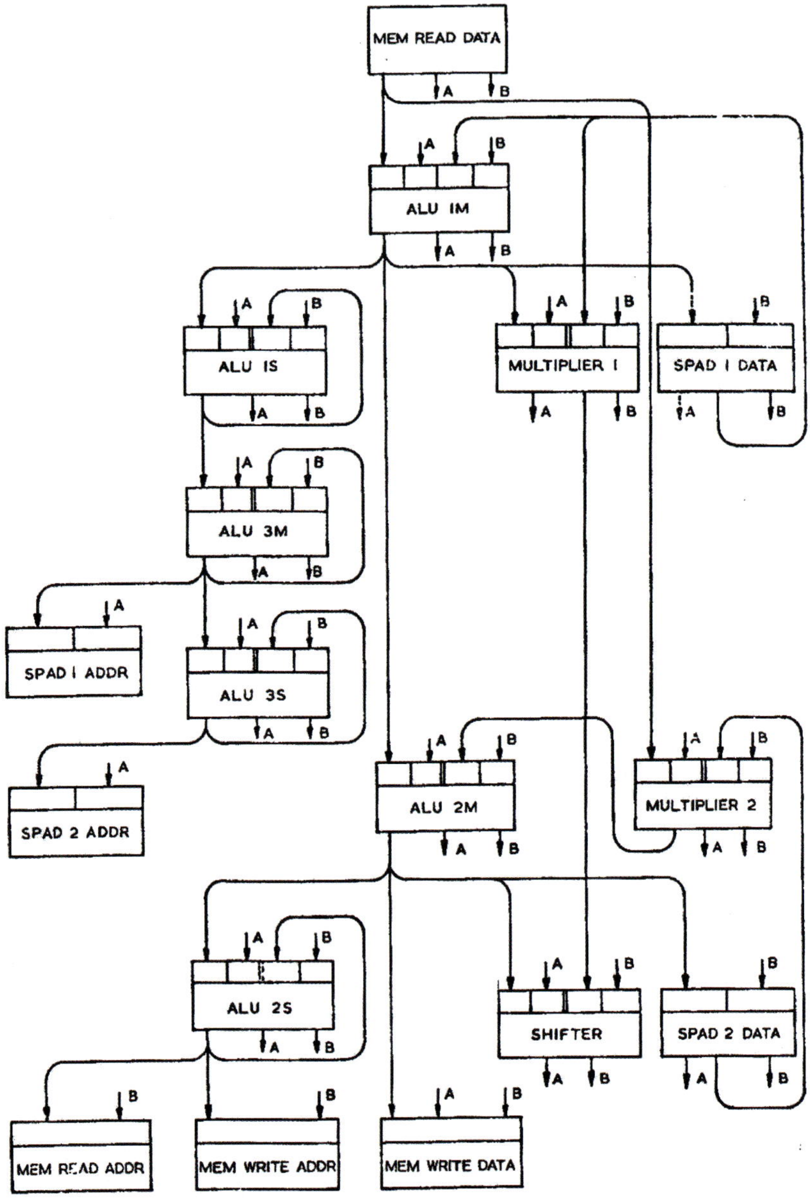

Image processor diagram
(Copyright EMI Music)

Appendix 9
EMIDEC and Austin computer architecture

The Austin computer processed bits serially, fetching them from the magnetic drum. Every instruction involved reading from the drum and writing the result back to it. The magnetic drum was used because it was better than the alternatives. Using valves to store data would be more expensive and less reliable, and mercury delay lines would give less storage capacity, although they would give faster access to the data.

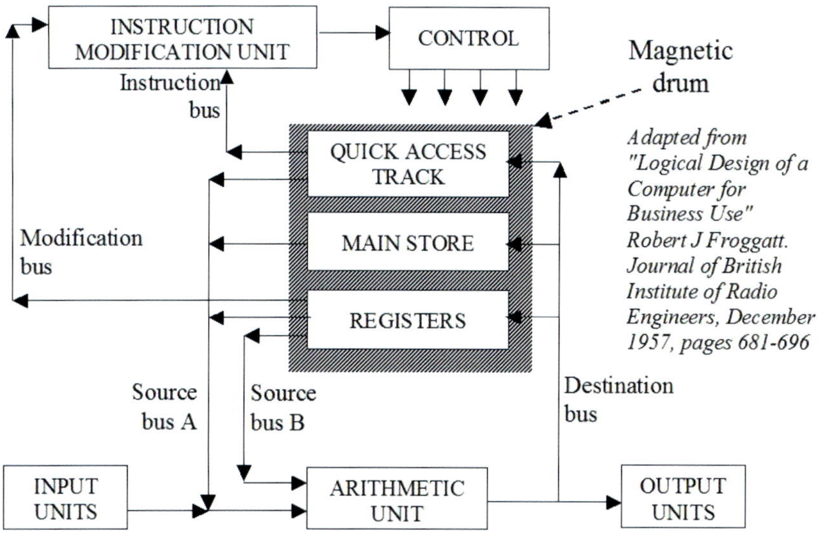

Austin computer diagram

The EMIDEC 1100 processed bits in parallel, processing the whole thirty-six-bit word at once. It used magnetic core memory for the fastest part of the memory hierarchy. This is shown in the next diagram as "immediate access core store".

The drum still played an essential role as a clock source and for storing data at faster speeds than magnetic tape. But the drum was relegated to become a second-level store. The data had to be moved into the core store before any arithmetic or other work was done on it. So blocks of data were moved from the drum into the core when they were needed. The computer could contain four drums, each eight inches diameter and thirteen inches long, storing 16,384 words.

The core memory was faster than the drum because waiting for the drum to rotate could take up to a fiftieth of a second.

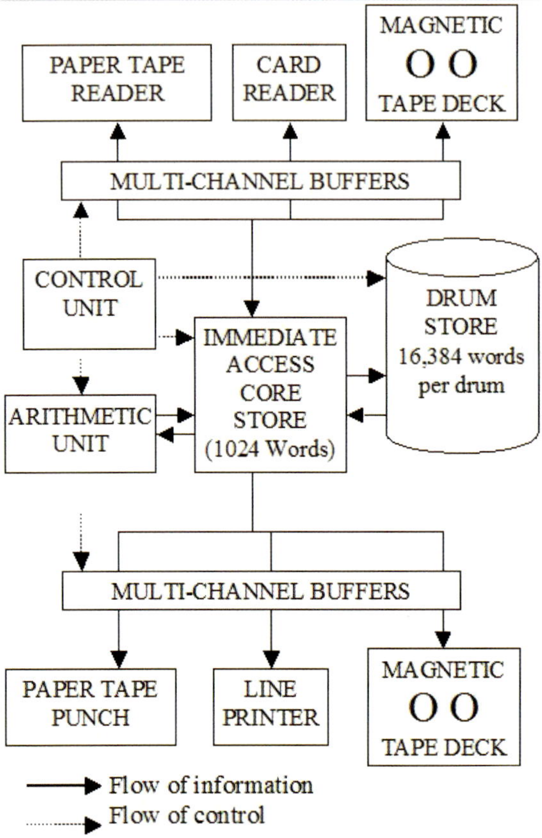

EMIDEC 1100

A typical EMIDEC 1100 used 10,000 transistors and 60,000 ferrite cores. About sixty per cent of the cores were in the immediate access store, which performed the same function as RAM in a modern PC. The core memory was bought in as a unit from Mullard. Ferrite cores were also used in the microprogram store, which defined the instruction set of the central processor, and in the mult-channel buffers that connected the computer to the tape decks, printers, etc

David Robinson says, *The principal logical designers of the 1100 were Mike Symons and myself. Mike designed the system for controlling the Samastronic printer (a nightmare logical problem!) and I think I did all the central processor and the drum control. The core of the control unit was a rectangular array of 2mm ferrite cores, mounted in a protective sandwich of Perspex. The microprogram for each function was set up by threading wires in and out of this array, and I think I designed all the functions by laying out the threading routes on a series of large sheets of paper. These sheets were then used by the girls who actually threaded the wires. I built a simple pantograph device so that they could easily relate the drawing directly to the matrix and get the wires through the right holes.*

Regarding the buffer store that is shown in the "frightful tangles" photo in Chapter 4, David Robinson recalls, *It was accessed differently from the core memory, it was accessed serially. You pulsed along the rows one at a time, one after another, and pulsed along the columns at the same time. But because the number of rows and columns were mutually prime you covered the whole thing.* This explains why there are twelve columns and nineteen rows.

Each computer program was a sequence of very low-level instructions, as shown in the following fragment.

0	1		0		8				Clear Register 8
1	1		11		9				Put 1 in Register 9
2	1		0		7				Clear Register 7
3	7		11		7				Add 1 to Register 7
4	9		20		9				Multiply Reg.20 by Reg.9
5	8	R	10		7				Subtract 10 from Reg.7
6	11		7	R	9				Test Register 7 zero
7	7	R	10		7				If Reg.7 non-zero add back 10
8	11		0	R	3				Return to Instruction 3
9									Proceed if Reg.7 zero above
10	90						1	0	

EMI had two teams developing computers during the years 1957–60. The Austin computer and the EMIDEC 1100 started because Clifford Metcalfe at EMI happened to be a friend of Leonard Lord who was the chairman of BMC. The EMIDEC 2400 design was started because the government offered funding, and Charles Kramskoy recruited a new team for the work. That team also worked on an EMIDEC 3400, which did not reach production.

The EMIDEC 2400 was larger and more powerful than the 1100 computer, but only four were sold. It was developed by EMI in conjunction with the National Research Development Corporation (NRDC). The 2400 machine took longer to design, and by the time it was ready the EMIDEC 1100 was already well established.

From 1949 onwards the NRDC had a major role in encouraging and supporting the computer industry in the UK, and in helping companies to work together or merge to compete with overseas companies such as IBM. Eventually all of the British mainframe computer manufacturers merged to become ICL in 1968. The NRDC looked after many patents from pioneering computer design work at Manchester University and elsewhere.

Professor John Hendry studied the NRDC in his 1989 book "Innovating for Failure: Government Policy and the Early British Computer Industry". He recalls meeting Godfrey as follows: *I only met him once, when I was researching that book, but I got an impression of immense creativity, rather appealingly combined with much humility. Having spent most of my career in Cambridge, I'm used to bright people, but he was exceptional.*

John Hendry read the detailed NRDC archives and interviewed ex-EMI staff including Godfrey, Bob Froggatt, Charles Kramskoy, Norman Hill, and Sir Joseph Lockwood. Hendry says that *EMI had two computer projects: the 1100 which enjoyed full management support and was treated as a commercial project, and the 2400, which was treated much as a one-of-a-kind defence contract.* (In the sense that it was funded like a defence contract.) The projects had different funding and separate design teams. The 1100 had an immediate order from BMC to focus the minds, with no need to wait while a consensus specification was evolved with the NRDC.

It may seem surprising that EMI had two independent design teams. Alan Thomson of the Computer Conservation Society and the British Computer Society has a lot of experience of attempting to look back more than fifty years, and offers a wise caveat: *it is easy to paint rational and coherent pictures, but the reality was more chaotic, and the chances are that it wasn't always logical.* Each design team chose its own path, one funding most of its product development from the NRDC and the other by selling commercial products. There were few links between them except that they shared the EMIDEC name.

Index

We have omitted many titles in the index for brevity. This includes medical, military, or academic titles (for example, Ambrose, Broadway, Bull, Cassidy, Clore, Cormack, Dix, Doyle, Evens, Firmin, Foxley, Green, Hendry, Isherwood, Johnson, Klioze, Kreel, Lavington, Lennon, Moseley, Oldendorf, Powell, Sagel, D&E Shoenberg, Sibbald, Slark, Solomon, Süsskind, Stanley, Taveras, Thomas, Voles, Watson, Webb, White). We apologise for any titles that may be missing or inaccurate.